STUDENT NOTEBOOK AND STUDY GUIDE TO ACCOMPANY

The Human Body:
CONCEPTS OF ANATOMY AND PHYSIOLOGY

Patty Bostwick-Taylor

Florence-Darlington Technical College

Wolters Kluwer | Lippincott Williams & Wilkins
Health

Philadelphia · Baltimore · New York · London
Buenos Aires · Hong Kong · Sydney · Tokyo

Executive Editor: David Troy

Development Editor: Laura Bonazzoli

Senior Product Manager: Eve Malakoff-Klein

Marketing Manager: Sarah Schuessler

Designer: Holly McLaughlin

Art: Body Scientific International

Compositor: Aptara, Inc.

351 West Camden Street   Two Commerce Square

Baltimore, MD 21201   Philadelphia, PA 19103

Printed in China

9 8 7 6 5 4 3 2 1

ISBN 978-1-60913-869-1

DISCLAIMER

Care has been taken to confirm the accuracy of the information present and to describe generally accepted practices. However, the authors, editors, and publisher are not responsible for errors or omissions or for any consequences from application of the information in this book and make no warranty, expressed or implied, with respect to the currency, completeness, or accuracy of the contents of the publication. Application of this information in a particular situation remains the professional responsibility of the practitioner; the clinical treatments described and recommended may not be considered absolute and universal recommendations.

To purchase additional copies of this book, call our customer service department at (800) 638-3030 or fax orders to (301) 223-2320. International customers should call (301) 223-2300.

Visit Lippincott Williams & Wilkins on the Internet: http://www.lww.com. Lippincott Williams & Wilkins customer service representatives are available from 8:30 am to 6:00 pm, EST.

A Letter to Students

Dear student,

Do you want know the secret to success in your anatomy and physiology course? Read, study, practice, and repeat. This unique student notebook and study guide combines lecture notes based on the book with built-in practice problems. Through the combined use of this book and your textbook, you can read, study, and practice your way to a successful understanding of the human body!

I know it's easy to get lost in the volume of content in an anatomy and physiology course. In my own anatomy and physiology classes, I provide an integrated student notebook and study guide just like this one. Each chapter has multiple notebook sections, with blanks for you to complete, which will help keep you focused, engaged, and listening. Since these note sections are based strictly on the information in the textbook, you have an instant guide to the most important information on which you will be tested. These notes condense and highlight the key concepts from the textbook. You'll find the notebook best serves you when used to prepare ahead of each upcoming class. When you complete the blanks before attending class, you can use both your visual and auditory senses to absorb the day's content during class time. Listen during class so you know the topics your instructor emphasizes. Coming to class prepared is a much better use of your time than busily scrambling to keep up with every word your instructor says during class!

Lecture notes are a key component of the equation for success in an anatomy and physiology class. But, how do you know if you are really prepared for your upcoming assignments? I have found that some students are not really sure how to study the content we cover in anatomy and physiology. To determine if you are adequately prepared for the upcoming assignments in your class, use the "Review Time!" problems in this student notebook to assess your comprehension of the material. I have provided practice problems after every major concept. You won't cover more than a few pages of content before you have an opportunity to practice what you know. Spend time with your instructor, a study buddy, or a tutor if you have difficulty answering the practice questions. Take the time to write out the answers to all of these practice questions, as the physical process of writing will help you to commit the information to memory. Later, when it's time for your final exam, your own answers will provide for you an instant study guide to which you can refer when studying for the biggest test in your anatomy and physiology class.

Best of luck to you in your anatomy and physiology class!

—Patty Bostwick-Taylor

Reinventing the Study Guide

Too often, students in the classroom struggle to both learn the concepts presented and simultaneously record crucial information. *Student Notebook and Study Guide to Accompany The Human Body: Concepts of Anatomy and Physiology* reinvents the traditional study guide by giving students a tool to grasp information in class and reinforce learning outside of class. This *Student Notebook and Study Guide* provides a structure for preparing ahead of time for class, for checking your knowledge and recording in-class the material presented in lectures, and for reinforcing your learning outside of the classroom with supplemental review questions and exercises.

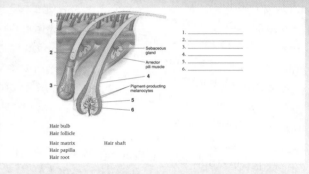

- **Tips for Success** provide suggestions to enhance your learning experience.
- Content is organized around the **Concept Statements** and **Learning Objectives** in *The Human Body: Concepts of Anatomy and Physiology* (available separately), simplifying notetaking and concept review.

- **Notetaking** sections help you organize lecture content.

> **Fibroblasts** and **macrophages**, phagocytic white blood cells, are also common in loose connective tissue. Macrophages are particularly numerous during _____
> Loose connective tissue that is found between skin and muscle is called **superficial fascia**.
>
> *Adipose Tissue*
> - **Structure:** Adipose tissue is composed of specialized fibroblasts called _____ that store energy as fat (triglycerides). Little extracellular matrix exists except for _____ fibers.
> - **Function:** Energy storage as fat, insulator to slow loss of _____ through the skin, padded cushion to absorb shocks to organs, fills body spaces. Subcutaneous fat is the most abundant location for adipose tissue. Adipocytes low in lipids trigger hunger sensations.
>
> *Dense Connective Tissue*
> **Overall structure:** Tightly packed fibers, mostly collagen, leave very little space for ground substance. Dense irregular and dense regular connective tissues vary in the direction of their collagen fibers.
> - **Dense irregular connective tissue:** _____ fibers branch extensively, ground substance is minimal, and fibroblasts are scattered.
> - **Function:** Forms scar tissue, wraps around _____ and _____ situated in the deep layer of the skin (known as the _____).

- **Modified art** from the text supports the needs of visual learners.

- **Review Time** questions test your recall and promote retention.

> **Review Time!**
>
> I. Using the terms in the list below, write the appropriate type of receptor in each blank. You may use a term more than once.
>
> Chemoreceptors   Mechanoreceptors   Nociceptors
> Photoreceptors   Thermoreceptors
>
> 1. Pain receptors
> 2. Smell and taste receptors
> 3. Hearing receptors
> 4. Detect temperature changes
> 5. Detect oxygen and carbon dioxide levels in the blood
> 6. Deep pressure receptors
> 7. Present only in the eye to detect light
> 8. Detect touch and pressure
> 9. Detect chemicals dissolved in fluid
> 10. Detect damage to nearby cells

- A searchable online *Student Notebook and Study Guide* is available free with the purchase of the print book.

- A complete Answer Key with all notes and responses is available online and free to purchasers of the print book.

To order a copy of the companion textbook, *The Human Body: Concepts of Anatomy and Physiology,* visit lww.com and reference ISBN 978-1-6091-3344-3.

Contents

Acknowledgments

Many thanks to Executive Editor David Troy for giving me an opportunity to create a one-of-a-kind student notebook and study guide for Bruce Wingerd's textbook, *The Human Body: Concepts of Anatomy and Physiology*. LWW Educational Sales Representative Jeanie Staton recognized my anatomy and physiology notebook as a possible ancillary during a visit to my office one day and placed me in contact with David. Thank you, Jeanie, for seeing potential in my work! Senior Product Manager Eve Malakoff-Klein has been my invaluable sounding board as we worked together on building this student notebook. Thank you, Eve, for your insight, attention to detail, and creative thinking. Last, much appreciation goes to my family, Rick and Cate, for allowing me the nightly quiet time to pursue this awesome opportunity!

Patty Bostwick-Taylor

Introduction to the Human Body

1

Tips for Success as You Begin This Class

Read Chapter 1 from your textbook before attending class. Listen when you attend lecture and fill in the blanks in this notebook. You may choose to complete the blanks before attending class as a way to prepare for the day's topics. The same day you attend lecture, read the material again and complete the exercises after each section in this notebook. For this chapter, you can facilitate your learning by making flash cards on the regional and directional terms.

CONCEPT 1

Anatomy and Physiology Defined

Concept: The study of the human body is an interdisciplinary science. It consists of fields that focus on structure or function at many levels.

LEARNING OBJECTIVE 1. Define anatomy and physiology.

Define **anatomy.** _____

_____

- **Gross anatomy:** The "big picture" of the body—anatomy visible with the naked eye.
- **Microscopic anatomy:** A microscope is needed to view the small structures of the body.

What key questions are answered by studies in anatomy?

1. _____
2. _____
3. _____

What are the two subdivisions of gross anatomy?

1. _____
2. _____

What are the two subdivisions of microanatomy?

1. _____
2. _____

List and describe the two primary approaches to studying anatomy.

1. _____

   _____

2. _____

   _____

Which approach does your textbook use? _____

_____

Define **physiology.** _____

_____

• What key question is answered by studies in physiology? _____

   _____

• How do we discover new information about physiology? _____

   _____

Review Time!

I. *Classify the following as studies in* anatomy *or* physiology.

   1. Where is the spleen located?   _____

   2. What is the shape of the kidney?   _____

   3. What is the function of the esophagus?   _____

   4. What does a neuron do?   _____

   5. How is a red blood cell shaped?   _____

II. *Classify the following studies to their correct subdivision of anatomy.*

   1. Study of cell structure.   _____

   2. Study of tissue locations.   _____

   3. Study of the overall shape of a leg bone.   _____

   4. Study of the shape of the foot.   _____

   5. Study of the location of the appendix.   _____

III. *Provide a brief answer for each of the following questions about anatomy and physiology.*

   1. Identify and list key words that will help you differentiate between studies of anatomy and physiology.

      _____

      _____

   2. How would you differentiate between studies in gross anatomy and microanatomy?

      _____

      _____

   3. What tool aids scientists in the pursuit of microanatomy knowledge? _____

      _____

   4. What is the key difference between the study of anatomy and physiology? _____

      _____

   5. In which study do scientists use a hypothesis to test new ideas? _____

      _____

CONCEPT 2

Structural Levels of Organization

Concept: The human body is composed of microscopic building blocks arranged into a series of increasingly complex structures. Health depends upon every level functioning properly.

LEARNING OBJECTIVE 2. **Describe the structural organization of the human body.**

LEARNING OBJECTIVE 3. **Identify the 11 systems that make up the human organism.**

List and describe the six structural levels of organization, starting with the most basic level.

1. **Chemical level:** Chemicals are composed of _____. The smallest quantity of an element is the _____. Atoms may combine to form _____.

2. **Cellular level:** Cells are composed of _____.

3. **Tissue level:** Tissues are organized groups of _____ working together. The four major tissue types are: (1) _____, (2) _____, (3) _____, and (4) _____.

4. **Organ level:** Organs are composed of two or more types of _____. What are some examples of organs? _____

5. **System level:** Systems are composed of two or more different _____. How many organ systems are in the human body? _____. Can you list those 11 organ systems?

   _____   _____   _____

   _____   _____   _____

   _____   _____   _____

   _____   _____

6. **Organism level:** The organism is composed of many different organ systems.

In summary, what is the structural level of organization from the smallest to the most complex?

Chemical → cells → tissues → organs → organ system → organisms

Review Time!

I.   Provide a brief answer for each of the following questions about structural levels of organization.

   1. Explain the relationship between atoms and elements. _____
   _____

   2. Describe the relationship between atoms and molecules. _____
   _____

   3. Discuss how cells and tissues are related structurally. _____
   _____

   4. Describe the role of the organ system in the human body. _____
   _____

   5. List in order, from the basic to the most complex, the structural levels of organization of a human being.
   _____
   _____

II. *Provide a brief answer for each of the following questions about organ systems.*

  1. Identify each of the organ systems pictured below.

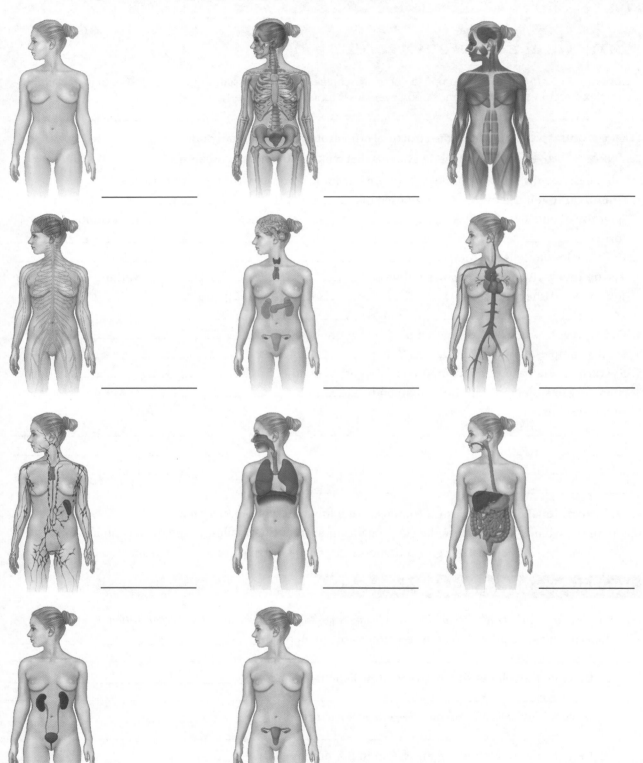

2. Which organ system houses the brain and spinal cord? _____

_____

3. Which organ system includes bones and joints? _____

_____

4. Which organ system releases hormones? _____

_____

5. Which organ system exchanges gasses between the external environment and the bloodstream?

_____

6. What are the major organs of the cardiovascular system?_____

_____

CONCEPT 3

The Characteristics of Life

Concept: All living cells are capable of organization, metabolism, movement, excitability, growth, and reproduction.

LEARNING OBJECTIVE **4. State the six characteristics of life.**

List and describe the six characteristics of life.

1. **Organization:** How can you relate organization to the human body? _____

_____

2. **Metabolism:** Metabolism is defined as the process by which the body obtains and uses

_____. Metabolism can be divided into two types: **catabolism** and **anabolism.**

   • Which type of metabolism breaks larger molecules apart? _____
   • Which type of metabolism is responsible for our growth? _____

3. **Movement:** What are some examples of things that move?_____

_____

4. **Excitability:** The capability of a cell to respond to changes in its environment is known as *excitability,*

   or _____. Changes in the environment that influence cells are called

   _____. What two systems respond to changes in the human body?

_____

_____

5. **Growth:** Enlargement of a cell or the whole body is known as *growth.*
6. **Reproduction:** On what two structural levels do humans reproduce?

_____

_____

Review Time!

I.   *Write the appropriate characteristic of life in each space.*

   1. Digestion   _____

   2. Molecules enter a cell   _____

3. Cell division   _____

4. Cells become larger in size   _____

5. Nervous system responds to changes in body temperature   _____

6. Muscles cause the elbow to bend and move the arm   _____

7. Anabolism   _____

8. Endocrine system responds to changes in blood calcium   _____

II. *Provide a brief answer for each of the following questions about the characteristics of life.*

1. Describe how you would differentiate between anabolism and growth. _____

_____

2. On what two levels does growth occur? _____

_____

3. What two systems respond to stimuli? _____

_____

4. Name and describe the two types of metabolism. _____

_____

5. Identify the two levels on which reproduction occurs. _____

_____

CONCEPT 4

Basic Terminology

Concept: The language used to describe the human body is universal, with an established set of terms.

LEARNING OBJECTIVE 5. Discuss the location of body parts using proper directional terms.

Describe what is meant by **anatomical position.** _____

_____

Why is anatomical position used by health care professionals? _____

_____

Directional Terminology

Directional terminology is the set of terms used to describe the location of one body structure relative to another.

> **TIP!** To learn directional terms, place the terms and definitions on flash cards. Notice how each term is paired with another term of opposite meaning. Practice using these terms by incorporating them into your everyday language.

• **Superior (cranial)** means toward the _____ or upper part of the body.

• **Inferior (caudal)** means away from the _____ or toward the lower end of the body.

• **Anterior (ventral)** means toward the _____ or belly side.

• **Posterior (dorsal)** means toward the _____.

- **Medial** means toward the _____ of the body. The midline is an imaginary line extending vertically down the middle of the body.
- **Lateral** means away from the _____ of the body.

- **Superficial (external)** means toward the _____ of the body.
- **Deep (internal)** means away from the surface of the body.

- **Proximal** means toward a structure's origin or closer to the point of attachment to the trunk.
- **Distal** means away from a structure's origin or farther from the point of attachment to the trunk.

Review Time!

I. *Write the appropriate directional term in each blank. You may find that more than one directional term will be appropriate for some statements.*

> **TIP!** Remember that your statements should reflect a person who is in anatomical position.

1. The hand is _____ to the elbow.
2. The shoulder is _____ to the wrist.
3. The belly button, or navel, is _____ to the spine.
4. The breast bone, or sternum, is _____ to the shoulder socket.
5. The skin is _____ to the muscles.
6. The neck is _____ to the head.
7. The nose is _____ to the ears.
8. The ears are _____ to the eyes.
9. The heart is _____ to the rib cage.
10. The fingers are _____ to the wrist.
11. The eyes are _____ to the nose.
12. The nose is _____ to the mouth.
13. The ankle is _____ to the knee.
14. The waist is _____ to the neck.
15. The skull is _____ to the brain.
16. The fingertips are _____ to the elbow.
17. The nose is _____ to the chin.
18. The knee is _____ to the ankle.
19. The stomach is _____ to the skin.
20. The ears are _____ to the nose.
21. The ear is on the _____ surface of the head.
22. The navel is on the _____ surface of the trunk.
23. The elbow is on the _____ surface of the arm.
24. The breasts are on the _____ side of the trunk.
25. The knee cap (patella) is on the _____ surface of the leg.

Sectional Planes

Sectional planes are flat surfaces that result from a section through the body.

The three main planes are:

1. The _____ or _____ plane divides the body into anterior and posterior portions. This type of section divides the body along its long axis.

2. The _____ plane divides the body into left and right portions. This type of section divides the body along its long axis.
   - If the portions are *equal* in size, the plane is _____.
   - If the portions are *unequal,* the plane is _____.

3. The _____ or _____ or _____ section divides the body into superior and inferior portions.

List and identify four diagnostic techniques that give us an idea of the interior of the human body.

_____

_____

_____

Review Time!

I.   Label the image below with the appropriate sectional plane.

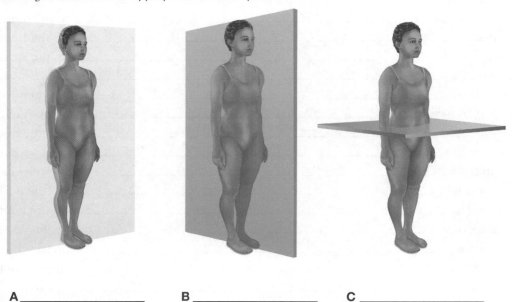

A_____   B_____   C_____

II.   In the space provided, write the appropriate sectional plane.

1. Charmaine's left arm has been amputated at the shoulder due to injuries sustained during a motorcycle accident. What type of sectional plane is created by the amputation?

_____

2. Charlie's leg below the knee was surgically removed due to diabetes mellitus. What type of sectional plane was used in this surgery? _____

_____

3. Intervertebral discs present between the vertebrae of the spine create a superior and an inferior division between adjacent vertebrae. What type of plane is created by the disc?

_____

4. Open heart surgery for Juan was accomplished by creating an incision with equal left and right halves. What type of sectional plane was used in his surgery? _____

_____

5. Gina needs to obtain an image of the liver showing anterior to posterior views. What type of sectional plane should be used? _____

CONCEPT 5

The Body Plan

Concept: The human body is divided into regions. Some regions contain spaces called cavities that house organs.

LEARNING OBJECTIVE   6. Describe the organization of the human body.

Body Regions

What are the five main regions of the human body? List them below.

1. _____
2. _____
3. _____
4. _____
5. _____

What three regions belong to the anterior trunk?

1. _____
2. _____
3. _____

What two regions belong to the posterior trunk?

1. _____
2. _____

Label the body's regions on the images below and on the next page using the terms from the corresponding lists.

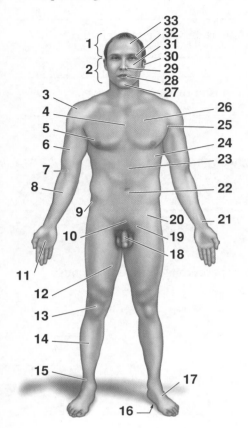

A Anterior view

1. _____
2. _____
3. _____
4. _____
5. _____
6. _____
7. _____
8. _____
9. _____
10. _____
11. _____
12. _____
13. _____
14. _____
15. _____
16. _____
17. _____

18. _____
19. _____
20. _____
21. _____
22. _____
23. _____
24. _____
25. _____
26. _____
27. _____
28. _____
29. _____
30. _____
31. _____
32. _____
33. _____

For the anterior view, use the following terms:

Abdominal	Carpal	Genital	Otic	Sternal
Acromial	Costal	Inguinal	Palmar	Tarsal
Antebrachial	Coxal	Mammary	Patellar	Thoracic
Antecubital	Cranial	Mental	Pedal	Tibial
Axillary	Facial	Nasal	Pelvic	Umbilical
Brachial	Femoral	Oral	Plantar	
Buccal	Frontal	Orbital	Pubic	

1 {

2 — — 15

14

13

3 —

12

4

5   9

10

11

6

7

8

B Posterior view

1. _____
2. _____
3. _____
4. _____
5. _____
6. _____
7. _____
8. _____
9. _____
10. _____
11. _____
12. _____
13. _____
14. _____
15. _____

For the posterior view, use the following terms:

Calcaneal	Femoral	Olecranal or cubital
Cervical	Gluteal	Perineal
Cranial	Lumbar	Popliteal
Digital or phalangeal	Manual	Sacral
Dorsal	Occipital	Vertebral

Review Time!

I. *Write the appropriate directional term in each blank. You may find that more than one directional term will be appropriate for some statements.*

> **TIP!** Remember that your statements should reflect a person who is in anatomical position.

1. The sternal region is _____ to the vertebral region.
2. Where is the palmar region relative to the manual region? _____
3. Where is the popliteal region relative to the patellar region? _____
4. The cubital (olecranal) region is _____ to the antecubital region.
5. The femoral region is _____ to the tibial region.
6. Where is the nasal region relative to the mental region? _____
7. The umbilical region is _____ to the abdominal region.

8. On what surface of the body is the plantar region? _____

9. On what surface of the body is the gluteal region? _____

10. The brachial region is _____ to the antebrachial region.

Body Cavities

Body cavities are usually lined with a membrane. If present, the membrane has two layers: an inner _____ layer and an outer _____ layer.

• Which layer wraps the visceral organ? _____

• Which layer contacts the wall of the cavity? _____

The two main body cavities and their subdivisions are:

1. **Dorsal:** The dorsal body cavity is located _____

   The two subdivisions of the dorsal body cavity are:

   • The _____ houses the brain. What bone(s) protect the brain and create the cranial cavity? _____

   • The _____ houses the spinal cord. What bone(s) protect the spinal cord and create the vertebral canal?_____

   What bone(s) border the thoracic cavity? _____

2. **Ventral:** The ventral body cavity is located. _____.

   The two subdivisions of the ventral body cavity are:

   • The _____ houses the heart and lungs.

   • The _____ houses the digestive organs.

What muscle separates the thoracic and abdominopelvic cavities? _____

Let's focus on the lungs and the thoracic cavity.

• In what narrow cavity within the thoracic cavity is each of the lungs housed?

_____

• What membrane surrounds the lungs? _____

• What is the name of the outer pleural membrane? _____

• What is the name of the inner pleural membrane? _____

Let's focus on the heart and the thoracic cavity.

• In what small cavity within the thoracic cavity is the heart housed? _____

• What membrane surrounds the heart? _____

• List the organs situated in the mediastinum. _____

_____

Let's focus on the abdominopelvic cavity.

• What organs are housed in the abdominal cavity? _____

_____

• What organs are housed in the pelvic cavity? _____

_____

• What membrane surrounds the organs of the abdominopelvic cavity? _____

• Where is the peritoneal cavity located? _____

• Why is the abdominopelvic cavity subdivided into four quadrants and nine regions?

_____

List the four quadrants of the abdominopelvic cavity.

1. _____   3. _____
2. _____   4. _____

List the nine regions of the abdominopelvic cavity.

1. _____   4. _____   7. _____
2. _____   5. _____   8. _____
3. _____   6. _____   9. _____

Review Time!

I.   Label the images below with the appropriate quadrants and regions of the abdominopelvic cavity.

A Abdominopelvic quadrants   **B** Abdominopelvic regions

1. _____
2. _____
3. _____
4. _____
5. _____
6. _____
7. _____
8. _____
9. _____
10. _____
11. _____
12. _____
13. _____

II.   In the space provided, write the appropriate directional term to complete the statement.

1. The umbilical region is _____ to the epigastric region.
2. The right hypochondriac region is _____ to the epigastric region.
3. The hypogastric region is _____ to the epigastric region.
4. The right inguinal region is _____ to the right hypochondriac region.
5. The right lumbar (lateral) region is _____ to the umbilical region.
6. The right upper quadrant is _____ to the right lower quadrant.
7. The right lower quadrant is _____ to the left lower quadrant.
8. The hypogastric region is _____ to the left inguinal region.

III. *Provide a brief answer for each of the following questions about the body cavities.*

1. List the organs housed in the thoracic cavity. _____

_____

2. Name the two ventral cavities separated by the diaphragm. _____

_____

3. The liver, stomach, pancreas, and intestines are in the _____ cavity of

the _____ body

cavity.

4. What two cavities belong to the dorsal body cavity? _____

_____

5. Which organs are covered by visceral pleura? _____

_____

6. Explain where the mediastinum is located. _____

_____

7. Explain where the peritoneal cavity is found. _____

_____

8. What is the relationship between the pleural cavities, thoracic cavity, and ventral cavity?

_____

_____

9. What bones create the thoracic cavity? _____

10. What bones create the dorsal body cavities? _____

_____

11. Name the three medial regions of the abdominopelvic cavity. _____

_____

12. What three regions of the abdominopelvic cavity are the most inferior?

_____

CONCEPT 6

Homeostasis: The Balance of Life

Concept: Homeostasis is the process by which the internal environment of the body is kept relatively stable despite changes in the world within and around us.

LEARNING OBJECTIVE 7. **Discuss the process of homeostasis and provide an example of negative and positive feedback in human functioning.**

LEARNING OBJECTIVE 8. **Define disease and its relationship to homeostasis.**

The process used by the body to maintain internal _____ within a relatively narrow range despite changes within and around it is known as *homeostasis.*

What are the two ways in which homeostasis is maintained?
1. Negative feedback
2. Positive feedback

Negative feedback: Once the body perceives a change, the body _____ the direction of the change until homeostasis is restored. **An example of negative feedback is**

_____.

_____

Positive feedback: Once the body perceives a change, the body _____ more of the change. **An example of positive feedback is** _____.

_____

Disease is a reduction from the ideal state of optimal health.

Review Time!

I. *Provide a brief answer for each of the following questions about homeostatis.*

1. Which type of feedback is most commonly used by the body to restore homeostasis?

    _____

2. What does negative feedback accomplish? _____

    _____

3. How does negative feedback restore homeostasis? _____

4. Does negative feedback accomplish the same goal as positive feedback? Explain.

    _____

5. Consider your response to an itch. Do you think this process is considered negative *or* positive feedback? Explain. _____

    _____

6. Consider the production of breast milk by a mother who is nursing a 4-month-old baby. As long as that baby suckles from its mother's breast, milk production must be maintained to nourish the child. Do you think the process of milk production by the mother is negative *or* positive feedback? Explain.

    _____

    _____

7. Consider what you do in response to being thirsty. As long as you are thirsty, you will drink to replenish your fluids. Explain why thirst is controlled by negative feedback.

    _____

    _____

2

The Chemical Foundation of Life

Tips for Success as You Begin

Read Chapter 2 from your textbook before attending class. Listen when you attend lecture and fill in the blanks in this notebook. You may choose to complete the blanks before attending class as a way to prepare for the day's topics. The same day you attend lecture, read the material again and complete the exercises after each section in this notebook. For this chapter, you can facilitate your learning by making flash cards on the topics you have the most difficulty remembering.

CONCEPT 1

Atoms, Elements, and Molecules

Concept: Matter is the stuff of life. Its most basic unit is the atom, which combines chemically with other atoms to form molecules.

Matter and Energy

LEARNING OBJECTIVE 1. Define element, atom, molecule, and compound, and distinguish between them.

_____ is anything that occupies space and has mass. List the three forms of matter.

1. _____

2. _____

3. _____

_____ is the amount of matter an object contains. Mass is similar to the concept of weight.

_____ is the capacity to do work. List the two forms of energy below.

1. _____ energy is the energy of motion.

2. _____ energy is the stored energy.

Atomic Structure

Atoms compose everything on earth, both living and nonliving. Atoms are the simplest units of

_____. The identity of the atom is lost when it is broken down into smaller

components known as subatomic particles.

Subatomic Particles

Complete the following blanks by supplying information about subatomic particles.

Protons

      Mass _____

      Charge _____

      Position _____

Neutrons

      Mass _____

      Charge _____

      Position _____

Electrons

      Mass _____

      Charge _____

      Position _____

Because the number of protons in an atom is equal to the number of electrons, the atom is always

considered to be electrically _____.

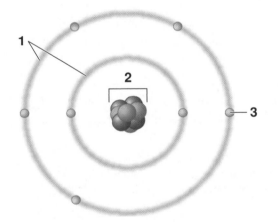

1. _____

2. _____

3. _____

Label the illustration of the atom with the following terms:

Electron   Energy level   Nucleus

Elements

Elements are composed of only one type of _____.
- What are some characteristics of elements? _____
- What do chemical symbols represent? _____
- How many naturally occurring elements are found on the Periodic Table of Elements?

_____

- What are the four most common elements in the human body? List them here in order from *most common* to *least common* in the human body.
  1. _____
  2. _____
  3. _____
  4. _____
- What other two elements complete the list of the six most common elements in the human body, accounting for 99% of the body's weight?
  5. _____
  6. _____

An additional 20 elements make up the remaining 1% of the body's weight.

Atomic Number and Weight

TIP! The atomic number as the **identification number** for **atoms of a particular element**.

The **atomic number** of an atom is determined by the number of _____ in that atom.
The **atomic weight** of an atom is the sum of the numbers of _____ and
_____ in that atom. Why do electrons not contribute significantly to the calculation for atomic weight? _____
Isotopes are atoms of the same element with differing numbers of _____.
Radioactive isotopes, or **radioisotopes**, release, or emit, subatomic particles in an effort to become more
_____.

TIP! Do you know how to determine the number of neutrons in an atom if you are given the atomic number and the atomic weight? Subtract the atomic number from the atomic weight. The difference will be the number of neutrons in an atom of an element. For instance, the atomic number of sodium is 11, while the atomic weight is 23. There are 12 neutrons in an atom of sodium.

Molecules and Compounds

Molecules are usually combinations of two or more _____. Atoms of the same element can combine to form molecules, such as O_2.
Compounds result when molecules are formed from atoms of different elements, such as water (H_2O).

Review Time!

I. *Briefly answer the following questions.*

1. How does potential energy differ from chemical energy? _____

_____

2. Explain how the concepts of matter and mass are similar. _____

_____

3. Explain how the concepts of matter and mass are different. _____

_____

4. Describe atomic structure. _____

_____

5. List the three subatomic particles associated with an atom, their mass, charge, and position.

_____

_____

6. List the names of the four most common elements found in the human body and their chemical

symbols._____

_____

_____

_____

7. Atoms that are electrically neutral have equal numbers of _____

and _____.

8. Which subatomic particle provides the atomic number of an atom? _____

_____

9. The sum of which two subatomic particles provides the atomic weight of an atom?

_____

10. What is the atomic weight of an atom with 6 protons and 7 neutrons? _____

_____

11. Explain what is meant by the following chemical shorthand:

^{14}N _____

$_{19}K$ _____

12. What type of atoms of the same element has different number of neutrons?

_____

13. How can we confirm isotopes are atoms of the same element? _____

_____

14. Will the atomic weight be the same for all isotopes of the same element? Explain.

_____

15. Explain how molecules and compounds are similar. _____

_____

16. Glucose is a chemical represented by the formula $C_6H_{12}O_6$. How would you classify glucose: as an

element or a *compound*? Explain your choice. _____

_____

II. *Using the portion of the Periodic Table shown below, answer the following questions.*

IA

1	
H	IIA
3	4
Li	**Be**
11	12
Na	**Mg**
19	20
K	**Ca**

1. Which element is represented by the symbol Na?   _____

2. Is the element represented by the symbol K one of the most common
    elements of the body?   _____

3. Which element is represented by the symbol H?   _____

4. Is the element represented by the symbol H one of the most common
    elements of the body?   _____

5. Which element is represented by the symbol Ca?   _____

6. What is the atomic number of sodium?   _____

7. How many protons are housed in the nucleus of an atom of magnesium? _____

8. What is the atomic number of hydrogen?   _____

9. How many protons are housed in the nucleus of a potassium atom? _____

10. Which element has an atomic number of 11?   _____

III. *Practice your knowledge of the elements and their symbols by writing the names of the elements represented in each of the following compounds. As you work through these questions, note which compound contains one or more of the four most common elements.*

	Name	**Contains one or more of the four most common elements**
1. KCl	_____	_____
2. $MgCl_2$	_____	_____
3. NaOH	_____	_____
4. $NaNO_3$	_____	_____
5. H_2CO_3	_____	_____
6. MgS	_____	_____
7. CH_4	_____	_____
8. CO_2	_____	_____
9. NaCl	_____	_____
10. H_2SO_4	_____	_____

CONCEPT 2

Chemical Bonds

Concept: Chemical bonds are formed between atoms when the electrons in their outer energy levels are gained or lost, or shared.

LEARNING OBJECTIVE 2. Describe how chemical bonds are formed.

LEARNING OBJECTIVE 3. Distinguish between ionic and covalent bonds.

Electrons and Chemical Bonding

Recall that electrons are housed in **energy levels** in the atom.

- The energy level closest to the nucleus has the lowest energy and holds _____ electrons.
- The second energy level holds _____.

> **TIP!** To recall how most energy levels are filled, think of sports cars and minivans. The first energy level holds two electrons, like a sports car holds two riders. The second energy level, like a minivan, holds eight electrons (or riders).

- When are atoms considered **inert** or stable? _____
  _____
- When are atoms considered **reactive**? _____
  _____
- Which types of atoms seek to fill their outer electron energy levels? _____
  _____

Review Time!

I. *Provide a short answer to the following questions. For the purpose of these questions, consider a carbon atom with six electrons.*

1. How many energy levels does this carbon atom have? _____
2. How many of carbon's electrons are in the lowest energy level? _____
3. How many of carbon's electrons are located in the second energy level? _____
4. Would you consider carbon an *inert* or *reactive* atom? _____
   Explain your choice. _____
   _____
5. How many *more* electrons are needed to stabilize carbon's second energy level?
   _____

6. Determine how many electrons are present in the outer energy level of an atom with an atomic number of 8. _____

_____

7. Calculate how many electrons are present in the outer energy level of an atom with 6 protons in its nucleus. _____

_____

Types of Chemical Bonds

• Which of the following types of atoms form chemical bonds: *inert* atoms or *reactive* atoms?

_____

• Why does that particular type of atom form chemical bonds? _____

_____

• What are two ways in which atoms can form a chemical bond to achieve stability?

   1. _____

   2. _____

Name the two types of chemical bonds that result from your previous two answers.

   1. _____

   2. _____

Ionic Bonds

Atoms that gain or lose electrons to achieve stability are said to be _____.

• Atoms that gain electrons will have an overall _____ charge. This atom will now be an *ion* with a negative charge. This ion is an _____.

• Atoms that lose electrons will have an overall _____ charge. This atom will now be an *ion* with a positive charge. This ion is a _____.

What happens to the ions in an ionic compound when placed in water? _____

_____

What happens when a compound *ionizes*? _____

_____

An example of this is _____

_____

Ionic bonds result when the positive ion and negative ion are held together due to electrostatic forces.

_____

Why do atoms form ionic bonds? _____

TIP! To help you remember the difference between cations and anions, notice the "t" in the word cation. The "t" can remind you of the + (positive) charge carried by the cation. Likewise, the prefix "an" is a reminder the anion has a negative charge.

Covalent Bonds

Atoms that share electrons to achieve stability are said to be _____.

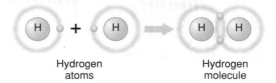

Hydrogen   Hydrogen
atoms   molecule

- Atoms sharing one pair, or two, electrons have formed a(n) _____ covalent bond.
  An example of this is _____

  _____

- Atoms sharing two pairs, or four, electrons have formed a(n) _____ covalent bond.
  An example of this is _____

  _____

  Why do atoms form covalent bonds? _____

  _____

Polar molecules result from the unequal distribution of electrons among atoms participating in a covalent bond.

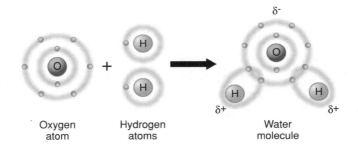

Oxygen   Hydrogen   Water
atom   atoms   molecule

> **EXAMPLE**
> Water, H_2O, is an example of a polar molecule.
> Due to the unequal distribution of electrons, which atoms in the water molecule carry a slightly positive charge? _____
> Which atom in the water molecule carries a slightly negative charge? _____

Hydrogen Bonds

Hydrogen bonds are the attraction of a slightly positive-charged _____ atom and an atom or molecule with a strong negative charge. Hydrogen bonds influence the three-dimensional shape of large molecules, such as _____ and _____ Hydrogen bonds are weak bonds and are similar to _____ bonds.

- What is **surface tension**? _____

  _____

- How does surface tension relate to hydrogen bonds? _____

  _____

Review Time!

I. *Practice your comprehension of chemical bonds. Complete the blanks in the following statements with one of the following terms:*

covalent   ionic   hydrogen

1. Electrons in the outer energy level are shared by atoms in _____ bonds.
2. An example of a(n) _____ bond is O_2.
3. _____ bonds are weak bonds.
4. Cations and anions form _____ bonds.
5. Polar molecules are _____ bonds.
6. _____ bonds result when a slightly positive-charged hydrogen atom is attracted and bonds with an atom or molecule with a strong negative charge.
7. Table salt (NaCl), is formed by a(n) _____ bond.
8. The type of bond that occurs when a positive ion and a negative ion are held together by electrostatic forces is called _____.
9. Name the type of bond that influences the three-dimensional shape of proteins and DNA.

    _____

10. Water molecules are polar molecules and are held together by _____ bonds.
11. Which type of bond is present in compounds that ionize when the chemical is placed in water?

    _____

12. Which type of chemical bond holds together these two atoms of oxygen, O=O?

    _____

13. The two types of bonds that form between or among reactive atoms are

    _____ and _____.
14. Identify the type of bond formed between these two hydrogen atoms, H—H.

    _____

15. The hydrogen atoms and oxygen atom within a water molecule are held together because electrons are shared. What type of bond is formed when these atoms share electrons?

    _____

CONCEPT 3

Chemical Reactions

Concept: Atoms and molecules react with one another when chemical bonds are formed or broken, resulting in new products.

LEARNING OBJECTIVE   4. **Compare and contrast synthesis reactions, decomposition reactions, and exchange reactions.**

Basic terminology to help you understand chemical reactions:

> **TIP!** You will often see an arrow used in a chemical reaction. If the arrow has only one point, that particular kind of arrow always points toward the products.

- **Reactants** are the atoms involved in the chemical reaction.
- **Products** are the newly formed substances resulting from the chemical reaction.

In the following chemical reaction, identify the reactants and the products.

$$AB + CD \rightarrow AC + BD$$

- Reactants _____
- Products _____

Types of Chemical Reactions

Name the three types of chemical reactions discussed in this chapter:

1. _____
2. _____
3. _____

1. **Synthesis reactions** are the combinations of new atoms, ions, or molecules to form new molecules. In a synthesis reaction, new bonds must be formed between the reactants.
   - Complete this synthesis reaction by providing the products:

     $$A + B \rightarrow \text{_____}$$

   - What are some examples of synthesis reactions in the body? _____
     _____
     _____

2. **Decomposition reactions** are opposite to synthesis reactions and involve the breakdown of molecules into simpler molecules, atoms, and ions. Instead of new bond formation as seen with synthesis reactions, what happens to the bonds between the reactants in decomposition reactions?

   _____

   - Complete this decomposition reaction by providing the products:

     $$AB \rightarrow \text{_____} + \text{_____}$$

   - What are some examples of decomposition reactions in the body? _____
     _____
     _____

3. **Exchange reactions** occur when chemical bonds are both formed and broken. In essence, molecules trade positions. Molecules are broken apart from one another as reactants and rearranged as new bonds form, creating the newly arranged products.
   - Complete this exchange reaction by providing the products:

     $$AB + CD \rightarrow \text{_____} + \text{_____}$$

   - What are some examples of exchange reactions in the body? _____
     _____
     _____

Reversible Chemical Reactions

What type of arrow is used to demonstrate that a chemical reaction is reversible? _____

Complete the following equation by providing the correct type of arrow to indicate chemical equilibrium:

$$A + B \text{_____} AB$$

List and briefly explain three factors that influence the direction in which the reaction will proceed.

1. _____
2. _____
3. _____

Review Time!

I.   Provide a short answer to the following questions about chemical reactions.

   1. Which type of chemical reaction forms new molecules? _____

_____

   2. Describe why digestion is classified as a type of decomposition reaction. _____

_____

   3. As we grow from infants into children, our bodies increase in size. Which type of chemical reaction do you think is responsible for our growth? _____

_____

   4. What is a catalyst? _____

_____

   5. What effect do catalysts have on reaction rates? _____

_____

   6. Which type of chemical reaction both breaks chemical bonds and forms new ones?

_____

CONCEPT 4

Chemical Compounds of the Cell

Concept: Inorganic compounds do not contain chains of carbon atoms, whereas organic compounds are composed of chains of carbon and form the primary structural and functional units of the body.

LEARNING OBJECTIVE 5. Distinguish between organic and inorganic compounds.

LEARNING OBJECTIVE 6. Identify the important features of water.

LEARNING OBJECTIVE 7. Describe salts, acids and bases, and pH.

What are the two categories of chemical compounds common in cells?

   1. _____

   2. _____

Inorganic Compounds

Inorganic compounds do not contain chains of _____ atoms and are usually held together by _____ bonds.

List the important inorganic compounds in the human body.

   1. _____

   2. _____

   3. _____

   4. _____

Water comprises approximately _____ of your body's mass. Water is the most important inorganic compound in the body and its importance is due to these four properties.

1. *Water is a universal* _____. Solvents dissolve (break down) solutes, resulting in a solution.

EXAMPLE

NaCl, table salt, is dissolved in water to form a solution. How should we classify NaCl, as the *solute* or the *solvent*? _____

2. *Water is an important transport medium.* Water transports tiny solutes such as _____ and _____ . Blood plasma is more than 90% water and can transport items such as _____ and _____.

3. *Water has a high* _____ *capacity.* Water absorbs and releases _____ quite slowly and, thus, temperature changes are gradual.

> **TIP!** Think of high heat capacity like this: If your body did not resist temperature changes, what would happen to you on a very hot day with an outside temperature of 105°F? Likewise, have you visited a lake or beach in the spring, when the air temperature is warm, yet the water is still freezing cold? Why is that the case? Both the homeostasis of your body temperature and a lake's resistance to change temperature are due to water's high heat capacity.

4. *Water is an effective lubricant.* Water reduces friction between moving body parts.

Name several places where water acts as a lubricant in the body. _____
_____
_____

Salts are inorganic compounds that dissolve and separate into freely moving ions when placed into a liquid solvent like water. Ionization is a _____ reaction that results in the formation of ions. Since these ions can conduct an electrical current, they are referred to as
_____.

Name these common electrolytes.

Na^+ _____

Cl^- _____

K^+ _____

Mg^{2+} _____

Ca^{2+} _____

PO_4^{3-} _____

CO_3^{2-} _____

HCO_3^- _____

Acids are molecules that release one or more _____ ions (H^+) when it ionizes in water.
- Strong acids, such as HCl, ionize *completely* to release all the hydrogen ions they contain.
- Weak acids ionize *partially,* only releasing some of the hydrogen ions they contain.
- When strong acids accumulate abnormally in the body, what condition results?
_____

Bases are molecules that reduce the amount of hydrogen ions in a solution. In water, bases release negatively charged ions, called hydroxyls (OH^-), which tend to combine with positively charged ions, if present. When hydroxyl ions are released by bases, they tend to combine with hydrogen ions and form water.

• Strong bases, such as NaOH, ionize _____.

• Weak bases ionize _____.

• When strong bases accumulate abnormally in the body, what condition results?

_____

How do **buffer systems** help maintain homeostasis? Explain. _____

_____

_____

Measuring Acids and Bases: The pH Scale

The **pH scale** is based on the concentration of hydrogen ions, measured in *moles,* per liter of solution. The pH scale we use converts these moles/Liter values into whole numbers.

In the space below, sketch the pH scale, while we notate the important points about the scale.

• The **pH scale** is numbered from _____ to _____

• What number on the pH scale is the **neutral point**? _____

• What two ions are released *equally* by substances at the **neutral point**?

   1. _____   2. _____.

• What substance is neutral? _____

• Solutions that contain many hydrogen ions have a pH less than 7, and are referred to as
   _____. (*The lower the number, the stronger the acid.*)

• Solutions that contain few hydrogen ions have a pH greater than 7, and are referred to as
   _____. (*The higher the number, the stronger the base.*)

• Each whole number on the scale represents a _____-fold difference in hydrogen ion concentration from the adjacent whole number.

TIP! If asked to calculate the difference in hydrogen ion concentration between two numbers on the pH scale, simply set up a difference and subtract the smaller number from the larger number. For instance, how many more hydrogen ions are released by a pH of 2 in comparison to a pH of 6? Subtract 2 from 6; your answer is 4. Now you have the number of zeros (4) to place behind 1. There is a 10,000-fold difference between a pH of 2 and a pH of 6 in terms of hydrogen ion concentration.

Review Time!

I. *For each of the following statements or descriptions, indicate the appropriate inorganic compound group. You may use a term more than once.*

acid   base   water

1. pH below 7   _____

2. Chemical that reduces hydrogen ion concentration   _____

3. Universal solvent   _____

4. Chemical with a pH of 7   _____

5. High heat capacity   _____

6. Ionizes and releases hydrogen ions in water   _____

7. NaOH   _____

8. Ionizes and releases hydroxyl ions in water   _____

9. HCl   _____

10. pH above 7   _____

II. *Provide a short answer to the following questions about inorganic compounds.*

1. Explain how strong acids and weak acids differ. _____
_____

2. Describe the organization of the pH scale. _____
_____

3. At what number is the neutral point of the pH scale? What is significant about this number?
_____

4. What are electrolytes? Provide some examples. _____
_____

5. Describe the high heat capacity of water. _____
_____

6. Explain how buffer systems maintain homeostasis. _____
_____

7. What is the most common inorganic compound in the human body? _____
_____

8. What ions are released when acids are placed into a solvent such as water?
_____
_____

9. How much of the human body is composed of water? _____
_____

10. What does the pH scale measure? _____
_____

11. Define acidosis. _____

12. Define alkalosis. _____

13. Although most inorganic compounds are formed from _____ bonds, what type of bond holds together the atoms of water molecules?

_____

_____

14. Recall that most inorganic compounds are held together by ionic bonds. Describe ionization.

_____

15. How many times more acidic is urine with a pH of 5, compared to urine with a pH of 7?

_____

16. Inorganic compounds do not contain long chains of _____ atoms.

_____

Organic Compounds

LEARNING OBJECTIVE 8. **Compare and contrast carbohydrates, lipids, proteins, and nucleic acids on the basis of their chemical structures and the roles they play in the body.**

Organic compounds typically contain one or more _____ atoms that are usually held together by _____ bonds. Carbon forms four covalent bonds with other atoms, such as _____, _____, and _____. Larger organic molecules are stabilized by _____ bonds.

List the four primary types of organic compounds below.

1. _____

2. _____

3. _____

4. _____

You will encounter two types of chemical reactions, usually reversible, as you read through the information on organic compounds. Those two reactions are:

1. **Dehydration synthesis:** Water is removed from reactants so a more complex molecule can be formed.

2. **Hydrolysis:** The addition of water causes larger compounds to break into its subunits.

Carbohydrates

Carbohydrate structure: Carbohydrates contain carbon, hydrogen, and oxygen in a ratio of 1:2:1. Carbohydrates are organized into rings or chains of carbon atoms and are water soluble (they dissolve in water).

Carbohydrate function: What is the main job of the carbohydrates? _____

_____

Types of carbohydrates: Carbohydrates are classified into three types on the basis of the number of

_____ atoms they contain.

1. **Monosaccharides** are simple sugars that contain between _____ and _____ carbon atoms. What function do monosaccharides serve? _____

What are three examples of monosaccharides?

1. _____

2. _____

3. _____

What is special about glucose? _____

_____

2. **Disaccharides** are formed when two monosaccharides join together through a chemical reaction known as _____. What are three examples of disaccharides and the monosaccharides from which they form?

1. _____ = glucose + fructose

2. _____ = glucose + galactose

3. _____ = glucose + glucose

3. **Polysaccharides** are formed when more than two carbohydrate molecules join together through a chemical reaction known as _____. What are two examples of polysaccharides and their functions?

1. _____ is a plant polysaccharide composed of glucose molecules. What is the function of starch for the plant?

2. _____ is an animal polysaccharide composed of glucose molecules. What is the function of glycogen for humans?

Which organs store glycogen in humans?_____

_____

Lipids

Lipid structure: Lipids are composed of carbon, hydrogen, and oxygen atoms, but not in the 1:2:1 ratio of carbohydrates. Lipids are not water soluble.

Lipid function: What are the main jobs of the lipids? _____

_____

Types of lipids: Lipids are classified into three groups: triglycerides, phospholipids, and steroids.

1. **Triglycerides** (neutral fats) are known as fats in the solid form and oils in the liquid form. The two building blocks of triglyceride are _____ and _____. The ratio of building blocks is 3:1 (fatty acids to glycerol). Fatty acids are composed of long chains of carbon atoms with hydrogen atoms attached.

   • When the fatty acid chains contain the maximum number of hydrogen atoms bonded to the chain of carbon atoms, the fatty acid chains are called _____. The carbon atoms are held together by single covalent bonds when the fatty acid chain is saturated. Animal fats such as butter are semisolid at room temperature.

   • However, when the fatty acid chains have less than the maximum number of hydrogen atoms bonded to the carbon chain, the fatty acid chain is said to be _____. Carbon atoms are held together by double bonds.

   Triglyceride functions: List the three functions of the triglycerides.

   A. Energy source

   B. _____

   C. _____

2. **Phospholipids** are structurally similar to neutral fats, but they have _____ fatty acid chains rather than three. What replaces the third fatty acid chain?

   _____ Phospholipids are major components of cell membranes.

3. **Steroids** form ring structures rather than fatty acid chains. What is the most well-known steroid?

   _____. Why is cholesterol important?_____

_____

Proteins

Protein structure: Proteins contain carbon, hydrogen, nitrogen, and oxygen and sometimes _____ and _____. Proteins are built from building blocks known as _____. When amino acids combine through dehydration synthesis, they are held together by _____ bonds. The sequencing of amino acids creates different types of proteins in the human body. Proteins are the most abundant organic compound in the body since they account for about 20% of the body's total weight.

- **Dipeptides** result when two amino acids join.
- **Polypeptides** result when a chain contains _____ or more amino acids.
- **Proteins** result when more than _____ amino acids join together.

Protein function: The role a protein plays is determined by its _____. The six primary roles of proteins are listed below. Add a description of each of these roles.

1. Structural support _____
   _____

2. Transport _____
   _____

3. Movement _____
   _____

4. Metabolism _____
   _____

5. Regulation _____
   _____

6. Communication _____
   _____

Enzymes are proteins that serve as catalysts for cells. What is a catalyst?_____
_____

Let's summarize how enzymes work.
- Enzymes work on a substance, known as _____
- New molecules that result from the chemical reaction are known as _____
- The special region where the substrate binds to the enzyme is the _____
- What are the three reactions that enzymes participate in?
  1. _____
  2. _____
  3. _____

Nucleic Acids

Nucleic acid structure: Nucleic acids contain carbon, hydrogen, nitrogen, oxygen, and phosphorus. These combine to form the building blocks of nucleic acids, known as _____. The three components of a nucleotide are:

1. A 5-carbon sugar
2. A phosphate group
3. _____

Nucleic acid function: Nucleic acids carry information that determines the structure and function of the cell. **The two main types of nucleic acids** are DNA and RNA.

- **DNA (deoxyribonucleic acid)** contains the hereditary information of life known as **genes.** Genes are segments of DNA that determine the structure of _____ molecules. What is found in a nucleotide of DNA?
  1. A 5-carbon sugar known as _____
  2. A phosphate group
  3. One of four nitrogenous bases: adenine, cytosine, guanine or _____.

DNA is wound into a double helix (*think spiral staircase*) held together by hydrogen bonds. The bases pair with one another in this pattern: adenine pairs with _____ while cytosine pairs with _____.

- **RNA (ribonucleic acid)** is structurally different from DNA. Let's start by examining the parts of the nucleotide:
  1. A 5-carbon sugar known as _____
  2. A phosphate group (same as DNA)
  3. One of four nitrogenous bases: adenine, cytosine, guanine, or _____

High-Energy Compounds

ATP (adenosine triphosphate) is a high-energy compound that provides the source of energy for our cells. ATP captures energy from the breakdown of larger molecules such as _____.

ATP structure: Which nucleic acid is similar in structure to ATP?

_____

What is the difference between RNA and ATP?_____

_____

Complete this equation:

ATP ↔ _____ + phosphate group + energy

What is the difference between ATP and ADP? _____

_____

Which molecule is the high-energy form, *ADP* or *ATP*? _____

_____

Review Time!

I. *For each of the following statements or descriptions, indicate the appropriate organic compound group. You may use a term more than once.*

carbohydrate   lipid   protein   nucleic acid

1. Polysaccharide _____

2. Amino acid _____

3. Peptide bond _____

4. DNA, RNA _____

5. Enzyme _____

6. Cholesterol _____

7. Glucose _____

8. Dipeptide _____

9. Most abundant organic compound in the body _____

10. Triglyceride _____

11. 1:2:1 ratio of carbon:hydrogen:oxygen _____

12. Phospholipid _____

13. Nucleotide _____

14. Glycogen _____

15. Saturated fatty acid chain _____

II. *Briefly answer the following questions about organic compounds.*

1. Explain how inorganic compounds differ from organic compounds. Provide at least two well-explained differences. _____

_____

_____

_____

2. What is the building block of proteins? _____

_____

3. List the three types of carbohydrates and provide two examples for each type.

_____

_____

_____

_____

_____

4. List the three types of lipids and briefly explain the structure for each.

_____

_____

_____

5. Describe how saturated fatty acid chains are structurally different from unsaturated fatty acid chains. Provide at least three well-explained differences. _____

_____
_____
_____
_____
_____

6. List the three components of a nucleotide of DNA. _____

_____
_____
_____

7. Discuss two structural differences between DNA and RNA. _____

_____
_____

8. Which of the following is the high-energy form: *ADP* or *ATP*? _____

Why?_____
_____

9. What is the building block of a nucleic acid? _____

_____

10. Which organic compound group provides the body with a source of energy to fuel the body's activities? _____

_____

11. What does the hydrolysis of proteins produce? _____

_____

12. Glucose, galactose, and fructose are examples of what type of carbohydrate?

_____

13. Explain how a phospholipid differs from a triglyceride in terms of structure.

_____

14. Enzymes are known as biological catalysts. What is a catalyst? _____

_____

15. What type of nucleic acid carries hereditary information as genes? _____

_____

16. Structurally, how does ATP differ from RNA? _____

_____

17. In which organic compound group do peptide bonds hold together the building blocks?

_____

18. What nitrogenous base replaces thymine in RNA? _____

19. How many fatty acid chains are found in a triglyceride? _____

20. What is the ratio of carbon to hydrogen to oxygen in a typical carbohydrate?

_____

21. How many strands are wound together in a molecule of DNA? _____

22. Between _____ and _____ carbon atoms create a monosaccharide.

23. Dipeptides are constructed from _____ amino acids while a polypeptide may have _____ or more amino acids.

24. Which organic compound group is *not* water soluble? _____

25. Which type of lipid is a major component of cell membranes? _____

26. Into which organic compound group is cholesterol classified? _____

27. Enzymes and their substrates bind together at a special region known as the

_____

28. What type of carbohydrate is starch? _____

_____

29. Describe the structure of a steroid. _____

_____

30. What building blocks are necessary to form a triglyceride through dehydration synthesis?

_____

_____

31. Identify the two monosaccharides that join through dehydration synthesis to form sucrose.

_____

_____

32. Name the most well-known steroid. _____

33. Into which organic compound group are enzymes placed? _____

34. Describe the function of enzymes in the body. _____

_____

_____

35. List the six functions of proteins. _____

_____

_____

_____

_____

_____

36. What molecule serves as a source of energy for our cells? _____

37. List the three functions of triglycerides. _____

_____

_____

38. What type of bond holds together most organic compounds? _____

39. List the six elements commonly found in proteins. _____

_____

_____

_____

_____

_____

40. Which organic group is the most abundant and accounts for approximately 20% of your body's weight? _____

Cells: The Basis of Life

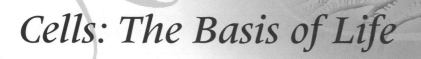

Tips for Success as You Begin

Read Chapter 3 from your textbook before attending class. Listen when you attend lecture and fill in the blanks in this notebook. You may choose to complete the blanks before attending class as a way to prepare for the day's topics. The same day you attend lecture, read the material again and complete the exercises after each section in this notebook. For this chapter, you can facilitate your learning of the organelles by making flash cards of their structures, functions, and locations (use Table 3.3 in your text book for a quick reference).

CONCEPT 1

The Environments of the Cell

Concept: Cells are bathed in a watery extracellular environment. Cells, in turn, are mostly water, bordered by a limiting membrane and filled with functional subunits called organelles.

LEARNING OBJECTIVE 1. Describe the compartments within and surrounding the cell.

Cells are mostly _____ and their external environment is also

_____. Functional subunits inside the cell are _____.

In fact, how much of your body is composed of water? _____

The Extracellular Environment

The **extracellular environment** is found outside the cell and includes **extracellular fluid (ECF).**

1. Besides water, what else will you find in the ECF? _____

_____

2. What cellular products are in the ECF? _____

_____

Two types of ECF are:

1. **Plasma** is the liquid medium used in the transport of substances in the _____.
   - Where is plasma found? _____
   _____

2. **Interstitial fluid** provides a liquid freeway through which substances can travel between cells.
   - Where is interstitial fluid located? _____
   _____
   - What other fluids qualify as interstitial fluids? _____
   _____

The **intercellular environment** is a part of the extracellular environment found directly between adjacent cells. This space may contain molecular bridges that _____.

The Intracellular Environment

The **intracellular environment** is found within the cell and includes **intracellular fluid (ICF)**. _____ physically separates the intracellular and extracellular environments.

- What will you find in ICF? _____
_____

- What percentage of the ICF is water? _____
_____

Two parts of the intracellular environment are:

1. **Cytoplasm** houses many small, highly organized structures known as _____.
2. **Nucleus** is a large, oval structure that houses _____. What does DNA control?
   _____

Review Time!

I.   *For each part in the list below, write the appropriate environment (extracellular or intracellular) in the blank.*

   1. ICF   _____
   2. Plasma   _____
   3. Nucleus   _____
   4. Cytoplasm   _____
   5. ECF   _____
   6. Intercellular environment   _____
   7. Organelles   _____
   8. Lymph   _____
   9. Interstitial fluid   _____
   10. Cellular products   _____

II. *Briefly answer the following questions about the intracellular and extracellular environments.*

   1. Specifically, where is ICF found? _____
   _____

   2. The cytoplasm and nucleus are the two parts of which environment? _____
   _____

3. In what compartment of what environment are organelles found? Be as specific as possible.

_____

4. What are the two types of ECF? _____

_____

_____

5. In which environment is plasma found? _____

_____

6. How would you classify interstitial fluid? _____

_____

7. Specifically, where is the intercellular environment found? _____

_____

8. What is the function of plasma? _____

_____

9. Approximately what percentage of your body is composed of water? _____

_____

10. What physically separates the intracellular and extracellular environments?

_____

CONCEPT 2

Cell Structure and Function: The Cell Membrane

Concept: The cell membrane separates the extracellular and intracellular compartments of the body. It regulates the movement of materials among these compartments.

LEARNING OBJECTIVE 2. Describe the structure of the cell membrane.

What piece of technology can we use to observe cells? _____

Cells vary in size and shape, which is a reflection of the various roles cells play in the body. Cells do share a few features in common, such as the cell (plasma) membrane, cytoplasm, and nucleus.

Cell Membrane Structure

The **cell membrane (plasma membrane)** provides a physical barrier that separates the intracellular environment from the _____ environment. The cell membrane regulates the movement of materials in and out of the cell. The term _selectively permeable_ is used to describe the cell membrane.

• Explain what _selectively permeable_ means. _____

_____

The **fluid mosaic model** is also used to describe the cell membrane. This model describes the cell membrane as an extremely thin barrier with nearly equal parts (in weight) of

_____ and _____ with a small amount of

_____. The roles of the two main components, the lipids and proteins, are

_____ and _____.

- **Lipids** create an oily sheet of molecules that creates the basic framework of the membrane. This barrier prevents the passage of most substances. Do you recall why from your studies in Chapter 2? Explain. _____

- **Proteins** are either anchored within the membrane to other cell structures, or float freely in the lipid sheet. Proteins can serve as "gatekeepers" or receptors.

Membrane Lipids

The three types of lipids found in the cell membrane are:

1. Phospholipids
2. _____
3. _____

Phospholipids are the most abundant lipids in the cell membrane. Each phospholipid contains a glycerol "head" portion and fatty acid chains, or "tails." *You may want to review the discussion of phospholipids from Chapter 2*. Two layers of phospholipids exist, creating a **phospholipid bilayer**. The "head" ends of the phospholipid are attracted to water and are called _____ while the "tails" repel water and are known as _____.

- Explain why the heads and tails orient so that the heads are outward and the tails are sandwiched on the inside. _____

TIP! To visually imagine the phospholipid bilayer, think of a sandwich. The "bread" of the sandwich is created by the phospholipid heads while the "meat" of the sandwich is created by the phospholipid tails oriented to the inside of the bilayer.

In the space below, sketch a few phospholipids of a cell membrane. Pay close attention to the way in which the heads and tails are oriented in your phospholipid bilayer. Label the heads and tails of the phospholipids, and label the hydrophilic and hydrophobic regions of the phospholipid bilayers.

Considering the cell membrane is in an oily state, what chemicals are prevented from traveling through the phospholipid bilayer? _____

What are some examples of chemicals that can pass through the phospholipid bilayer? _____

Cholesterol is interspersed among the phospholipid bilayer. Cholesterol has a stabilizing influence on the cell membrane.

Glycolipids are lipids with a _____ group attached. On which surface of the membrane are they situated (the surface that contacts the ECF or the ICF)? _____

Membrane Proteins

The proteins of the cell membrane are categorized into two types, **peripheral proteins** and **integral proteins.** Can you differentiate between the locations of each of these proteins?

1. Peripheral proteins are attached to either the *outside* surface or the *inside* surface of the cell membrane.

2. Integral proteins (more numerous) have at least some portions of their structures within the _____. Integral proteins that are completely within the bilayer are known as _____ proteins. **Transmembrane proteins** may serve as pores for the passage of certain substances such as water or as **ion channels** for the transport of certain ions.

Glycoproteins are the union of either a peripheral or an integral protein, and a _____ molecule.

• What are some of the functions of a glycoprotein? _____ _____ _____

Membrane Carbohydrates

Carbohydrates can form complexes with lipids; the union is known as a _____.
Carbohydrates can form complexes with proteins; the union is known as a _____.
The combinations of these carbohydrate complexes on the outer surface of the cell membrane create a very thin layer known as the **glycocalyx**. The function of the glycocalyx brings us back to the functions of the glycolipids and glycoproteins. As a unit, the function of the glycocalyx is to:

1. Lubricate and provide _____ for the cell.
2. Anchor the cell to adjacent structures.

Review Time!

I.   *Briefly answer the following questions about the cell membrane.*

1. Describe the fluid mosaic model of the cell membrane. _____ _____ _____

2. What part(s) of the phospholipid bilayer is/are hydrophobic? _____ _____

3. What part(s) of the phospholipid bilayer is/are hydrophilic? _____ _____

4. Explain why some items cannot travel across the phospholipid bilayer. _____ _____

5. Besides phospholipids, what are the two other types of lipids found associated with the cell membrane? _____ _____

6. With what two organic compound groups do carbohydrates bind? _____ _____ _____

7. What are the two types of proteins associated with the cell membrane? _____ _____ _____

8. What type of cell membrane protein forms pores or ion channels? _____
_____

9. What are the two components of a glycolipid? _____
_____

10. What is the function of a glycoprotein? _____
_____

11. What type of protein is attached either to the outside surface or the inside surface of the cell
membrane? _____
_____

12. What components form the glycocalyx? _____
_____

13. What are the two functions of the glycocalyx? _____
_____
_____

14. What are the two examples of substances that cannot pass through the phospholipid bilayer?
_____
_____

15. What two environments are physically separated by the cell membrane? _____
_____
_____

II. *Use the following terms to label the sections of the cell membrane shown below.*

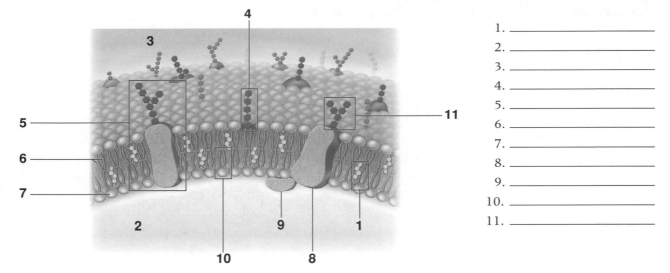

1. _____
2. _____
3. _____
4. _____
5. _____
6. _____
7. _____
8. _____
9. _____
10. _____
11. _____

Cholesterol	Glycoprotein	Peripheral protein
Cytoplasm	Hydrophobic tail	Phospholipid
Extracellular fluid	Hydrophobic head	Sugar
Glycolipid	Integral protein	

Movement Across Cell Membranes

LEARNING OBJECTIVE 3. Identify the ways in which materials move across the cell membrane.

Cells transport materials across the cell membrane in various ways. There are two categories of transport.

- **Passive processes:** Powered by kinetic energy that causes molecules to move about randomly, but energy is not required from the cell. Molecules move *along* a _____ _____ from areas of _____ concentration to areas of _____ concentration. What are the four types of passive processes we will discuss?

  1. _____

  2. _____

  3. _____

  4. _____

  > **TIP!** Think of a concentration gradient like a slide at the playground. The tendency for molecules is to move from areas of higher concentration to areas of lower concentration, similar to the effortless ride of a child from the top of the slide to the bottom of the slide.

- **Active processes:** Molecules move against the concentration gradient from lower areas of concentration to higher areas of concentration. Active processes require energy, or _____. What are the two types of active processes we will discuss?

  1. _____

  2. _____

Four Types of Passive Processes

Diffusion

Molecules collide with one another in a region of **higher** concentration which tends to move the molecules to a region of **lower** concentration. The molecules eventually reach a state of even distribution, or balance known as _____.

List three examples of diffusible substances in the human body.

1. _____

2. _____

3. _____

Diffusion can occur in two different ways. Molecules that are soluble in _____ can diffuse directly through the phospholipid bilayer. Small molecules, such as water and most ions, can pass through the tiny pores in the membrane created by *channel proteins.*

Facilitated Diffusion

Large, water-soluble (lipid-insoluble) molecules cannot travel through the phospholipid bilayer. These molecules must use *carrier proteins.*

These molecules are still transported along (or down) a _____ from a region of higher concentration to a region of lower concentration without the use of ATP. As with diffusion, movement occurs until equilibrium is reached.

To be transported, the molecule must first bind to a _____ in the cell membrane. The protein changes shape and the molecule is transported to the inside of the cell.

List two examples of substances that move by facilitated diffusion.

1. _____.

2. _____.

The rate of transport across the membrane depends on the speed the carrier proteins can move the molecules into the cell.

Osmosis

Osmosis is a special type of _____ that moves water molecules through channel proteins across a permeable membrane from a region of higher *water* concentration to a region of lower *water* concentration without the use of ATP. (The higher the *water* concentration, the lower the *solute* concentration.) As with diffusion, water molecules move across a membrane until _____ is reached. Osmosis occurs whenever two compartments containing water, each with different amounts of dissolved solutes, are separated by a barrier (membrane) that prevents the movement of the solutes.

Osmotic pressure is the force required to oppose the movement of water molecules across a membrane. This force depends on the concentration gradient created by the unequal distribution of solutes on either side of a membrane.

> **TIP!** In other words, the presence of solutes in a particular environment (either intracellular or extracellular) creates osmotic pressure. Water is attracted to those solutes and is "pulled" toward them. Keep in mind the following phrase: water follows salt (solutes).

Let's consider three extracellular environments and their impacts on the movement of water either into or out of a cell. Imagine placing a blood cell into a beaker full of a solution.

1. **Isotonic solutions** are ones in which the ECF is said to be in equilibrium with the ICF of the red blood cell. The concentration of water molecules is the _____ on either side of the cell membrane. The cell is said to be in _____ with its environment. Water flows into and out of the cell at an equal rate.

2. **Hypotonic solutions** are ones in which the ECF has a *lower* or *smaller* concentration of solutes than the ICF. To achieve equilibrium, water enters the cell and the cell swells up like a water balloon. *Remember, water follows salt (solutes).* Some cells will rupture or _____, in red blood cells it is called _____.

3. **Hypertonic solutions** are ones in which the ECF has a *higher* or *greater* concentration of solutes than the ICF. To achieve equilibrium, water leaves the cell and the cell dehydrates, shrinks, and shrivels, a process known as _____. *Remember, water follows salt (solutes).*

> **TIP!** A quick way to recall that cells bloat when placed in hypotonic solutions, remember the "O" in hyp**O**tonic solutions bl**O**at cells. Likewise, in a hypertonic solution, cells will shrivel. Remember the "R" in hype**R**tonic causes sh**R**iveling or c**R**enation.

Filtration

Filtration occurs when water, and sometimes solutes, is forced across a permeable membrane. Solutes will travel with the water if (1) they are small enough to penetrate membrane pores and (2) a pressure gradient is present.

• Where does filtration occur in the body? _____

_____

Review Time!

I. *Using the terms in the list below, write the appropriate passive environment in each blank. You will use the terms more than once.*

   Diffusion   Facilitated diffusion   Osmosis   Filtration

   1. Requires carrier proteins for transport of substances _____
   2. Movement of water across the cell membrane from a region of higher water concentration to a region of lower water concentration _____
   3. Movement of glucose across the cell membrane _____
   4. Movement of lipid-soluble substances across the cell membrane _____
   5. Water and some solutes are forced across the cell membrane _____
   6. Rate of transport depends on the speed of carrier proteins _____
   7. Transport of water-soluble substances _____
   8. Forced movement of water through capillary walls _____
   9. Solutes will travel with water across a membrane if a pressure gradient is present _____
   10. Water moves in response to osmotic pressure _____

II. *Briefly answer the following questions about passive processes.*

   1. Describe the similarities between diffusion and facilitated diffusion. _____
   _____
   _____

   2. Explain how facilitated diffusion is different from diffusion. Include two well-explained differences. _____
   _____
   _____

   3. When a cell has been placed into a hypertonic solution, what happens to that cell? _____
   _____

   4. Explain which passive processes utilize channel proteins for transport and why. _____
   _____
   _____

   5. Describe why an isotonic solution is equilibrium for a cell. _____
   _____
   _____

   6. Explain why a patient receiving an intravenous (IV) drip of a hypotonic solution can experience hemolysis. _____
   _____
   _____

   7. Explain why a patient receiving an IV drip of a hypertonic solution will experience cell crenation. _____
   _____

8. You are stranded on an island and have two sources of water: the salty ocean and fresh water (possibly contaminated with microbes). Which water do you choose to drink and why?

_____

_____

9. Testosterone, a sex hormone formed from cholesterol, travels along its concentration gradient into a cell. Name and explain the passive process you think this cell uses to incorporate this hormone.

_____

_____

_____

10. Carbon dioxide molecules move along their concentration gradient into a cell. Name and explain the method you think a cell will use to transport this blood gas. _____

_____

_____

11. Drinking too much water over a short period of time can disrupt the electrolyte balance in the body (a problem called _water intoxication_ or _hypotonic hydration_). Explain how cells respond to being placed in an environment with a lower concentration of solutes than their ICF.

_____

_____

_____

12. Describe how the size and composition of a substance influences the type of passive process used.

_____

_____

13. Using what you know about the structure of the cell membrane, explain why water must use channel proteins to move across the membrane. _____

_____

_____

14. Using what you know about the structure of the cell membrane, explain why a carrier protein must be used during facilitated diffusion. _____

_____

_____

15. Are _solutes_ or _water_ moved across a membrane during osmosis? Explain your choice. How does this movement help the cell achieve equilibrium with its environment? _____

_____

_____

_____

Two Types of Active Processes

Active Transport

Active transport carries substances *against* the concentration gradient across a selectively permeable cell membrane.

Carrier proteins, or **ion pumps**, must be used in the transport of solutes such as sodium (Na^+), potassium (K^+), calcium (Ca^{2+}), magnesium (Mg^{2+}), chloride (Cl^-) and iodide (I^-). The most common pump is the _____. This pump moves Na^+ ions out of the cell and K^+ ions into a cell to maintain the cell's homeostasis.

- Energy, or _____, must be used to power the carrier proteins.

Vesicular Transport

Vesicular transport is used to move large volumes of fluids or particles across the cell membrane.

Vesicles are formed from the existing membrane when the membrane buds off and creates a sac filled with fluids or particles. Vesicles may be moved within the cell's interior, or from cell to cell.

The two types of vesicular transport are **endocytosis** and **exocytosis**.

Endocytosis

Endocytosis is a type of vesicular transport in which large volumes of fluid or large particles are brought into a cell. Here's how endocytosis is accomplished.

1. The cell extends a segment of the cell membrane around the material and encloses it.
2. Once enclosed, the segment buds off inside the cell, forming a vesicle.

There are three types of endocytosis.

1. **Receptor-mediated endocytosis** begins when a molecule binds a receptor on the cell membrane. As a result, the cell membrane folds around the molecule and forms a sack-like vesicle that brings the molecule inside the cell.
   - What are some examples of specific substances that can move by receptor-mediated endocytosis? Viruses such as HIV, _____.
     _____

2. **Phagocytosis** ("cell eating") begins when a particle binds to a receptor in the cell membrane. A segment of the membrane, known as a _____, moves outward by streaming cytoplasm and surrounds the particle and engulfs it. Digestive enzymes from lysosomes ingest the particle in its vesicle.
   - What types of cells can perform phagocytosis? _____
     _____
   - What kinds of particles can be phagocytized? _____
     _____

3. **Pinocytosis** ("cell drinking") begins when a segment of the cell membrane folds inward around a droplet of ECF, forming a vesicle. The vesicle detaches from the membrane and enters the cytoplasm. Like phagocytosis, enzymes from lysosomes enter the vesicle to break down engulfed materials.
   - What are some examples of cells that can perform pinocytosis? _____
     _____

Exocytosis

Exocytosis is a type of vesicular transport used by cells to move bulk materials out of the cell into the extracellular environment. Here's how exocytosis is accomplished:

1. Bulk materials such as waste products are packaged into vesicle inside the cell.

2. Vesicles fuse with the cell membrane and the contents are dumped into the extracellular environment.

   • **Excretion** is the exocytosis of _____ products through exocytosis.

   • **Secretion** is the exocytosis of _____ molecules through exocytosis.

Review Time!

I. *For each action in the list below, write the appropriate active process (*active transport *or* vesicular transport*) in the blank.*

   1. Receptor-mediated endocytosis   _____

   2. Pinocytosis   _____

   3. Sodium–potassium pump   _____

   4. Exocytosis   _____

   5. Cells engulf bacteria   _____

   6. Excretion of wastes   _____

   7. Substances are carried against the concentration
      gradient by an ion pump   _____

   8. Secretion of hormones   _____

   9. Large volumes of fluid are brought into the cell in vesicles   _____

   10. The cell uses a pseudopod to engulf particles   _____

II. *Briefly answer the following questions about active processes.*

   1. Differentiate between secretion and excretion. _____

      _____

      _____

   2. Describe how receptor-mediated endocytosis is different from pinocytosis. _____

      _____

      _____

   3. Provide two well-explained similarities between pinocytosis and phagocytosis.

      _____

      _____

   4. Why is the sodium–potassium pump an important ion pump? _____

      _____

      _____

   5. Explain why a cell could not perform active transport without ATP. _____

      _____

      _____

   6. Molecules moved against their concentration gradient must be pumped into the cell by a carrier protein. Identify this active process and describe how it works. _____

      _____

      _____

7. White blood cells phagocytize bacteria. Explain how this process occurs. _____
_____

8. List the three types of endocytosis. How are these processes different? Explain.
_____
_____

9. When might a cell utilize a pseudopod to perform endocytosis? _____. Explain
how the pseudopod assists with this particular type of endocytosis. _____
_____
_____

10. What is a vesicle? Describe. _____
_____
_____

CONCEPT 3

Cell Structure and Function: The Cytoplasm and Its Organelles

Concept: Organelles are structures in the cytoplasm that provide the cell with a division of labor.

LEARNING OBJECTIVE 4. Distinguish between the cellular organelles on the basis of their structure and function.

Recall that the cytoplasm of a cell is situated between the cell membrane and the nucleus. Most of the volume of the cytoplasm is a thickened gel-like ICF known as _____.
• What is found in the cytosol?_____
_____
_____

Suspended within the cytosol are **organelles**. Some organelles are in direct contact with the cytosol because they are not surrounded by a membrane. List these six organelles.

1. _____.
2. _____.
3. _____.
4. _____.
5. _____.
6. _____.

Other organelles house particular sets of enzymes and are enclosed by selectively permeable membranes. List these five organelles.

1. _____.
2. _____.
3. _____.
4. _____.
5. _____.

TIP! To devise a mental image of the cytoplasm of a cell, visualize a bowl of jelly with fruit pieces interspersed within the jelly. The jelly symbolizes the cytosol while the fruit pieces exemplify the organelles.

Cytoskeleton

- **Structure:** The cytoskeleton is a network of three main proteins (microfilaments, intermediate filaments, and microtubules) that form a complex scaffold within the cytoplasm.
  1. **Microfilaments** (thin filaments) are formed from the protein _____. Microfilaments may cause a cell to move for those cells that are mobile or change shape.
  2. **Intermediate filaments** are intermediate in size between microfilaments and microtubules. Two proteins that can serve as intermediate filaments are _____ and _____. Intermediate filaments help stabilize the position of organelles within the cell, secure the cell's shape, and give the cell strength and durability.
  3. **Microtubules** are long, hollow tubes that help to maintain the shape of the cell. Microtubules are composed of the protein _____, which undergoes constant rearrangement. When located near the nucleus, microtubules form organelles known as _____. Likewise, microtubules form structures that extend away from the cell known as _____ and _____.
- **Function:** The cytoskeleton provides structural strength and flexibility, and helps determine a cell's shape.

Centrioles

- **Structure: Centrosomes** are a dense network of protein fibers that also contain **centrioles**, cylindrical structures composed of nine groups of three microtubules.
- **Function:** Centrioles are found in all cells that divide by a process called mitosis; centrioles also play a role in the formation and regeneration of _____ and _____.
- **Location:** Near the nucleus as part of a centrosome.

Cilia and Flagella

- **Structure:** Although **cilia** are not found on all cells, cells that do have cilia may have hundreds of them. Cilia originate from the cytoplasm just deep to the cell surface and their exposed portion is covered by the cell membrane. **Flagella** are similar to cilia, but are much _____.
- **Function:** Cilia beat in coordination with one another to move fluids along a cell's surface. Flagella move in a whip-like manner to provide movement to the cell itself.
- **Location:** Cilia in the respiratory tract beat in unison to move mucus upward from the lungs. A single flagellum is found only on human _____.

Microvilli

- **Structure:** Microvilli are fingerlike projections formed from tiny folds of the _____ of certain cells.
- **Function:** Microvilli increase surface area of the cell and the amount of material that can pass across the cell membrane.
- **Location:** Microvilli are in cells that absorb substances, such as the small intestine.

Ribosomes

- **Structure:** Ribosomes are smaller than other organelles and composed of about 60% _____ and 40% _____.
- **Function:** Ribosomes serve as the site for protein synthesis.
- **Location: Free ribosomes** are dispersed through the _____ of the cell while **fixed ribosomes** are attached to the endoplasmic reticulum (ER).

Endoplasmic Reticulum

- **Structure:** The ER is a series of branching and rejoining hollow tubules. The walls, formed from phospholipid bilayer membrane, create an enclosed sac. The **rough ER** appears rough due to the presence of numerous fixed _____. The **smooth ER** lacks ribosomes.
- **Function:** Rough ER is responsible for protein synthesis. The proteins are sent to the Golgi apparatus to be prepared for export. Smooth ER is responsible for lipid synthesis of organic compounds such as _____ and _____ that build the cell membrane, _____ that form certain hormones, and _____ that are stored in the liver for energy. Glycogen, a carbohydrate, is also synthesized in the smooth ER. The smooth ER also detoxifies poisonous substances such as alcohol.
- **Location:** The ER is found through the cytoplasm and is continuous with the membrane surrounding the nucleus.

Golgi Apparatus

- **Structure:** The Golgi apparatus is constructed of flattened disc-shaped sacs known as _____, resembling a stack of pancakes. Each of the 5 to 6 cisterna that composes a single Golgi apparatus is enclosed by a single phospholipid bilayer membrane.
- **Function:** The Golgi apparatus contains enzymes that modify proteins, lipids, and carbohydrates that are synthesized by the _____. **Secretory vesicles**, containing molecules, pinch off the cisternae and migrate toward the cell membrane in the process of exocytosis.
- **Location:** The Golgi apparatus is normally found near the nucleus.

Mitochondria

- **Structure:** Each mitochondrion is uniquely bound by two layers of phospholipid bilayer membrane. The inner of the two membranes folds into convolutions known as _____ which provide an attachment site for enzymes. The space formed by the inner membrane is known as the **matrix** which contains enzymes and _____. Since mitochondria have their own DNA, they can replicate themselves when energy demand increases.
- **Function:** Mitochondria are often called the "energy powerhouses" of cells because they break down nutrients molecules, commonly glucose, to supply the cell with energy, primarily in the form of _____. The process of ATP production is a metabolic function and is known as **cellular respiration**.
- **Location:** Mitochondria are located randomly through the cytoplasm, but are not found in all cells.

Lysosomes

- **Structure:** Originating from the _____, lysosomes are similarly enclosed by a single phospholipid bilayer membrane.

- **Function:** Lysosomes have several functions.
  1. Since lysosomes house numerous hydrolytic enzymes, they are active in breaking apart intracellular particles, nutrient molecules, ingested microorganisms, or dead body cells. For this reason, lysosomes are often known as the "_____ system of the cell."
  2. Lysosomes also have the nicknames of "self-destruct bags" and "suicide packets" because of the role in the recycling process that follows cell death. Upon death of the cell, **autolysis** occurs as lysosomes rupture and release enzymes into the cytoplasm so that the components of the cell are digested for reuse by other cells.
  3. Lysosomes release enzymes into the extracellular environment by the process of _____ so that the enzymes can break down materials outside the cell.
- **Location:** Lysosomes are randomly distributed through the cytoplasm.

Peroxisomes

- **Structure:** Smaller than lysosomes, peroxisomes are similar spherical structures that contain enzymes.
- **Function:** The enzymes found in a peroxisome detoxify molecules such as _____ from alcoholic beverages.
- **Location:** Peroxisomes are randomly distributed throughout the _____.

Review Time!

I.   For each of the following statements or descriptions, indicate the appropriate organelle or structure. You may use a term more than once.

Centrioles	Cilia and flagella	Cytoskeleton
Golgi apparatus	Lysosomes	Microvilli
Mitochondria	Peroxisomes	Ribosomes
Rough ER	Smooth ER	

1. Synthesizes lipids _____
2. Performs autolysis _____
3. Makes ATP _____
4. Makes the lysosome _____
5. Appearance resembles a stack of pancakes _____
6. Houses both DNA and enzymes in the matrix _____
7. Site of cellular respiration _____
8. Found fixed on the surface of the rough ER _____
9. Long, slender projections _____
10. Synthesizes glycogen _____
11. Located freely in the cytoplasm or fixed to the rough ER _____
12. Found only in cells that undergo cell division (mitosis) _____
13. Fingerlike projections that increase surface area _____
14. Microtubules, microfilaments, and intermediate filaments form a scaffold within the cytoplasm of a cell _____
15. The only organelle to have two layers of the phospholipid bilayer _____
16. "Energy powerhouse" of the cell _____

17. Inner membrane is folded into cristae _____
18. Site of protein synthesis _____
19. "Self-destruct bag" of the cell _____
20. Described as "free" or "fixed" _____
21. Forms packages known as secretory vesicles _____
22. Exists as part of a centrosome _____
23. Commonly found in cells that absorb substances _____
24. Composed of nine groups of three microtubules _____
25. "The digestive system of the cell" _____
26. Rhythmic movements _____
27. Modifies and packages cellular products for exocytosis _____
28. Often attached to the nuclear envelope _____
29. Releases enzymes into the extracellular environment _____
30. Named for the presence, or absence, of ribosomes _____

II. *Briefly answer the following questions about the parts of a cell.*

1. Describe the unique structure of the mitochondrion. _____

2. Compare and contrast the functions and structures of the two types of ER. _____

3. Explain the relationship between the functions of the ER and the Golgi apparatus. _____

4. Explain how these terms are related: cytosol, cytoplasm, and ICF. _____

5. Differentiate among the structures of the three proteins that compose the cytoskeleton. _____

6. Differentiate among the functions of the ribosome, lysosome, and peroxisome. _____

7. How do microvilli differ from cilia and flagella? Explain. _____

8. Discuss how the peroxisomes and smooth ER are similar in some of their functions.

_____

_____

_____

9. Besides the nucleus, in which organelle is DNA housed? What role does the DNA play for that organelle? _____

_____   _____

_____

10. Using a microscope, how would you distinguish between rough and smooth ER?

_____

_____

_____

CONCEPT 4

Cell Structure and Function: The Nucleus

Concept: The nucleus is the "control center" of the cell because it contains DNA, which controls the synthesis of proteins according to instructions in the genes.

LEARNING OBJECTIVE 5. Explain why the nucleus is the control center of the cell.

LEARNING OBJECTIVE 6. Identify the structural components of the nucleus.

Nucleus

- **Structure:** The nucleus is a large structure in the cell, supported by the cytoskeleton.
- **Function:** The nucleus is often called the "control center" of the cell because of the genetic material it contains. The primary function of the nucleus is to regulate _____ which is controlled by DNA and its genes.
- **Location:** Mostly spherical in shape, the nucleus is usually situated near the center of the cell.

Nuclear Envelope

- **Structure:** The nuclear envelope is a double membrane that separates the _____ from the _____. The nuclear envelope is similar to the cell membrane since both are constructed of a selectively permeable phospholipid bilayer. Unlike the cell membrane, the nuclear envelope contains perforations known as **nuclear pores**.
- **Function:** The nuclear pores permit the movement of ions and small molecules and allow for chemical communication between the nucleus and other parts of the cell.

Nucleoplasm

- **Structure:** Similar to cytosol, the **nucleoplasm** is a gel-like fluid that contains water, ions, enzymes, _____ and _____ nucleotides, small amounts of DNA and RNA, and a network of protein filaments that support the DNA. Several **nucleoli** house enzymes, structural proteins, and RNA.

- **Function:** Nucleoli assemble _____. DNA provides instructions for the assembly of amino acids to form _____ during protein synthesis. When a cell is not dividing, DNA appears as threadlike filaments called **chromatin**. In a dividing cell, DNA organizes into 23 pairs of _____, or a total of 46 chromosomes. Each chromosome contains segments of DNA, known as _____.

CONCEPT 5

Protein Synthesis

Concept: The genetic code in the DNA of cells determines body structure and function because of its central role in protein synthesis, which occurs through two processes: transcription and translation.

LEARNING OBJECTIVE 7. Explain the function of DNA.

LEARNING OBJECTIVE 8. Describe how proteins are produced through transcription and translation.

First, let's review information about DNA before we start with the two-step process of protein synthesis (transcription and translation). DNA:

- Provides the basis for heredity.

- Regulates the synthesis of _____ in the cell. It determines the exact structure and function of each protein. It provides the message that directs the sequence of amino acids to form a protein.

- Is located in the nucleus of the cell and is unable to leave the nucleus.

- Resembles a long, twisted ladder composed of _____ subunits, each consisting of a sugar group, phosphate groups, and one of four nitrogen bases (adenine, thymine _____, or _____). Do you recall the way the nitrogen bases form complementary pairs? Adenine always pairs with _____ while cytosine always pairs with _____.

- Codes for amino acids in the form of a **triplet code** (three nitrogen bases along one strand of the DNA molecule) create a **codon**. Genes are a section of DNA that contains the triplet codes for the amino acids forming a complete protein.

Transcription

Transcription is the process of forming messenger RNA (mRNA). Since DNA is housed in the nucleus and cannot leave the nucleus, the DNA code must somehow be passed to the cytoplasm. Recall that proteins are assembled at the ribosomes in the cytoplasm. An intermediary messenger, called **mRNA**, will take the code from DNA to the cytoplasm.

- During transcription, the triplet code from _____ is copied (transcribed) to form an mRNA molecule within the _____.

- Transcription begins when a section of DNA is unraveled, exposing a specific group of DNA nucleotides to the nucleoplasm. RNA nucleotides are bound to the DNA nucleotides with the assistance of an enzyme known as RNA _____.
- A new chain of RNA nucleotides is formed that is complimentary to the original DNA nucleotide sequence. Cytosine on DNA pairs with the free nucleotide _____, guanine on DNA strand pairs with the free nucleotide _____. Thymine on the DNA strand pairs with the free nucleotide adenine, and adenine on the DNA strand pairs with the free RNA nucleotide _____.
- Once the new mRNA molecule is formed, it detaches from the DNA and leaves the nucleus through _____ in the nuclear envelope.
- Upon reaching the cytoplasm, the mRNA attaches to ribosomes in preparation for translation, the next step.
- Each triplet code of DNA is now a complimentary set called a _____ on the mRNA. Each codon corresponds to a section of DNA; the sequence of nucleotide bases is preserved in the mRNA molecule.

Translation

Translation is the process of interpreting the codons from mRNA into a specific sequence of amino acids. During translation, the nucleotide base sequence is transformed into an amino acid sequence. The process can be summarized as:

$$DNA \rightarrow RNA \rightarrow \text{_____}$$

- Translation begins when mRNA attaches to a _____ in the cytoplasm.
- Molecules of **transfer RNA** (tRNA) read the mRNA instruction, bind to the corresponding _____ in the cytoplasm, and transport them to the ribosome.
- The ribosome moves along the mRNA, and tRNA brings the next amino acid into place.
- Amino acids are joined by peptide bonds to form a polypeptide, or protein.
- A stop command will bring an end to this process and the completed polypeptide is released from the ribosomal complex.

> **TIP!** To remember which process of protein synthesis comes first, use this trick: transCription is alphabetically before transLation. Also, to keep track of what is made during each process, use this trick: RNA is made during transcRiption ("R" for RNA). Amino acids result from translAtion ("A" for amino acids).

Review Time!

I. *Briefly answer the following questions about the nuclear functions.*

1. Differentiate between the nucleolus and nucleoplasm. _____
_____
_____

2. Differentiate between chromatin and chromosomes. Which form is used during protein synthesis?
_____
_____
_____
_____

3. Explain how DNA serves as the basis for proteins. _____

_____

_____

4. Discuss how the triplet code is related to the codon. _____

_____

_____

5. Identify the two steps of protein synthesis and briefly summarize the events of each step.

_____

_____

6. What RNA nitrogen base is complimentary to thymine in DNA? _____

_____

7. What bonds hold together the amino acids of a protein? _____

_____

8. Through what part of the nuclear envelope does the mRNA molecule travel on its way to the
   cytoplasm? _____

_____

9. Describe the function of mRNA. _____

_____

_____

10. Predict how membrane transport would be affected if protein synthesis failed to occur.

_____

_____

_____

11. Why must DNA be rewritten into RNA during transcription? _____

_____

12. What is the role of RNA polymerase? _____

_____

13. Transcribe this strand of DNA into mRNA:

A T C T C G G T C A

_____

14. Describe the role of tRNA during translation. _____

_____

_____

15. Relate DNA to genes. _____

_____

_____

CONCEPT 6

Life Cycle of the Cell

Concept: Most of a cell's lifetime is spent producing new molecules and energy, and duplicating DNA in preparation for cell division. Cell replacement and body growth are achieved by cell division, which includes mitosis and cytokinesis.

LEARNING OBJECTIVE   9. Describe the role of cell division in maintaining health.

LEARNING OBJECTIVE   10. Describe the phases of mitosis.

The **cell life cycle** includes the changes that occur during the life of a cell. The moment a new cell is formed by cell division marks the beginning of the cell's life cycle. The two phases of a cell's life are _____, the time during which the cell grows and performs its functions and _____, the time when the cell reproduces itself.

Interphase

Interphase is the time of a cell's life between cell divisions and occupies most of the cell's life (more than 90%). There are three subphases or periods of interphase.

1. **G1:** The first growth phase during which the cell is actively manufacturing new molecules for growth and secretion, making new organelles, producing energy, and performing roles for the body.
2. **S phase:** The time when DNA replication occurs.
3. **G2:** The second growth period during which time the cell prepares for division if it is to divide. If cell division is to occur, it will follow this phase.

Cell Division (Mitosis)

Cell division comprises two major events.

1. **Nuclear division** occurs when the _____ divides.
2. **Cytoplasmic division**, or **cytokinesis**, occurs with the division of the cytoplasm.

Nuclear division may proceed through either mitosis or meiosis (meiosis is studied in Chapter 18). Mitosis occurs in _____ cells (nonreproductive cells) when new cells are needed for growth or replacement. Meiosis occurs in _____ cells during sperm or egg production.

Mitosis is the division of the replicated DNA that is packaged inside two newly formed nuclei resulting in the formation of two identical daughter cells. There are four stages of mitosis.

1. **Prophase** is the first stage of mitosis. Visual clues to look for include the presence of visible chromosomes. Each strand of a chromosome is known as a **chromatid**. The two chromatids are connected at the _____. Centrioles migrate to opposite ends of the cell and microtubules develop around each centriole. Later in prophase, the microtubules form a network of bundles, the **spindle**, that extend from one side of the cell to the _____ of each chromatid.
2. **Metaphase** is recognizable by the presence of the chromosomes lined up in the center of the cell. The nuclear envelope has completely disappeared and the spindle is well developed by the end of this stage.

3. **Anaphase** is the third stage and is characterized by the movement of the _____ toward opposite poles of the cell. Shrinking spindle fibers separate the chromatids. Late in this stage, **cytokinesis** begins with the appearance of a line of division, called the **cleavage furrow**, through the cytoplasm.

4. **Telophase** is the last stage of mitosis. The two groups of chromatids reach the opposite poles of the cell and clump together to form chromosomes. A nuclear _____ reforms around each set of chromosomes. The spindle _____ while the nucleoli within each newly formed nucleus reappears. The cleavage furrow divides the cytoplasm completely to form two new daughter cells. Chromosomes eventually uncoil to resume the chromatin state.

> **TIP!** The life cycle of the cell can easily be remembered in the correct order as IPMAT where I stands for Interphase, and PMAT are the four stages of mitosis (Prophase, Metaphase, Anaphase, and Telophase).

Cytokinesis

Although mitosis is complete at the end of telophase, cell division is only complete with the separation of the parent cell into two daughter cells. **Cytokinesis**, or cytoplasmic division, begins during late _____ with the appearance of the **cleavage furrow**.

Review Time!

I. Using the terms in the list below, write the appropriate stage of mitosis in each blank. You may use a term more than once.

Anaphase   Metaphase   Prophase   Telophase

1. Cleavage furrow begins to form   _____
2. Cytokinesis is complete and the cell divides into two new daughter cells   _____
3. Chromosomes line up in the center of the cell   _____
4. Centrioles migrate to each end of the cell and microtubules start to develop the spindle   _____
5. Chromosomes are separated by shrinking spindle fibers   _____
6. Cleavage furrow begins to appear late in this stage   _____
7. Nuclear division is complete during this stage   _____
8. Nuclear envelope reforms around each set of chromosomes   _____
9. By this stage, the nuclear envelope has completely disappeared   _____
10. The spindle disappears   _____

II. Briefly answer the following questions about cell reproduction.

1. Is mitosis the same as the cell cycle? Explain. _____
   _____
   _____

2. How many cells are created by the process of mitosis? Are these cells genetically identical?
   _____
   _____

3. What part of the life cycle does a cell enter after the completion of telophase and mitosis?

_____

_____

4. What types of cells undergo mitosis—*somatic* cells or *sex* cells? _____

_____

5. Which process makes sex cells—*mitosis* or *meiosis*? _____

_____

6. Does a cell spend more of its life in interphase or mitosis? _____

_____

7. Explain what occurs during cytokinesis. _____

_____

8. During what part of the life cycle is the DNA replicated? _____

_____

9. Explain what is involved in the formation of the spindle. _____

_____

10. Is the cleavage furrow involved in cytoplasmic division or nuclear division? Explain.

_____

_____

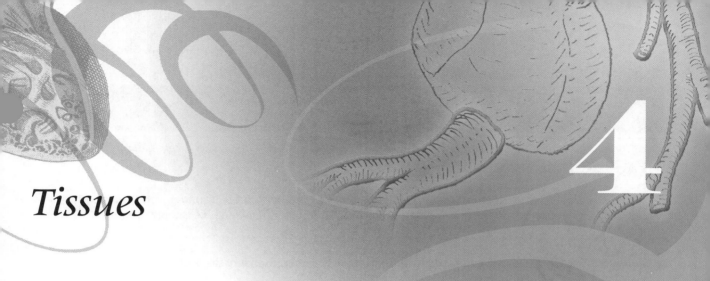

Tissues

Tips for Success as You Begin

Read Chapter 4 from your textbook before attending class. Listen when you attend lecture and fill in the blanks in this notebook. You may choose to complete the blanks before attending class as a way to prepare for the day's topics. The same day you attend lecture, read the material again and complete the exercises after each section in this notebook. Spend time every day with this chapter as it will help you make sense of the material. For this chapter, you can facilitate your learning by making flash cards of the tissues. Place a picture of the tissue on one side of your flash card and the name and/or function on the reverse side. Learn the names of the tissues first. As you become familiar with the names, add the functions, locations, and structures.

Introduction

LEARNING OBJECTIVE 1. Define the term *tissue* and indicate the four main types in the body.

Tissues are cooperative groups of _____ sharing a common function that are united to perform a particular function. Tissues also include the cellular products and extracellular fluids that are found outside the cells.

The four primary types of tissues are:

1. _____
   _____

2. _____
   _____

3. _____
   _____

4. _____
   _____

CONCEPT 1

Epithelial Tissues

Concept: Epithelial tissue is composed of cells packed close together. It protects underlying tissues and controls permeability due to the physical barrier that is formed. Often, it includes cells that secrete.

LEARNING OBJECTIVE 2. Describe the structural characteristics of epithelial tissue and indicate its common functions.

LEARNING OBJECTIVE 3. Distinguish between the various types of epithelium, providing an example of where each is found in the body.

- **Overall structure of epithelial tissue:** Epithelial tissues are tightly packed cells with little or no intercellular material between the cells. For this reason, epithelial tissues lack blood vessels, known as _____.

- **Functions:** Epithelial tissue covers body surfaces, lines the inside of body cavities and organs, and forms _____. The three functions of epithelial tissues are:

  1. _____: Epithelial tissues form a barrier to protect the underlying cells from the sun's radiation, infection, or physical injury.

  2. _____: The cells of the epithelial tissue form a filter to regulate what can travel from one side of the tissue to the other.

  3. _____: Some commonly secreted products are enzymes, hormones, and mucus.

Features of Epithelial Tissues

Cell junctions are present between the cells of epithelial tissues that lock together the cells. The two cell junctions most commonly associated with epithelial tissues are:

  1. _____: Lock together two cells by protein filaments and intercellular cement.

  2. _____: Fuse the lipid bilayers of two adjacent cells to create a chemically resistance barrier.

Epithelial tissues are anchored by a **basement membrane** that attaches the epithelial tissue to an underlying tissue. Epithelial tissues also have a free surface that may face the lumen (interior cavity) of a body cavity or organ.

Covering and Lining Epithelium

Covering and lining epithelium covers body and organ surfaces and lines internal organs and body cavities. The tightly packed cells form a blanket and a barrier.

Epithelial tissues are classified in two ways:

  1. **Cell shape**
     - **Squamous** cells are flattened.
     - **Cuboidal** cells are _____ shaped.
     - **Columnar** cells are _____.
  2. **Layered arrangement of cells**
     - **Simple** implies a *single* layer of cells.
     - **Stratified** indicates *multiple* layers of cells.

Simple Squamous Epithelium
- **Structure:** A single layer of flattened cells with a centrally located nucleus; all cells contact the basement membrane. From above, this tissue looks like floor tiles.
- **Function:** The thinness of this tissue allows rapid influx and outflow of substances.
- **Locations:** Lines the inside wall of _____ vessels and _____ vessels, and forms the walls of tiny capillaries, the walls of the air sacs in the lungs, and the lining of the body cavities.

Simple Cuboidal Epithelium
- **Structure:** A single layer of cube-shaped cells with a centrally located nucleus. Cells may contain cilia, _____, or both along their free surface.
- **Function:** Forms the walls of small tubes, or _____, that carry secretions.
- **Locations:** Kidneys, _____, and many glands.

Simple Columnar Epithelium
- **Structure:** A single layer of elongated, cylindrical cells with nuclei near the basement membrane.
- **Function:** Secrete cellular products.
- **Locations:** Lining the inside wall of the uterus, and digestive organs such as the _____ and _____.

Stratified Squamous Epithelium

> **TIP!** Pay attention only to the shape of the surface layer of cells as they are squamous (flat) in shape.

- **Structure:** Multiple-layered arrangement of cells.
  Why should we ignore the cells closer to the basement membrane when naming this tissue?
  _____
  _____
- **Function:** Protect body parts from wear and tear.
- **Locations:** Forms the outer layer of the skin and dips into all of the openings of the body to protect them from injury.

Pseudostratified Columnar Epithelium
- **Structure:** Composed of a single layer of cells; each cell touches the basement membrane, but not all reach the free surface. The name of the tissue comes from the illusion created by the lack of uniformity among cells' shapes and locations of nuclei.
- **Function:** If ciliated to move along _____, this tissue will be named *pseudostratified ciliated columnar (PSCC) epithelium.*
- **Locations:** Lines part of the respiratory tract such as the _____ and _____.

Transitional Epithelium
- **Structure:** Composed of multiple layers of cells that alternate between two shapes: _____-shaped cells and _____-shaped cells.

- **Function:** Transitional means "to _____" and this tissue has the ability to change its shape. Two functional features of transitional epithelium:
    1. **Elasticity:** The tissue can stretch.
    2. **Extensibility:** The tissue can return to its original shape after stretching.
- **Locations:** Urinary bladder and ureters (accommodate the passage of urine)

Glandular Epithelium

Glandular epithelium consists of closely packed cells that are specialized to make and secrete products. A particular type of glandular epithelium is referred to as a **gland**. Glands secrete one or more products.

- **Some examples of glands are** _____

_____

We will now discuss two types of glands, *exocrine* and *endocrine*.

Exocrine Glands

Exocrine glands "secrete outside" and empty their products into tiny tubes, or _____ onto the body surface or into a cavity.

- **Some examples of exocrine glands are** _____

_____

Exocrine glands are classified as organs because they are supported by connective tissue and supplied by blood vessels and nerves.

Endocrine Glands

Endocrine glands "secrete within" and place their products into the extracellular space. These products move by diffusion into the bloodstream for transport throughout the body.

- **Some examples of endocrine glands are** _____

_____

Endocrine glands are also classified as organs because:

_____

_____

_____

Review Time!

I. *Using the terms in the list below, write the appropriate covering and lining epithelium in each blank. You may use a term more than once.*

Glandular epithelium	*Simple squamous epithelium*	*Simple cuboidal epithelium*
Simple columnar epithelium	*Stratified squamous epithelium*	*Pseudostratified columnar epithelium*
Pseudostratified ciliated columnar epithelium	*Transitional epithelium*	

1. Single layer of flattened cells _____
2. Functions to stretch and recoil _____
3. Multiple layers of flattened cells _____
4. Found in the trachea _____
5. Forms the outer layer of the skin _____
6. Falsely appears stratified, but is in fact a single layer of cells _____

7. Lines the innermost wall of the uterus and some digestive organs

   _____

8. Lacks uniformity because all cells do not reach the free surface

   _____

9. Single layer of elongated, cylindrical cells

   _____

10. Located in the digestive tract, such as the lining of the stomach

    _____

11. Forms the glands of the endocrine system

    _____

12. Free surface may contain cilia or microvilli

    _____

13. Lines the wall of blood vessels

    _____

14. Protects from wear and tear

    _____

15. Formed from a single layer of cube-shaped cells

    _____

CONCEPT 2

Connective Tissue

Concept: Connective tissue consists of a vast amount of intercellular material secreted by interspersed cells. It supports and protects body parts, forms connections that facilitate communication, and stores energy molecules and minerals.

LEARNING OBJECTIVE 4. Describe the structural characteristics of connective tissue that make it distinct from epithelial tissue.

LEARNING OBJECTIVE 5. Distinguish between the types of connective tissue on the basis of their structural and functional differences.

- **Overall structure of connective tissue:** Connective tissue is usually composed of widely scattered cells that are interspersed in a large amount of nonliving extracellular matrix. Connective tissue is the most abundant type of tissue in the body.
- **Functions:** Connective tissue mainly supports other body structures and keeps our tissues "glued" together and our organs in place. The six functions of connective tissue are:

1. _____: Connective tissues provide a structural scaffold that anchors and supports the soft tissues and organs of the body.

2. _____: Connective tissues protect soft, inner organs and tissues from physical injury, and the _____ blood cells it contains help to protect the body from infection.

3. _____: Connective tissues form connections between body parts; blood transports materials throughout the body.

4. _____: Connective tissues store energy-containing molecules in adipose tissue while bone tissue stores _____ and _____.

5. _____: Connective tissue, such as red marrow, produces blood cells.

6. _____: Connective tissues contain cells that quickly respond to tissues in need of repair that have been damaged.

- **Organization of connective tissues:** The cells of connective tissue fall into one of the two categories.

1. Cells that produce and maintain the extracellular matrix include fibroblasts, _____,
   and chondrocytes. The extracellular material is a mixture of sugar–protein molecules and interstitial
   fluid known as **ground substance**. Several types of protein fibers are suspended within the ground
   substance that forms a mesh known as the **extracellular matrix** (in most types of connective tissue).
   The three major types of protein fibers are collagen fibers, elastic fibers, and reticulin fibers (listed next
   in the order of abundance in the body).

   - **Collagen fibers** are the most abundant form of protein fibers in the extracellular matrix, making
     up nearly _____ percent of total body weight. Strands are thick and wavy.
     Collagen fibers are flexible yet provide great tensile strength (in other words, collagen fibers resist
     _____). Collagen is also used by the body for tissue repair by forming the
     main part of _____ tissue that forms over a wound.

   - **Elastic fibers** are composed of _____. How are elastic fibers different from
     collagen fibers? _____
     _____
     _____
     Elastic fibers are characterized by two features: elasticity and _____
     (the ability to strength and return to the original shape).
     _____

   - **Reticular fibers** are the least abundant of the proteins in connective tissue matrix.
     How are these fibers similar to collagen fibers? _____
     _____
     How are these fibers different from collagen fibers? _____
     _____
     These fibers resist _____ and anchor organs to body parts, in the walls of
     blood vessels, and in the interior of organs such as the _____,
     _____, and _____.
     In addition to fibers, blood vessels present in connective tissue makes them **vascular**. This blood
     supply brings nutrients and oxygen to tissues for growth and repair.

2. The second group is white blood cells that protect the tissue from _____.

Connective Tissue Proper

Connective tissue proper is common between and within most organs of the body. It is characterized
by abundant extracellular matrix produced by **fibroblasts** which produce extracellular material. Four
subtypes vary by the amount and type of fibers found in the matrix:

1. Loose connective tissue
2. Adipose tissue
3. _____ tissue
4. Dense connective tissue

Loose Connective Tissue

Loose connective tissue (areolar tissue) is the most widespread of all connective tissues. What types of
protein fibers are found here? _____
_____
_____

Fibroblasts and **macrophages**, phagocytic white blood cells, are also common in loose connective tissue. Macrophages are particularly numerous during _____.
Loose connective tissue that is found between skin and muscle is called **superficial fascia**.

Adipose Tissue

- **Structure:** Adipose tissue is composed of specialized fibroblasts called _____ that store energy as fat (triglycerides). Little extracellular matrix exists except for _____ fibers.
- **Function:** Energy storage as fat, insulator to slow loss of _____ through the skin, padded cushion to absorb shocks to organs, fills body spaces. Subcutaneous fat is the most abundant location for adipose tissue. Adipocytes low in lipids trigger hunger sensations.

Dense Connective Tissue

Overall structure: Tightly packed fibers, mostly collagen, leave very little space for ground substance. Dense irregular and dense regular connective tissues vary in the direction of their collagen fibers.

- **Dense irregular connective tissue:** _____ fibers branch extensively, ground substance is minimal, and fibroblasts are scattered.
- **Function:** Forms scar tissue, wraps around _____ and _____, situated in the deep layer of the skin (known as the _____).
- **Dense regular connective tissue:** Collagen fibers extend in regular, parallel lines, ground substance is minimal, and fibroblasts may be linearly arranged.
- **Function:** This tissue is tough and withstands physical stress; it is the primary component of tendons (connect muscles to _____) and ligaments (connect bones to _____ across joints).

Cartilage

- **Overall structure:** Cartilage is flexible despite its thickened gel-like ground substance which is hardened and stabilized by protein fibers in the matrix. Blood vessels cannot invade the extracellular material, but diffusion carries nutrients and oxygen to the cells in this tissue from a dense connective tissue layer that surrounds the cartilage (called the **perichondrium**). **Chondrocytes** are "cartilage cells" and lie embedded within small spaces known as _____ ("small lake"). Adults have three types of cartilage that we'll explore next.

Hyaline Cartilage

Hyaline cartilage is the most abundant of the three types of cartilage.

- **Structure:** Hyaline cartilage has a smooth, glassy texture formed by glycoproteins and carbohydrate molecules that form the ground substance. _____ fibers and chondrocytes in their lacunae are also present.
- **Function:** Hyaline cartilage covers the ends of bones that form some joints; forms the connection between the ribs and sternum; and forms the soft part of the nose, part of the respiratory tract, and the fetal skeleton.

Elastic Cartilage

Elastic cartilage is characterized by the presence of elastic fibers.

- **Structure:** Elastic cartilage contains chondrocytes within lacunae and elastic fibers. This type of cartilage has less ground substance than _____ cartilage.
- **Function:** This type of cartilage is more elastic than other types; it forms the supportive framework of the ears and the epiglottis.

> **TIP!** Keep in mind the "E" letters here—*e*ar and *e*piglottis are formed from *e*lastic cartilage.

Fibrocartilage

Fibrocartilage is characterized by the presence of wavy collagen fibers.

- **Structure:** Abundant collagen fibers have embedded chondrocytes within their

  _____

- **Function:** Fibrocartilage serves as a shock-absorbing cushion for many of the body's joints, such as

  _____

> **TIP!** To differentiate between fibrocartilage and dense regular connective tissue, look for chondrocytes. They are present in the fibrocartilage but not present in the dense regular connective tissue.

Bone

Bone (osseous tissue) contains cells called _____ embedded in lacunae, protein fibers such as _____, and ground substance in addition to mineral salts embedded in extracellular matrix. Blood vessels originate from the **periosteum** and penetrate through the hard matrix and bring nourishment, by diffusion, to the osteocytes. **Compact bone** and **spongy bone** are two types of bone tissue.

Compact Bone

Compact bone is a densely packed combination of mineral salts and collagen fibers.

- **Structure:** The hard matrix of bone is arranged like the layers of an onion, called the **lamellae**, around a **central canal** (haversian canal) that houses _____. Osteocytes in their enclosed lacunae are sandwiched between layers of lamellae. Tiny canals, called **canaliculi**, penetrate through the hard matrix so that the long cytoplasmic extensions of the osteocytes can receive materials diffused directly from the blood vessels of the central canal. A(n) _____ is the lamellae, osteocytes, and central canal.
- **Function:** Compact bone covers the surfaces of all bones of the body.

Spongy Bone

Spongy bone is not dense like compact bone; rather, spongy bone consists of a network of bony plates with spaces in between.

- **Structure:** Spongy bone is composed of bony plates of hard matrix with osteocytes inside their _____. The spaces in between are filled with **red marrow**.
- **Function:** Blood cell formation takes place inside the red marrow of spongy bone cavities.

Fluid Connective Tissue

Ground substances may be hard, as with compact bone, or fluid, as with blood or lymph. Both blood and lymph have cells suspended in a fluid ground substance with proteins in a dissolved state.

Blood

Blood is composed of cells, or _____, suspended in a watery ground substance known as _____. The three cell types are:

1. **Red blood cells**, which transport _____
2. **White blood cells** (most types), which provide protection from _____
3. **Platelets** (cell fragments), which help prevent _____ during injury.

Lymph

Lymph also has a watery ground substance like blood, but it lacks _____ and _____. Some white blood cells are present that are essential in protecting the body from _____. Lymph travels with lymphatic vessels to circulate the fluid back into the bloodstream.

Review Time!

I. *Using the terms in the list below, write the appropriate type of connective tissue in each blank. You may use a term more than once.*

Adipose tissue	*Dense irregular tissue*	*Elastic cartilage*
Dense regular tissue	*Loose connective tissue (areolar tissue)*	*Fibrocartilage*
Hyaline cartilage	*Lymph*	*Spongy bone*
Blood	*Compact bone*	

1. Fluid tissue with red blood cells, white blood cells, and platelets _____

2. Collagen fibers extend in regular, parallel lines _____

3. Adipocytes store energy in the form of triglycerides _____

4. Type of cartilage with elastic fibers _____

5. Hard tissue with bony plates and red marrow _____

6. Tissue forming the structure of the ear and epiglottis _____

7. Most widespread of all connective tissues _____

8. Most abundant type of cartilage _____

9. Tissue characterized by osteons _____

10. Shock-absorbing type of cartilage _____

11. Forms tendons and ligaments _____

12. Tissue with a smooth, glassy ground substance _____

13. Chondrocytes embedded in densely packed wavy collagen fibers _____

14. Tissue in the dermis of the skin _____

15. Fluid tissue with some white blood cells _____

16. Tissue forming the fetal skeleton _____

17. Red blood cell formation occurs in spaces in this tissue _____

18. Central canal, lamellae, osteocytes within lacunae characterizes this tissue   _____

19. Extensively branching collagen fibers with scattered fibroblasts   _____

20. Forms superficial fascia between skin and muscle   _____

CONCEPT 3

Muscle Tissue

Concept: Muscle tissue is specialized to produce movement by contracting. It includes three types: skeletal muscle attached to bones, smooth muscle in the walls of hollow organs, and cardiac muscle in the heart wall.

LEARNING OBJECTIVE   6. Describe the characteristics of muscle tissue and its three types.

Overall structure and function of muscle tissue: Muscle cells have large filaments of protein within their cytoplasm that can contract (shorten) to produce movement.

Skeletal (Striated) Muscle Tissue

- **Structure:** Found attached to bones, skeletal muscle tissue is composed of large, long cylindrical cells with many nuclei. Muscle cells are also called muscle _____. Alternating bands of light and dark are called _____.
- **Function:** Contracts voluntarily (through conscious thought) to produce the movement of bones.

Smooth (Visceral) Muscle Tissue

- **Structure:** Found forming parts of the walls of many hollow organs such as blood vessels, stomach, small and large intestines, blood vessels, and urinary bladder, smooth muscle consists of spindle-shaped cells without _____.
- **Functions:** Contracts involuntarily to coordinate contractions of cells that create muscular movements.

Cardiac Muscle Tissue

- **Structure:** Found only in the heart, the striated, rectangular cells of cardiac muscle tissue join end-to-end at a thickened region of the cell membrane known as the **intercalated disc**. What function does the intercalated disc serve? _____

- **Function:** Contracts involuntarily to produce pulsations that push blood out of the heart and into blood vessels.

Review Time!

I.   Using the terms in the list below, write the appropriate type of muscle tissue in each blank. You may use a term more than once.

Skeletal   Cardiac   Smooth

1. Lacks striations   _____

2. Voluntary   _____

3. Many nuclei   _____

4. Attached to bones   _____

5. Found only in the heart   _____

6. Contractions produce pulsations of the heart wall   _____

7. Large, long cylindrical cells   _____

8. Intercalated discs   _____

9. Spindle-shaped cells   _____

10. Contractions produce muscular movements in walls
    of some hollow organs   _____

II. Sort the muscle tissues by each characteristic. Place the name of the muscle tissue (skeletal, cardiac, or smooth) under each appropriate column.

Striations	Intercalated discs	Voluntary

CONCEPT 4

Nervous Tissue

Concept: Nervous tissue is composed of neurons, which are specialized cells that respond to change and conduct impulses, and neuroglia, which support the neurons.

LEARNING OBJECTIVE ▸ **7.** Describe the organization of nervous tissue and explain its primary function.

- **Structure:** Two cells make up nervous tissue.
  1. **Neurons:** Cells specialized to conduct _____. The three parts of each neuron are **cell body** (houses the nucleus), **dendrites** (branched extensions of the cell body), and **axon** (often a very long extension of the cell body).
  2. **Neuroglia:** Support cells that maintain, protect, and support neurons, especially those in the brain and spinal cord.
- **Function:** Nervous tissue can conduct electrochemical signals rapidly. It is characterized by two properties:
  1. **Excitability:** The capacity to respond to a _____.
  2. **Conductivity:** The ability to transmit _____ from one place to another.

Review Time!

I. *Using the terms in the list below, label the parts of nervous tissue.*

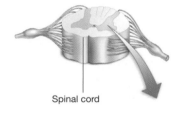

Spinal cord

1. _____
2. _____
3. _____
4. _____
5. _____
6. _____

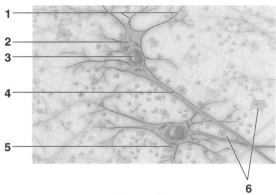

Axon	Neuroglia
Dendrites	Neurons
Cell membrane	Nucleus

CONCEPT 5

Membranes

Concept: Membranes are simple combinations of tissues, usually epithelial and connective tissues, that form sheets that support, partition, and protect parts of the body.

LEARNING OBJECTIVE 8. Describe the four types of membranes of the body and where they are found.

A membrane is the simplest combination of _____ in the body to form a functional unit.

- **Overall structure:** Most membranes, called **epithelial membranes**, consist of a layer of epithelial tissue associated with _____ tissue and other structures such as blood and lymphatic vessels and nerves. Synovial membranes do not contain epithelium; they line joint cavities.
- Epithelial membranes include three different types:
  1. **Mucous membranes**
  2. **Serous membranes**
  3. **Cutaneous membranes**
- **Function:** Membranes divide areas of the body or organs, line internal surfaces of hollow organs and body cavities, and anchor organs to other structures.

Mucous Membranes

- **Location:** Line the internal walls of the:
  1. _____ tract from mouth to anus
  2. _____ tract from nasal cavity to the air sacs of the lungs
  3. _____ tract of the ureters, urinary bladder, and urethra
  4. *Reproductive* tracts of males and females (all reproductive organs)
- **Structure: Mucus** is secreted by the epithelium that covers the outer surface. Describe mucus.

  _____

- **Function:** The function of mucus is _____

  _____

  _____

Serous Membranes

- **Location:** Lines the internal surfaces of the _____ and
  _____ cavities and cover most of the organs in those cavities. For example:
  1. **Pericardium** surrounds the _____.
  2. **Pleurae** line the thoracic cavity and surround each _____.
  3. **Peritoneum** lines the *abdominal cavity* and *covers abdominal organs*.
- **Function:** Epithelium that lines the outer surfaces secretes a clear, watery fluid that provides lubrication.

Cutaneous Membrane

The **cutaneous membrane** is the _____.

Synovial Membranes

- **Location:** Lines the wall of cavities of certain joints such as the knee, elbow, and shoulder.
- **Structure:** Synovial membranes lack _____ tissue and are not regarded as epithelial membranes. They are composed of loose _____ tissue and some fat.
- **Function:** Cells secrete a clear, watery fluid, called *synovial fluid,* to lubricate the opposing bones of the joint as they move. Synovial fluid also nourishes _____ at the ends of bones with oxygen and nutrients.

Review Time!

I.   *Using the terms in the list below, write the appropriate membrane type in each blank. You may use a term more than once.*

   Cutaneous membrane   *Mucous membrane*   *Serous membrane*   *Synovial membrane*

   1. Surrounds each lung   _____
   2. Lines joint cavities such as the knee and elbow   _____
   3. Lines the digestive tract from mouth to the anus   _____
   4. Cells secrete synovial fluid to lubricate bones of a joint   _____
   5. Mucus is secreted by the outer epithelium   _____
   6. Skin   _____
   7. Surrounds the heart   _____
   8. Lines the internal surfaces of the thoracic and
      abdominopelvic cavities   _____
   9. Lacks epithelial tissue   _____
   10. Only composed of connective tissue and some fat   _____

II. *Provide a brief answer for each of the following questions.*

   1. What secretions are released by cutaneous membranes? _____
   _____

   2. Why are synovial membranes not classified as epithelial membranes? _____
   _____

   3. What do the pericardium and pleurae share in common? _____
   _____
   _____

   4. Name the type of epithelial membrane that secretes serous fluid. _____
   _____

   5. Sometimes, people think they are having a heart attack, but in fact have pericarditis. What is inflamed in cases of pericarditis? _____
   _____

   6. List some organ systems that are lined with mucous membrane. _____
   _____
   _____

7. Describe the function of mucus. _____
_____

8. Describe the function of synovial fluid. _____
_____

9. List the three types of membranes that are classified as epithelial membranes.
_____
_____
_____
_____

10. Name the two body cavities with serous membranes. _____
_____
_____

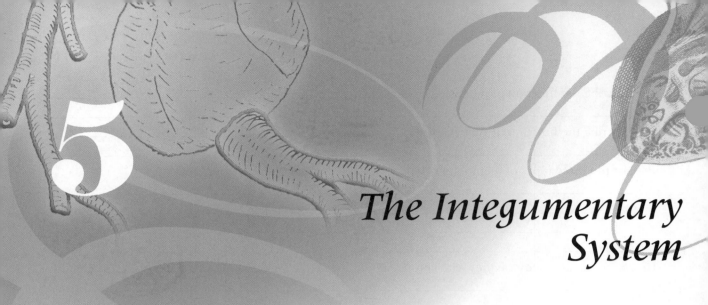

5

The Integumentary System

Tips for Success as You Begin

Read Chapter 5 from your textbook before attending class. Listen when you attend lecture and fill in the blanks in this notebook. You may choose to complete the blanks before attending class as a way to prepare for the day's topics. The same day you attend lecture, read the material again and complete the exercises after each section in this notebook.

Introduction to the Integumentary System

LEARNING OBJECTIVE 1. Identify the basic functions of the integumentary system.

The integumentary system covers the body and has a surface area of about 2 square meters (20 square feet). The primary organ of this system is the skin, but it also includes smaller accessory organs such as hair, ——————————————, glands, and receptors.

The functions of the integumentary system include:

- **Protection:** The skin creates a physical barrier that protects against loss of fluids, damage to the body due to physical injury or ultraviolet light, and invasion by microorganisms.
- **Communication:** The sensory receptors in the skin react to stimuli such as heat, ——————————————, touch, and pain. This information is relayed to the brain and spinal cord.
- **Excretion of wastes:** ——————————————— glands in the skin release small amounts of metabolic waste materials.
- **Vitamin D production:** Exposure to ultraviolet light (sunlight) allows the skin to produce vitamin D, which facilitates calcium absorption through the digestive tract.
- **Regulation of body temperature:** The skin contains ——————————————— glands whose secretions provide evaporative cooling. The blood supply to the skin can be regulated to help cool or warm the body when needed.

CONCEPT 1

The Skin

Concept: The skin includes a superficial epidermis, composed of layers of epithelial cells that are pushed toward the skin surface to regenerate the skin, and a deep dermis, which is a highly vascular region of connective tissue that houses the accessory structures.

LEARNING OBJECTIVE 2. Distinguish between the two primary layers of skin.

The primary organ of the integumentary system is the _____. The skin consists of two distinct layers: the *epidermis* (thin, superficial layer of epithelium) and the *dermis* (thicker, deep layer of connective tissue).

Epidermis

LEARNING OBJECTIVE 3. Describe the composition of the epidermis.

LEARNING OBJECTIVE 4. Describe the changes that occur in epidermal cells as they approach the skin surface.

- **Structure:** The epidermis is composed of stratified _____ epithelium with a basal layer of dividing columnar or cuboidal cells that push older cells toward the surface. The cytoplasmic content of the cells are gradually replaced by **keratin**, a tough, _____ protein. Keratinization occurs as cells progressively accumulate keratin. What is the benefit of keratin? _____

_____

- **Function:** The epidermis forms a _____-resistant protective wrap over the body's surface.

Layers of the Epidermis

Four primary types of cells are found in the epidermis:

1. **Keratinocytes** account for 99% of the cells in the epidermis. They undergo keratinization and produce vitamin _____.
2. **Dendritic cells** are located in the _____ layer of the epidermis and trap unwanted debris through phagocytosis. *What is phagocytosis?* _____

_____
3. **Basal cells** form the _____ layer of the epidermis (stratum germinativum) and undergo cell division continuously.
4. **Melanocytes** are occasionally interspersed between basal cells to produce the _____ in skin color.

Thick skin is composed of _____ to _____ rows (or more) of keratinocytes and found where there is frequent contact with rough surfaces. The keratinocytes form five distinct layers in the epidermis. The _____ of the hands and _____ of the feet have thick skin. **Thin skin** is found everywhere else and contains _____ rows of cells or less.

From the deepest layer to the most superficial layer, the five distinct layers of the epidermis in thick skin are:

- **Stratum germinativum (stratum basale)** is the deepest layer of the epidermis. It is a single layer of continuously dividing basal cells that are either _____ or _____ cells. The newly formed cells are pushed toward the surface as more are made.

- **Stratum spinosum** is a multiple-layered arrangement of _____ cells, mainly keratinocytes with some _____ cells present. Dendritic cells stimulate a defense mechanism against unwanted microorganisms and tumor cells. The keratinocytes contain _____, molecular bridges connecting them to adjacent cells; these give a spiny or prickly appearance to this layer (thus, *spinosum* = spiny). The nuclei of cells in the spinosum layer are darkened, an early sign of cell death. As cells reach the skin surface, the supply of nutrients and oxygen becomes exhausted.

- **Stratum granulosum** is formed of _____ to _____ rows of keratinocytes with granules in the cytoplasm (thus, *granulosum* = granules). The granules are in progress of transforming into _____. Cells in this layer are near death.

- **Stratum lucidum** is present only in the thick skin of the palms and soles. Thin skin lacks this layer. If present, it contains _____ to _____ rows of dead cells that are mostly transparent (thus, *lucidum* = clear). Keratin formation continues although these cells are dead.

- **Stratum corneum** is the most superficial layer of the epidermis consisting of _____ to _____ rows of flattened, dead cells. The layers of dead cells form a hardened outer layer (thus, *corneum* = pertaining to hard). The outermost dead cells are constantly lost by normal wear and tear, known as *desquamation,* and replaced by cells from the deeper layers. It takes _____ to _____ weeks for cells to migrate from stratum germinativum (basale) to the surface and dead cells will remain in stratum corneum an additional _____ weeks before they are shed.

TIP! To remember the layers of the epidermis in order from deep to superficial, keep this little saying in mind: **G**reat **S**tudents **G**ive **L**ove and **C**are (each letter corresponds to the stratum name—germinativum, spinosum, granulosum, lucidum, corneum). Or, if you use stratum basale instead of stratum germinativum, remember that **B**etter **S**tudents **G**ive **L**ove and **C**are. Likewise, from superficial to deep, remember that **C**orny **L**ucy's **G**randma **S**pent **B**illions. Or, **C**orny **L**ucy's **G**randma **S**ells **G**ators.

Skin Color

LEARNING OBJECTIVE   5. Explain the mechanisms that determine skin color.

Melanin is the dark-colored pigment produced by melanocytes that lie between the dividing cells of stratum _____.

- Skin color is determined by the amount of melanin present, not by the number of melanocytes that are present. Although melanin production is regulated by DNA, it can be modified by exposure to _____ light. In response, melanin secretion is increased and tanning results.

- The function of melanocyte activity is to protect body cells from the harmful effects of
_____ light, which can cause mutations. Overexposure to ultraviolet light
can cause sunburns or skin cancer.

Carotene is an orange-yellowish pigment that is normally present in stratum _____
and the dermis of lightly pigmented individuals.

Blood provides a pinkish tone among lightly pigmented individuals who have small amounts of melanin
and carotene. An increase in blood flow to the skin causes the skin color to become bright pink or red.

Dermis

LEARNING OBJECTIVE 6. Describe the composition of the dermis.

- **Structure:** The dermis is a region of _____ tissue located beneath the
epidermis. The cells are scattered, unlike the epidermis, and the extracellular material contains a
large amount of collagen. Blood vessels in the dermis supply stratum germinativum of the epidermis
as well as its own cells with nourishment and waste removal. Blood also helps regulate body
_____. Two areas of the dermis are:

1. **Papillary region:** A superficial area adjacent to the epidermis composed of loose connective tissue.
This region gains its name for the fingerlike projections, called _____,
that extend toward the epidermis. The papillae provide the dermis with a bumpy surface
(*think egg crate appearance*) that locks into the epidermis. **Friction ridges** are present in the

_____, _____, _____,
and _____, and help us to grasp objects. They are formed by contours of the
papillae projecting into the epidermis.

2. **Reticular region:** A deep, thicker area composed of dense _____
connective tissue. This region is named for the dense concentration of collagen,
_____, and _____ fibers that weave throughout it
and provide strength, extensibility, and elasticity to it. Accessory organs are located within or extended
through the reticular region.

Hypodermis

LEARNING OBJECTIVE 7. Describe the structure and function of the hypodermis.

The hypodermis (subcutaneous layer) is not part of the skin, but a region deep to the
_____.

- **Structure:** The hypodermis is composed of loose connective tissue and adipose tissue. It is often more
abundant in the abdomen and thighs and sparse in the chest and upper limbs.
- **Function:** The hypodermis connects the skin by collagen to underlying structures. The hypodermis also
insulates tissues from temperature extremes and provides a shock-absorbing cushion as well as a reserve
for _____ storage.

Review Time!

I. Using the terms in the list below, label the strata or cells on the epidermis illustration.

1. _____
2. _____
3. _____
4. _____
5. _____
6. _____
7. _____
8. _____
9. _____

Basal cell	Melanocyte	Stratum granulosum
Dendritic cell	Stratum corneum	Stratum lucidum
Keratinocyte	Stratum germinativum (basale)	Stratum spinosum

II. Using the terms in the list below, write the appropriate stratum of the epidermis in each blank. You may use a term more than once.

Glandular tissue	Simple squamous	Simple cuboidal
Stratum corneum	Stratum germinativum (basale)	Stratum granulosum
Stratum lucidum	Stratum spinosum	

1. Continuous mitosis occurs in this layer   _____
2. Layer only present in palms and soles   _____
3. Layer with small granules in the cytoplasm   _____
4. Transparent, dead cells populate this layer   _____
5. Most superficial layer   _____
6. Desmosomes bridge together adjacent keratinocytes
   in this layer   _____
7. Cells in this layer are columnar or cuboidal cells _____
8. Layer consisting of 20 to 50 rows of dead cells   _____
9. Layer lost to normal wear and tear   _____

10. Layer in which carotene may be present _____
11. Layer in which melanocytes are present _____
12. Oldest cells are found in this layer _____
13. Layer closest to the dermis _____
14. Layer receiving the most nourishment from the blood
    vessels in the dermis _____
15. Layer deep to stratum granulosum _____
16. Layer superficial to stratum basale _____
17. Single layer of cells is found in this stratum _____
18. Bottom layer of the epidermis _____
19. Layer with keratinocytes and dendritic cells present _____
20. Layer missing from thin skin _____

III. *For each of the descriptions below, indicate whether it is characteristic of the* epidermis *or the* dermis.

1. Composed of connective tissue _____
2. Houses melanocytes _____
3. Contains collagen, reticular, or elastic fibers _____
4. Contains carotene _____
5. Constructed of four or five layers called strata _____
6. Constructed of two regions _____
7. Lacks blood vessels _____
8. Desquamation occurs here _____
9. Keratinocytes _____
10. Dead, keratin-filled cells _____

IV. *Provide a brief answer for each of the following questions.*

1. What defenses are present in the epidermis to protect against microorganisms?

   _____

   _____

2. What is unique about the activity of cells in stratum germinativum (basale)?

   _____

   _____

3. What types of cells are present in the epidermis to provide protection to the underlying dermis?

   _____

   _____

   _____

4. Explain the function of friction ridges. _____

   _____

5. Explain two factors that influence how much melanin a person may produce.

   _____

   _____

   _____

6. While walking barefoot, Jill stepped on a splinter that pierced into the dermis. In order, name all of the layers of the epidermis that the splinter pierced. _____ _____

7. When we are dry or sunburned, the outer parts of our epidermis may peel off in sheets. What molecular bridge connects adjacent keratinocytes together? _____

8. Name the four primary types of cells in the epidermis and provide a brief role for each. _____ _____ _____ _____

9. Distinguish between the two regions of the dermis. What connective tissue is found in each region? _____ _____ _____ _____ _____

10. What layer is deep to the dermis? Identify three functions it serves. _____ _____ _____ _____

11. Into which layer of the skin is ink injected to form a tattoo? Explain why the particular layer of the skin you identified is important for the tattoo to survive. _____ _____ _____

12. Where are hypodermic injections placed? Explain why. _____ _____ _____

CONCEPT 2

Accessory Organs

Concept: Accessory organs are located mostly within the dermis, although they do not originate there. They play a variety of roles, including protection, communication, and excretion.

LEARNING OBJECTIVE 8. Describe the structure and function of the hair, sebaceous glands, sweat glands, nails, and receptors.

LEARNING OBJECTIVE 9. Explain how hair and nails are produced.

Although accessory organs (epidermal derivatives) are embedded within the _____ of the skin, they originated elsewhere during embryonic development.

Hair

Structure: Hair includes a **hair shaft**, which extends from the surface of the skin, and a **hair root**, which plunges below the skin surface to anchor the hair in the skin

- **Hair follicle** is a sheath of _____ cells that surrounds the hair root.
- **Hair bulb** is formed by the distal base of the hair _____ and the hair follicle. The hair bulb is nourished with blood from vessels in the dermis.
- The blood vessels push into the bulb to form the **hair papilla**.
- **Hair matrix** is a cluster of actively dividing cells in the hair follicle surrounding the bulb; these follicle cells arise from stratum _____ of the epidermis and are the *only* source of new hair.

As we discuss the parts of the hair, add labels to the illustration below. When you are done, you should be able to identify the parts of a hair listed below.

Sebaceous gland

Arrector pili muscle

Pigment-producing melanocytes

1. _____
2. _____
3. _____
4. _____
5. _____
6. _____

Hair bulb	Hair papilla
Hair follicle	Hair root
Hair matrix	Hair shaft

Function: Hair protects the skin from damage that may be caused by sunlight, foreign particles, and injury.

Hair growth: Hair growth is similar to the replacement of the epidermis: as cells divide by mitosis, new cells are pushed upward and away from the blood supply, resulting in gradual cell death and keratinization. Growth is limited to the hair _____. The shaft is composed entirely of _____ (*living* or *dead?*) cells composed mainly of _____. Hair grows at a rate of 1 millimeter every _____ days. As long as dividing cells in the matrix are healthy, the hair will continue to grow.

Hair loss: Shaving or cutting the hair has no effect on growth rate because only the shaft is being cut. We usually lose about _____ to _____ hairs a day from a normal adult scalp. A percentage of hair follicles are in a resting phase in which they do not produce hair. Hairs lost each day are replaced as other follicles return to their active phase. If follicles are damaged, hair normally lost will not be replaced and baldness, or *alopecia* results. Male hormones have been shown to inhibit follicle activity, leading to a break in the cycle of hair growth, loss, and replacement. A genetically determined condition known as _____ results.

Hair color: Differences in hair color result from varying concentrations of a pigment known as _____ and are mainly genetically determined. Blonde hair contains very little melanin while black hair contains a lot. Gray or white hairs come with age and as an increased accumulation of _____ in the hair shaft promotes the loss of color.

Associated structures: Two structures associated with the hair follicle are the (1) arrector pili muscle and the (2) sebaceous gland. The **arrector pili muscle** is a smooth muscle that extends at an angle from the hair follicle to the papillary region of the _____ and is responsible for standing hairs in a vertical position when cold or frightened (producing "goose bumps"). A small amount of heat is produced by this muscle, which increases the insulating effect of hair. This muscle also presses against the _____ gland to force the release of _____ onto the skin's surface.

Review Time!

I.   Using the terms in the list below, write the appropriate accessory organ or part in each blank. You may use a term more than once.

Hair bulb   Hair follicle   Hair matrix   Hair root   Hair shaft

1. Portion of the hair that projects from the surface of the skin   _____
2. Distal base of the hair root and follicle that is slightly larger than the rest of the root   _____
3. Actively dividing cells in the hair follicle that surround the bulb   _____
4. Sheath of epithelial cells that form a downward extension into the dermis   _____
5. Anchors the hair in the skin   _____
6. Growth region of the hair   _____
7. Portion of hair made up entirely of dead, keratinized cells   _____
8. Shaving removes this portion of the hair   _____
9. Androgens inhibit this part of the hair   _____
10. Hair papilla is part of this region of the hair   _____

Sebaceous Glands

Structure: Sebaceous glands, or **oil glands**, are exocrine glands that are nearly always associated with _____ follicles.

- Each sebaceous gland consists of a cluster of glandular epithelial cells that are connected to the hair follicle by a duct. Sebaceous glands are found throughout the skin except for the _____ and _____, and secrete an oily substance known as _____.
- **Sebum components:** Components of sebum include water, _____, cholesterol, protein, and _____. Sebum may be emptied into either a hair follicle, hair root, or directly onto the_____.

Sebum functions: The three primary functions of sebum are:

1. Keep hair and skin _____ and _____.
2. Provide a water-resistant layer to the skin's surface.
3. Inhibit the growth of bacteria.

Sebaceous gland activity: Sebaceous glands are relatively inactive until puberty, when rising levels of sex hormones begin to stimulate them. Sebum production continues at an elevated rate during puberty and for many years afterward. Despite its antibacterial properties, sebum can support colonies of bacteria, which enter the sebaceous glands and ducts to produce a local inflammation (pimple or *comedo*). Ducts blocked by bacteria and their byproducts can lead to a painful abscess (boil or *furuncle*).

Sweat Glands

Structure: A **sweat gland** (*sudoriferous gland*) is a second type of exocrine gland that originates as a tube that is tightly coiled into a ball in the dermis or _____.

Function: Sweat glands secrete a water substance called sweat (perspiration). The components of sweat are water, _____, and small amounts of metabolic waste material known as urea. Sweat helps maintain body _____ by cooling the body as the sweat evaporates. To a lesser degree, sweat helps the kidneys eliminate metabolic wastes (urea and excess salts). There are two types of sweat glands:

1. **Eccrine glands** function throughout life. They are distributed in all regions of the skin and secrete a watery sweat in response to _____ body temperatures. Sweat travels from the coiled tube into a winding duct that opens onto the skin's surface by way of a pore.
2. **Apocrine glands** begin functioning during puberty in response to sex hormones. The sweat released by apocrine glands is thickened and contains proteins, which promote the growth of microorganisms normally found on the skin. Microorganisms on the skin break down proteins and can create a pungent odor. Apocrine glands are active primarily during periods of emotional stress and are more numerous in the _____ and _____. Apocrine sweat is secreted into a duct that empties into the space between a hair _____ and a hair _____, and from there reaches the skin surface.

> **TIP!** If you have trouble remembering the different locations for eccrine sweat glands and apocrine sweat glands, keep this trick in mind: the term **AP**ocrine is reminiscent of a hairy "**AP**e." The apocrine sweat glands secrete sweat into a duct that empties into the small space between a hair follicle and a hair root before it reaches the skin.

Nails

Structure: Nails are formed from the outer layer of the epidermis, stratum _____.
Similar to stratum corneum, nails are composed of a waterproofing protein called
_____, but in a more compressed state.

- _____ is the visible surface of the nail.
- **Nail bed** is covered by the nail plate.
- **Free edge** is the distal end of the nail.
- _____ (eponychium) is a small flap of stratum corneum overlying the proximal edge of the nail.
- **Nail root** is deep to the cuticle.
- **Nail matrix** is an active stratum _____ layer in the nail root that produces new cells by mitosis.
- **Lunula** is a small part of the matrix that can be seen through the nail body as a light-colored crescent.

As we discuss the parts of the nail, add labels to the illustration below. When you are done, you should be able to identify the parts of a nail listed below.

Distal bone of finger

Growth region (nail matrix)

1. _____
2. _____
3. _____
4. _____
5. _____

Cuticle   Nail bed   Nail root
Lunula   Nail plate

Function: Nails protect the ends of fingers and toes from injury and help you pick up small objects.

Nail growth: Epithelial cells that continuously produce nails are influenced by blood circulation, metabolism, and diet. A deficiency in _____ results in thin, brittle nails while yellowed nails may indicate a _____ disorder, liver disease, or AIDS. Circulatory disorders can lead to pitted or concave nails.

Review Time!

I.   *Using the terms in the list below, write the appropriate accessory organ or part in each blank. You may use a term more than once.*

Cuticle	*Lunula*	*Nail bed*	*Nail root*
Nail follicle	*Nail matrix*	*Nail plate*	

1. Portion of the nail that undergoes mitosis   _____
2. Light-colored crescent of the nail matrix   _____
3. Nail plate overlies the nail   _____
4. Part of the nail root that contains active stratum germinativum   _____
5. Part of the nail that is deep to the cuticle   _____

6. Flap of stratum corneum that overlies the proximal edge
   of the nail _____
7. Visible surface of the nail _____
8. If damaged, the nail will no longer grow _____

Receptors

Receptors in the skin consist of the distal ends of _____ wrapped by a capsule of connective tissue. These neurons carry impulses toward the brain where the information is interpreted as *sensations* such as cold or heat, pressure, fine touch, and pain. In turn, the brain makes changes to maintain homeostasis. Thus, the skin functions as an important sense organ.

Skin receptors include:

• **Lamellar** (Pacinian) **corpuscles** are located in the deep _____ and respond to changes in _____.

• **Tactile** (Meissner) **corpuscles** in the _____ region of the dermis respond to slight changes in _____ or fine touch.

• **Free nerve endings** in the _____ respond to excessive temperature and pressure changes for the detection of _____.

Review Time!

I. *Provide a brief answer for each of the following questions.*

1. Gina wants to rid herself of some unwanted hair permanently. She has read about various methods for hair removal. What is the one part of the hair that must be damaged to guarantee no further hair growth? Explain. _____
   _____
   _____

2. Explain why hairs that have been plucked from the roots continue to grow back. What part of the hair has continued to provide growth? _____
   _____
   _____

3. Sam works at a barber shop and sometimes has customers ask for him to cut off all their dead shafts. Explain to his customers what Sam will be doing. _____
   _____

4. How are gray hairs structurally different from pigmented hairs? _____
   _____

5. Consider the hygiene habits of humans; bathing has become a daily occurrence for many of us. Browse the shelves of nearly any store, and you will likely find aisles of conditioners, creams, lotions, and moisturizers. What secretion are we removing every time we bathe and wash our hair? Why is this secretion important? _____
   _____
   _____

6. Which type of sweat gland is responsible for cooling us when we are too hot? What does sweat from this particular type of gland contain? _____
   _____
   _____

7. What type of secretion is targeted when we apply deodorant to the armpits? Why do secretions from these glands emit an odor? _____

_____

8. How are nails and hair similar in terms of structure? Compare their various parts.

_____

_____

_____

_____

9. Contrast the type of sweat produced by eccrine sweat glands and apocrine sweat glands.

_____

_____

_____

10. Compare the nail root to the hair root. How are these roots functionally similar? How are they structurally similar? _____

_____

_____

_____

CONCEPT 3

Repair Mechanisms of the Skin

Concept: A major function of the skin is to make repairs to prevent injury to underlying tissues and organs. Although cut injuries and burn injuries differ, repair mechanisms are similar.

LEARNING OBJECTIVE 10. Compare and contrast the process of skin repair for cuts and for burns.

The two most common skin wounds are cuts and burns. First, we explore the repair of cut skin.

Repair of Cut Skin

1. When an injury extends through the epidermis into the _____, bleeding occurs. A **blood clot** forms temporarily to cover the wound and to prevent bacteria from invading underlying tissue.

2. Tissue damage and blood loss stimulate a series of internal events known as **inflammation**. Inflammation causes increased pain, but its main function is to bring macrophages, other white blood cells, platelets, clotting proteins, and fibroblasts to the injury site.

   • What role do macrophages play in the inflammatory process? _____

   _____

   • What role do the platelets and clotting proteins play? _____

   _____

   • What is the function of a fibroblast in the site of injury? _____

   _____

- Increased blood flow brings these defensive substances to the site of injury. What two events promote an increase in blood flow? _____
_____

3. Epithelial tissue migrates into the wound and the blood clot hardens to form a
_____ within a few days of injury. The scab will dissolve or lift off the newly
formed skin, but in some cases _____ or _____
will be necessary to bring the edges of the injured skin together.

Major injuries: In major injuries, *granulation tissue* results because the skin is unable to be restored to the
original condition. What does granulation tissue contain? _____
_____

Damaged sweat and sebaceous glands, hair follicles, muscle fibers, and nerves are seldom repaired; these
accessory structures are replaced by *fibrous dermal tissue*. Inflexible, fibrous **scar tissue** results that becomes
more flexible over time with the continued activity of epidermal cells and fibroblasts.

Repair of Burns

A burn is a wound cause by any form of heat-producing energy, such as fire,
_____, radiation, or _____. Heat destroys proteins,
which can lead to cell death and the loss of the protective barrier function of the skin. The result is a loss of
body fluids and electrolytes and the entry of harmful bacteria.

Classification of Burns

1. Burns can be classified on the *extent* of the burn. The *Rule of Nines* divides the body into regions based
   on the number nine (see the figure below). Burns over 50% of the body are often fatal.

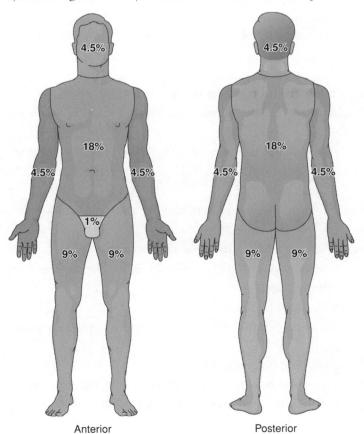

Anterior   Posterior

2. Burns can be classified by the *depth* of tissue damage.
   - First-degree or superficial thickness burns cause local redness.
   - Second-degree or medium thickness burns usually cause _____
     and _____.
   - Third-degree or full thickness burns irreversibly destroy the _____ and
     _____.

Healing process: For a first- or second-degree burn, the healing process is similar to that of a cut. If damage from a second-degree burn covers a large area, a surface scar results. In a third-degree burn, both layers of the skin cannot heal.

CONCEPT 4

Temperature Regulation

Concept: The integumentary system plays a key role in the homeostatic mechanism that regulates body temperature.

LEARNING OBJECTIVE   11. Discuss the role of the integumentary system in regulating body temperature.

The range of normal body temperature on the Celsius scale is _____
to _____. The range of normal body temperature on the Fahrenheit scale is
_____ to _____.

- Why is it important for body temperature to be maintained within this range?
  _____
  _____

How is body temperature maintained when we are too hot?

- Heat-sensitive receptors in the skin sense external temperatures and relay the information to the
  _____.
- The brain stimulates sweat glands to increase secretion. Sweat evaporates and your skin is cooled, When your skin cools, your body temperature lowers. A lower body temperature promotes the cooling of the
  _____ as well.
- The brain also signals blood vessels to dilate (relax and expand). More blood flows to the skin and heat loss is facilitated.

How is body temperature maintained when we are too cold?

- The brain stimulates blood vessels in the skin to constrict. Blood flow to the skin is reduced as well as the amount of heat lost through the skin.
- Skeletal muscles may be stimulated by the brain to _____ to generate heat.
- _____ muscles in the skin contract, increasing muscle metabolism and generating heat.

Other systems involved in regulating body temperature:

- **Cardiovascular system:** Heart beats faster when hot to push blood to the skin to facilitate heat loss.
- **Respiratory system:** Breathing rate increases to carry out more heat as you expire (exhale).

Review Time!

I. *Provide a brief answer for each of the following questions.*

1. Explain how you would differentiate between a first-, second-, and third-degree burn.

   _____

   _____

   _____

2. Explain why burns are harmful. _____

   _____

   _____

3. Explain what normal skin accessory organs are missing from scar tissue. _____

   _____

   _____

4. Describe how inflammation helps heal skin. _____

   _____

   _____

5. What are the two ways in which burns are classified? _____

   _____

   _____

6. Describe how the integumentary system assists with homeostasis of body temperature.

   _____

   _____

   _____

7. Explain how the integumentary system helps lower the body temperature when we are too hot.

   _____

   _____

8. Describe the skin's response to body temperature that has fallen. _____

   _____

   _____

9. Heat stroke can occur when a person no longer sweats and the body temperature rises above the normal range. Why is sweating a critical component of body temperature maintenance?

   _____

   _____

   _____

10. Calculate the percentage of the body burned (*Rule of Nines,* see figure on p. 89 or see Figure 5.10 in your text) if the anterior torso and anterior surface of both arms are burned. _____

   _____

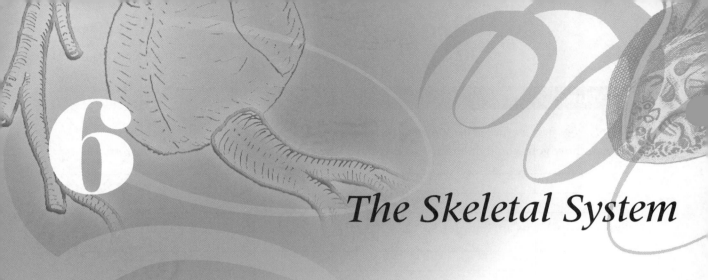

6

The Skeletal System

Tips for Success as You Begin

Read Chapter 6 from your textbook before attending the class. Listen when you attend the lecture and fill in the blanks in this notebook. You may choose to complete the blanks before attending the class as a way to prepare for the day's topics. The same day you attend the lecture, read the material again, and complete the exercises after each section in this notebook. For this chapter, you can facilitate your learning of the bone names by practicing spelling the bone names and working with a picture or a bone model to practice the bone names.

Introduction to the Skeletal System

LEARNING OBJECTIVE 1. Identify and describe the five functions of the skeletal system.

The skeletal system includes hard flexible bones and the joints between the bones. The functions of the skeletal system are:

- **Support:** The skeleton forms a structural frame that supports other body structures.
- **Protection:** Bones protect internal organs such as the _____ protected by the cranial bones and the _____ and lungs protected by the ribcage.
- **Required for movement:** Bones, with their attached _____ muscles, act as levers to provide movement.
- **Blood cell formation:** Hematopoiesis, the process of blood cell formation, occurs in blood-forming connective tissue called red marrow found within bone.
- **Storage:** Two important minerals, _____ and _____ are stored in bone tissue. Why are these minerals important? _____

_____

CONCEPT 1

Bone Structure

Concept: Bones come in many shapes and sizes, but they all share common features. Each one is composed mainly of bone tissue, which is a mixture of organic and inorganic materials that are highly organized to form either compact bone or spongy bone.

LEARNING OBJECTIVE 2. Distinguish between long bones, short bones, flat bones, and irregular bones, and provide examples of each.

Bones are dynamic organs in a constant state of change.

Types of Bones

The four major categories of bones, based on shape, are:

1. **Long bones** are longer than wide. The function of these bones is to absorb stress from the body weight.
   • **Examples of long bones are** _____
   _____

2. **Short bones** are cube shaped and are roughly equal in length and width.
   • **Examples of short bones are** _____
   _____

3. **Flat bones** are thin and flat.
   • **Examples of flat bones are** _____
   _____

4. **Irregular bones** do not fit into any of the other categories because of their complex shapes.
   • **Examples of irregular bones include the** _____ **and bones of**
   the _____.

Review Time!

I. *Using the terms in the list below, write the appropriate type of bone in each blank. You may use a term more than once.*

   Long bone   *Short bone*   *Flat bone*   *Irregular bone*

   1. Cube-shaped bone   _____
   2. Bones that form the wrist   _____
   3. Bones that have a complex shape and do not fit into other
      categories   _____
   4. Arm and leg bones   _____
   5. Bones of the face   _____
   6. Bones that form the cranium of the head   _____
   7. Thin and flat bones   _____
   8. Bones that are longer than they are wide   _____
   9. Ribs   _____
   10. Vertebrae   _____

Parts of a Long Bone

LEARNING OBJECTIVE 3. Identify the parts of a typical long bone.

As we discuss the parts of a long bone, add labels to the illustration below. When you are done, you should be able to identify the parts of the long bone listed below.

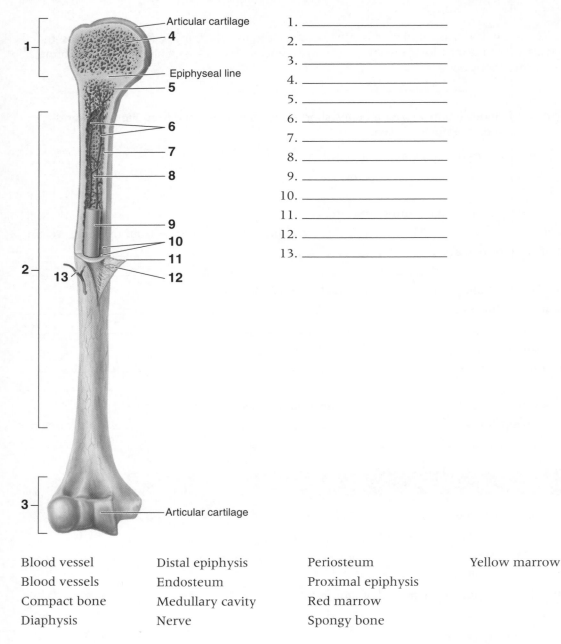

1. _____
2. _____
3. _____
4. _____
5. _____
6. _____
7. _____
8. _____
9. _____
10. _____
11. _____
12. _____
13. _____

Blood vessel	Distal epiphysis	Periosteum	Yellow marrow
Blood vessels	Endosteum	Proximal epiphysis	
Compact bone	Medullary cavity	Red marrow	
Diaphysis	Nerve	Spongy bone	

- **Diaphysis** is the shaft of the long bone composed of _____ bone.
- **Epiphysis** (singular; *epiphyses* for plural) is the end of the long bone that contributes to a joint (articulation).
- **Medullary cavity** is inside the _____ and houses yellow marrow.
- **Red marrow** is a special blood-forming connective tissue found in spongy bone. The function of red marrow is _____

- **Yellow marrow** fills the medullary cavity of the diaphysis and is composed of fatty tissue. The function of yellow marrow is _____
- **Articular cartilage** is a thin layer of hyaline cartilage that covers the _____.
- **Periosteum** is a membrane formed by a thin layer of dense connective tissue, rich in blood vessels, that covers the outer surface of the bone. The periosteum is anchored to the underlying bone by protein fibers. The periosteum provides an anchor for tendons, which connect bone to _____, and ligaments, which connect bone to _____.
- **Endosteum** is a membrane that lines the interior surface of the medullary cavity.

Review Time!

I.   *Using the terms in the list below, write the appropriate part of the long bone in each blank. You may use a term more than once.*

Articular cartilage	*Diaphysis*	*Endosteum*	*Epiphysis*
Medullary cavity	*Periosteum*	*Red marrow*	*Yellow marrow*

1. Shaft of the bone   _____
2. Connective tissue that covers the epiphyses   _____
3. Fatty tissue stored in the medullary cavity   _____
4. Lining of the inside of the medullary cavity   _____
5. Part of the bone constructed of hyaline cartilage   _____
6. Attachment site for tendons and ligaments   _____
7. Blood-forming connective tissue   _____
8. Space found inside the diaphysis   _____
9. Forms a joint, or articulation   _____
10. Dense connective tissue covering of the bone   _____

Chemical Composition of Bone Tissue

LEARNING OBJECTIVE   4. Describe the organic and inorganic components of bone tissue.

- **Inorganic components:** Mineral salts, mainly calcium _____, but also calcium _____ and calcium _____. The combination of calcium phosphate and calcium hydroxide forms hard and durable _____, which accounts for nearly two-thirds of the weight of bone and withstands the force of compression.
- **Organic components:** Collagen fibers provide slight flexibility and account for one-third of the weight of the bone. Collagen fibers weave threads through the _____ crystals in the bone's matrix that enables the bone to bend slightly without breaking and to resist against pulling forces.

Cells of Bone Tissue

LEARNING OBJECTIVE   5. Distinguish between the three types of bone cells based on their functions.

1. **Osteocytes** are the most abundant cells in bone. One osteocyte resides inside a tiny chamber, known as a _____. This chamber is filled with interstitial fluid that is refreshed by the diffusion of fluid from blood vessels that penetrate through the bone in tiny channels called **canaliculi**. The primary **function** of osteocytes is to _____.

2. **Osteoblasts** originate from osteogenic cells and mature to become osteocytes. Osteoblasts may migrate from one area of bone tissue to the next. Their **function** is to secrete _____ prior to the formation of hydroxyapatite crystals. They also secrete other substances that lead to the formation of bone matrix.

3. **Osteoclasts** are large, multinucleated cells that arise from a cell that also gives rise to blood cells in the red marrow of spongy bone. Osteoclasts are "bone destroyers" because they secrete _____ and _____ that break down the bone matrix during **osteolysis**. Osteolysis releases _____ and _____ into circulation of bodily fluids and is regulated by hormones.

Types of Bone Tissue

LEARNING OBJECTIVE 6. Compare and contrast the structure of compact bone versus spongy bone.

Two types of bone tissue will be discussed next: compact bone, which contains a relatively dense matrix, and spongy bone, which consists of a network of thin plates.

Compact Bone

Compact bone contains a dense matrix. It usually forms the outer walls of a bone. The following components can be seen with the aid of a microscope:

- **Lamellae** are rings (concentric circles) of dense bone matrix. Osteocytes can be seen in their _____ embedded in these rings.
- **Central canal** (haversian canal) is at the center of a set of concentric rings (lamellae).
- **Osteon** (haversian system) consists of one central canal, its lamellae, lacunae, and the osteocytes surrounding it.
- **Perforating** (Volkmann's) **canals** carry blood vessels perpendicularly from the periosteum into the bone and connect with central canals. Blood travels through vessels in (1) perforating canals, to (2) central canals, and then the blood diffuses through (3) _____ to the (4) osteocytes.

> **TIP!** Think of the perforating canals as "roads" that travel east and west. Central (haversian) canals are roads that run north and south. Canaliculi are alleys that carry you to a particular location—the osteocytes.

Spongy Bone

Spongy bone does *not* contain osteons. This tissue forms the interior of a bone or lines the marrow cavity of the bone. This tissue is *not* dense or thick, but contains many thin plates known as **trabeculae**. The trabeculae provide a latticework arrangement that gives the tissue a sponge-like appearance. _____ marrow is found between the trabeculae.

- Recall, what is the function of red marrow? _____

Osteocytes within lacunae are found in both compact bone and spongy bone; these osteocytes receive blood from the _____ by way of short canaliculi.

The three main functions of trabeculae and spongy bone are:

1. _____ provide **resistance** against stress arriving from different directions.
2. Spongy bone is **lighter** than compact bone, making it easier for muscles to move the skeleton.
3. Spongy bone provides a **protected** environment for _____ in the red marrow.

Review Time!

I. *Using the terms in the list below, write the appropriate term in each blank. You may use a term more than once.*

Collagen   Compact bone   Hydroxyapatite crystals   Osteocytes

Lamellae   Osteoblasts   Osteoclasts

Osteon   Spongy bone   Trabeculae

1. Type of bone tissue constructed from trabeculae   _____

2. Concentric circles, or rings, of bone matrix   _____

3. Bone destroying cells   _____

4. Mature bone cells that reside within a lacuna   _____

5. Type of bone tissue constructed from osteons   _____

6. Thin plates that form spongy bone   _____

7. Component that is the majority of bone matrix   _____

8. Enables bones to twist and bend slightly   _____

9. Cells that mature into osteocytes   _____

10. Type of bone tissue that provides a protected environment
    for hematopoiesis   _____

11. Lamellae, central canal, osteocytes, and lacunae   _____

12. Matrix of spongy bone are these little beams   _____

13. Type of bone with a dense matrix   _____

14. Formed when calcium phosphate combines with
    calcium hydroxide   _____

15. Type of bone tissue that forms the outer walls   _____

16. Cells that secrete calcium   _____

17. Cells that contribute to osteolysis   _____

18. Provides a hard and durable quality to bone   _____

19. Type of bone tissue forms the bone's interior   _____

20. Lighter of the two bone tissues   _____

II. *Provide a brief answer for each of the following questions.*

1. Through a microscope, you observe rings with a small canal in the center. You determine this type
   of tissue to be _____. Explain how you came to this decision.

   _____

   _____

   _____

2. Besides compact bone and spongy bone, what other types of connective tissues are associated with
   bone?_____

   _____

   _____

3. Explain why bone is considered an organ._____

   _____

   _____

4. While walking in the woods, you find a bone that is approximately 10 centimeters long and
   2.5 centimeters wide. How would you classify this bone by shape? _____

5. How are osteoblasts functionally different from osteoclasts? Explain._____
_____
_____

6. What is the main inorganic component of bone?_____

7. What is the main organic component of bone?_____

8. Which component creates the majority of the bone?_____

9. What is the role of osteoclasts in osteolysis?_____
_____
_____

10. What are three functions of spongy bone?_____
_____
_____
_____

11. Describe the following canals in bone: canaliculi, central canal, perforating canal.
_____
_____
_____
_____

12. Discuss the relationship among lamellae, central canal, lacunae, and osteocytes.
_____
_____
_____
_____

CONCEPT 2

Bone Development, Growth, and Remodeling

Concept: Bones begin developing at an early stage in life in two ways: from embryonic membranes, and from cartilage. After birth, bones grow in two directions, length and width, until body growth stops. Bones continue to change throughout adulthood through bone remodeling in response to the body's demands.

Bone development and growth is discussed next in three phases: (1) origins of bone during embryonic development; (2) growth of bone during fetal life, childhood, and adolescence; and (3) remodeling changes that occur in bone throughout life.

Bone Development

The process of bone development, or **osteogenesis**, begins about _____ weeks after fertilization. For some bones, it can occur into the early adult years until around age 25. Osteogenesis involves the replacement of preexisting _____ tissue with bone tissue by either intramembranous ossification or endochondral ossification (both processes are discussed next).

Intramembranous Ossification

LEARNING OBJECTIVE ▸ **7. Identify the intramembranous bones and explain how they are formed.**

Intramembranous ossification involves bone formation within a sheet of connective tissue in an embryo, called an embryonic membrane. Which bones form by intramembranous ossification?

_____

Next, we will explore the process of intramembranous ossification.

Intramembranous ossification for the formation of *spongy bone*

- Blood vessels carry blood to the _____ membrane beginning at the fifth week of life.
- Osteoblasts transform and begin producing new bone matrix.
- Thin plates of bone form that thicken and connect to form trabeculae of _____ bone.
- Some _____ become trapped in the matrix and become osteocytes.
- Red marrow fills the spaces between the trabeculae. Do you recall the function of red marrow?

_____

Intramembranous ossification for the formation of *compact bone*

- The outer areas of the embryonic membrane spaces do not fill with red marrow.
- _____ thicken due to osteoblast activity until spaces fill with bone matrix.
- Compact bone is formed over spongy bone, creating a "sandwich" of compact—spongy—compact bone.

Endochondral Ossification

LEARNING OBJECTIVE ▸ **8. Identify the endochondral bones and describe how they develop from hyaline cartilage.**

Endochondral ossification occurs when hyaline cartilage is replaced with bone. Which bones form by endochondral ossification? _____

_____

Next, we will explore the process of endochondral ossification.

- The process of endochondral ossification begins at 6 weeks of life when chondroblasts produce _____ cartilage in future bone areas.
- The cartilage template grows in the fetus in both length and width.
- Blood vessels grow into the cartilage template and bring _____ into an outer membrane, transforming it into a periosteum.
- Walls of the _____ are formed and thickened by osteoblasts, creating a **bone collar**.
- Blood vessels penetrate the center of the cartilage model and establish the _____ **center of ossification**. Chondrocytes die and degeneration leaves an early medullary cavity in the center of the diaphysis.
- More blood vessels penetrate the cartilage at the epiphyses. More osteoblasts migrate in and form _____ **ossification centers**.
- The secondary ossification center appears at different times for different individuals for various bones.
- Once the secondary ossification centers arise, the cartilage-to-bone conversion begins.
- The _____ becomes filled with spongy bone. A cap of original cartilage remains at the epiphyses to form articular cartilage, which remains throughout adulthood.
- A thin growth plate consisting of _____ cartilage persists through childhood and adolescence and is discussed next.

Bone Growth

LEARNING OBJECTIVE 9. Describe the process of bone growth in length and width.

Bones grow in size after ossification begins.

- *Flat bones* of the skull grow closer together after birth until they form tight joints (sutures). With age, the bones thicken to provide protection from injury.
- *Long bones* grow in length and width. Growth in length is called _____ *growth* while growth in width is called _____ *growth.*

Longitudinal growth occurs in a band of hyaline cartilage between the diaphysis and the epiphysis called the growth plate or **epiphyseal plate**. The plate consists of chondroblasts stacked in rows like coins.

- On the shaft side of the plate, osteoblasts are continually invading the cartilage and converting it to _____. Osteoclasts erode the new bone and expand the medullary cavity.
- On the epiphysis side of the plate, _____ continually add new cartilage. The shaft increases in length while the epiphyseal plate regenerates itself.

As the growing years end, chondroblast activity slows and finally ceases. The process of cartilage placement by bone on the shaft side of the plate catches up with the epiphysis and obliterates the plate. The bone is said to be in a state of *closure of the epiphyses* and an epiphyseal line is visible between the diaphysis and epiphysis.

Appositional growth is growth in the width of a bone by cells in the periosteum.

- Osteoblasts produce new bone matrix and cement themselves within lacunae along the outer surface of the bone. The osteoblasts are transformed into _____ as they become cemented within lacunae.
- With the addition of bone matrix to the outer surface, the medullary cavity in the bone's center expands by the activity of "bone-destroyers," known as _____.
- Normally, more bone matrix is added to the _____ than is removed from the inside of the bone, providing a thicker and stronger bone.

Bone Remodeling

LEARNING OBJECTIVE 10. Define the role of bone remodeling in maintaining homeostasis.

Bone remodeling is a normal part of bone maintenance, or homeostasis, that involves the osteolysis of bone matrix by "bone-destroyers" called _____ and the deposition of new bone matrix by cells known as _____. Bone remodeling depends on demands of the body; most bones are completely remodeled every 5 to _____ years. Factors that influence the rate of bone remodeling are hormones, _____, physical activity, injury (such as in response to a fracture), or _____.

The three main purposes of bone remodeling are:

1. **Helps maintain mineral homeostasis.** Two minerals are recycled: _____ and _____. If their levels are in excess in the blood stream, osteoblasts store them in newly produced bone matrix. If their blood levels drop, osteo- _____ remove them from bone matrix and return them to the blood.

2. **Strengthens bones when they are subject to prolonged stress.** The action of muscles pulling on _____ attached to bones creates stress on bones. Bones subjected to stress thicken with new matrix.

3. **Assists in healing of bone tissue.** Osteoblasts replace lost or damaged bone tissue by depositing new matrix after injury or infection.

Review Time!

I. *Using the terms in the list below, write the type of ossification or growth in each blank. You may use a term more than once.*

Appositional growth   Endochondral ossification   Intramembranous ossification   Longitudinal growth

1. Facial bones fuse together   _____

2. Bone growth in width   _____

3. Bone growth at the epiphyseal plate at the age of 7   _____

4. Formation of a primary ossification center   _____

5. Ossification beginning at 6 weeks of life with the production
   of hyaline cartilage by chondroblasts   _____

6. Ossification occurring in the femur, humerus, and other
   long bones   _____

7. Growth at the periosteum   _____

8. Cartilage to bone conversion at the secondary ossification
   center   _____

9. Bone formation within an embryonic membrane   _____

10. Ossification beginning at 5 weeks of life with arrival of blood
    vessels at embryonic membrane   _____

II. *Provide a brief answer for each of the following questions.*

1. Differentiate among the types of bones that are affected by intramembranous and endochondral
   ossification._____
   _____
   _____

2. Describe the role of chondroblasts in endochondral ossification. _____
   _____
   _____

3. At the age of 40, what type of bone growth can occur: longitudinal or appositional growth?
   Explain. _____
   _____
   _____

4. A 7-year-old child fell at the playground and broke her thigh bone along an epiphyseal plate. What
   concerns should her parents have about that broken bone? _____
   _____
   _____

5. Explain how osteoblasts and osteoclasts function to remodel bone. _____
   _____
   _____

6. Where is red marrow found and what is its function? _____
   _____
   _____

7. Describe how the medullary cavity forms. _____
   _____
   _____

8. From what existing structure does the articular cartilage arise during endochondral ossification?

_____

_____

9. What is the difference between an epiphyseal plate and an epiphyseal line?

_____

_____

_____

10. Outline the steps of endochondral ossification. _____

_____

_____

_____

_____

_____

_____

CONCEPT 3

Organization of the Skeleton

Concept: The skeleton provides a frame for the body and includes all bones and joints. It is organized into two regional divisions: axial and appendicular. Bones contain features, such as grooves, holes, and processes, that support the bones' various functions.

LEARNING OBJECTIVE 11. **Identify the two regional divisions of the skeleton.**

_____ (*how many?*) bones are in the **skeleton** of the human body. The two main regions of the skeleton are:

1. **Axial skeleton:** Contains the bones that lie along the axis of the body, from the skull to the base of the spine, such as the:
    - _____ consists of the *cranium* bones that border the cranial cavity to protect the brain and the *facial* bones that form the face.
    - **Hyoid bone** is a U-shaped bone in the _____.
    - **Vertebral column** consists of *vertebrae* separated by intervertebral discs, and the *sacrum.*
    - _____ includes 12 pairs of *ribs* and the *sternum.*

2. **Appendicular skeleton:** Contains the bones appended (or attached) to the axial skeleton, such as the:
    - _____ includes the *scapula* (shoulder blade) and *clavicle* (collar bone) on either side of the body.
    - **Upper limb** bones include the *humerus* (of brachium), *radius, ulna* (of antebrachium), _____ (wrist), *metacarpals* (hand), and *phalanges* (fingers).
    - _____ includes two *coxal* (hip) *bones* combined with the *sacrum* to form the pelvis.
    - **Lower limb** bones include the *femur* (of thigh), _____ (kneecap), *tibia* and *fibula* (lower leg), *tarsals* (ankle), *metatarsals* (foot), and *phalanges* (toes).

LEARNING OBJECTIVE 12. Describe the common features found in many bones.

Surface Features of Bones

Surface features are landmarks that distinguish one bone from another, but do not vary greatly from person to person. Projections and depressions typically serve as attachment points for _____ or tendons, to strengthen the bone, or for articulation with other bones. Openings, channels, and grooves permit the penetration of _____ or nerves and provide spaces for housing body structures.

CONCEPT 4

Bones of the Axial Skeleton

Concept: The axial skeleton contains the bones forming the skull, the vertebral column, and the thoracic cage. It also includes the hyoid bone in the neck.

LEARNING OBJECTIVE 13. Identify the bones of the axial skeleton.

LEARNING OBJECTIVE 14. Identify the prominent features of the axial bones.

List the bones of the axial skeleton:

1. _____
2. _____
3. _____
4. _____

The Skull

The skull contains _____ (*how many?*) bones held together by joints known as _____. In an infant, sutures are not yet established and fibrous membranes extend between the flat bones of the cranium. These membranes are known as **fontanels** and are an infant's "soft spots."

Paranasal Sinuses

Paranasal sinuses are air-filled chambers within the skull that are lined with mucous membrane. Inflammation of the mucous membrane is called _____. Functions of the sinuses are:

• Connect with the nasal cavity to drain fluids
• Decrease the weight of the skull
• Resonate sound from the voice

List the bones that house the five paranasal sinuses.

1. _____
2. _____
3. _____
4. _____

The bones of the skull include _____ (*how many?*) bones of the cranium and _____ (*how many?*) smaller facial bones. The lower jaw bone—the mandible—is a skull bone.

Cranium

The cranium encloses and protects the _____, and provides an attachment site for the muscles of the scalp, lower jaw, neck, and back. These eight bones belong to the cranium.

1. **Frontal bone** forms the anterior part of the skull above the eyes, or forehead.
   - **Orbits** are _____ sockets.
   - **Supraorbital foramen** is a hole above each orbit through which _____ and _____ pass.
   - **Frontal sinuses** are within the frontal bone—one above each orbit near the midline.
2. **Parietal bones** (2) form the lateral parts of the cranium.
   - _____ is the joint where the parietal bones meet at the top of the skull.
   - **Coronal suture** is the joint where the parietal bones meet the _____ bone.
3. **Occipital bone** forms the posterior wall and floor of the cranium.
   - **Lambdoid suture** is where the occipital bone meets the parietal bones.
   - **Foramen magnum** is a large opening on the inferior surface through which the _____ will pass.
   - **Occipital condyles** border each side of the foramen magnum; they articulate (form joints) with the first vertebra.
4. **Temporal bones** (2) are below the parietal bones on either side of the cranium.
   - **Squamous suture** is where each temporal bone unites with a _____ bone.
   - **External auditory meatus** is an opening which leads toward the _____.
   - **Mandibular fossa** is a depression anterior to the external auditory meatus which provides an articular (joint) surface for the _____.
   - **Zygomatic process** is a bridge-like extension of bone that projects anteriorly.
   - **Zygomatic arch** is formed by the zygomatic process of the temporal bone that joins the zygomatic bone to form the _____.
   - **Styloid process** is a pointed process projected below the external auditory meatus.
   - _____ is a blunt projection posterior to the styloid process that serves as an attachment site for muscles of the neck.
   - **Carotid canal** is an opening that allows the _____ artery to pass through the bone.
   - **Jugular foramen** is an opening that allows the passage of the _____ vein.
5. **Sphenoid bone** is a butterfly-shaped bone that forms the lower lateral walls and floor of the cranium and posterior walls of the orbits.
   - **Optic foramen** is a round hole that may be seen by looking through the orbits.
   - **Superior** and **inferior orbital** _____ are two crack-like openings lateral to the optic foramen that transmits blood vessels and nerves.
   - **Sella turcica** is a saddle-shaped process visible from within the cranial cavity that houses the _____ gland.
   - **Sphenoidal sinuses** are two small spaces within the bone.

6. **Ethmoid bone** is a small bone anterior to the _____ bone that forms part of the cranial floor, orbital walls, and nasal cavity walls.
   - **Cribriform plate** divides the cranial cavity from the nasal cavity.
   - **Crista galli** is the "rooster's comb" that serves as a point of attachment for the membranes enclosing the brain in the cranial cavity.
   - **Perpendicular plate** projects downward from the cribriform plate which forms most of the nasal septum dividing the nasal cavity into right and left halves.
   - **Conchae (superior, middle)** are projections in the lateral walls of the nasal cavity.
   - **Ethmoid sinuses** exist within the ethmoid body.

Facial Bones

The bones of the face include _____ (*how many?*) immovable bones and a movable lower jaw.

1. **Maxillary bones** (2) are on each side of the face and form the upper jaw. Portions form the floor of the orbits, the roof of the mouth, and the walls and floor of the nasal cavity.
   - **Maxillary sinuses** are located within these bones and drain into the nasal cavity.
   - **Alveolar margins** (processes) are ridges through which the upper teeth articulate with the maxillary bones.
   - **Palatine process** is the roof of the mouth; it fuses along the midline before birth. If fusion does not occur, a *cleft palate* results and an opening remains between the mouth and the nasal cavity.
2. **Palatine bones** (2) are located posterior to the _____ bones. They form the roof of the mouth, floor of the nasal cavity, and lateral walls of the nasal cavity.
3. **Zygomatic bones** (2) form the cheekbones and orbits.
   - **Temporal process** extends to the temporal bone on the side of the head to unite with the _____ process.
   - **Zygomatic arch** is the prominence of the cheekbone formed by the union of the temporal process of the zygomatic bone and the zygomatic process of the temporal bone.
4. **Nasal bones** (2) form the bridge of the nose. The anterior part of the nose is formed by _____ plates.
5. **Lacrimal bones** (2) form part of the orbit's medial walls.
6. **Vomer** is a bone located along the midline of the nasal cavity. Its posterior margin unites with the perpendicular plate of the ethmoid, forming the nasal _____.
7. **Inferior nasal conchae** (2) are attached to the lateral walls of the nasal cavity and situated below the superior and middle conchae of the _____ bone. The conchae are also known as turbinates.
8. **Mandible** is the lower jaw bone that articulates with the _____ bones. It is the *only* movable bone of the skull.
   - **Condylar process** articulates with the mandibular fossa of the temporal bone to form a joint known as the _____
   - **Alveolar margin** (process) is an arch containing sockets for teeth.

Review Time!

I. *Using the terms in the list below, write the appropriate bone in each blank. You may use a term more than once.*

Ethmoid bone   Frontal bone   Lacrimal bone   Vomer   Zygomatic bone

Maxillary bone   Nasal bone   Occipital bone   Mandible

Parietal bone   Sphenoid bone   Temporal bone   Palatine bone

1. Forms the nasal septum along with the ethmoid bone   _____

2. Forms part of the cheekbone along with the temporal bone   _____

3. Forms the posterior roof of the mouth   _____

4. Lower jaw bone   _____

5. Sella turcica belongs to this bone   _____

6. Cribriform plate belongs to this bone   _____

7. Upper jaw bones   _____

8. Only movable bone of the skull   _____

9. Forms the forehead   _____

10. Borders the squamous suture with the parietal bone   _____

11. Bone that houses the foramen magnum   _____

12. Bones that meet along the sagittal suture   _____

13. Bone that houses eye sockets known as orbits   _____

14. Pair of bones that form the medial walls of the orbits   _____

15. Perpendicular plate belongs to this bone   _____

16. Superior and middle nasal conchae belong to this bone   _____

17. Carotid artery passes through an opening in this bone   _____

18. Pair of bones that unite with the frontal bone at the
     coronal suture   _____

19. External auditory meatus belongs to this bone   _____

20. Bones that house the largest of the sinuses   _____

II. *Using the list of terms provided, label the illustration below of the skull, anterior view, with the appropriate bone names and markings.*

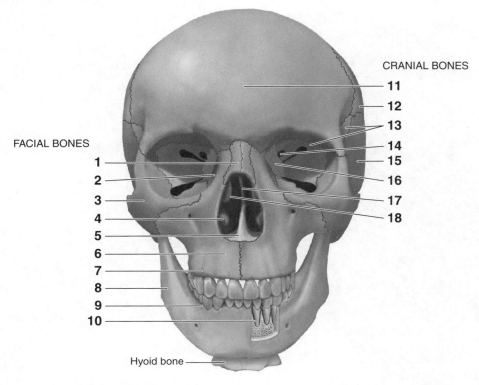

1. _____
2. _____
3. _____
4. _____
5. _____
6. _____

7. _____
8. _____
9. _____
10. _____
11. _____
12. _____

13. _____
14. _____
15. _____
16. _____
17. _____
18. _____

Ethmoid bone (include labels for the middle nasal concha and for the perpendicular plate)

Frontal bone

Inferior nasal concha

Lacrimal bone

Mandible (include label for the alveolus and for the alveolar margin)

Maxilla (include a label for the alveolar margin)

Nasal bone

Parietal bone

Sphenoid bone (include a label for the optic foramen)

Temporal bone

Vomer bone

Zygomatic bone

III. Using the list of terms provided, label the illustration below of the skull, lateral view, with the appropriate bone names and markings.

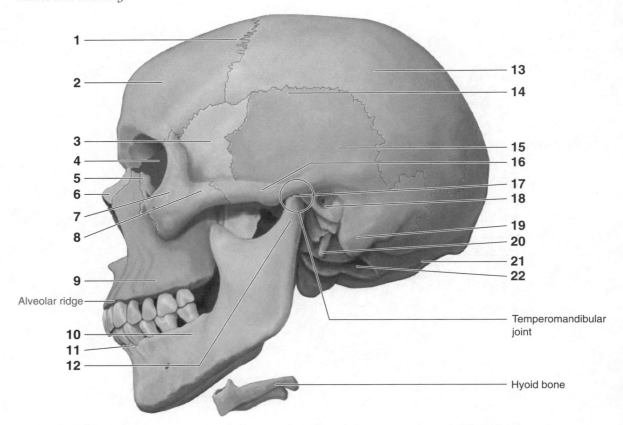

1. _____   9. _____   17. _____
2. _____   10. _____   18. _____
3. _____   11. _____   19. _____
4. _____   12. _____   20 ._____
5. _____   13. _____   21 ._____
6. _____   14. _____   22 ._____
7. _____   15. _____
8. _____   16. _____

Coronal suture

Ethmoid bone

Frontal bone

Lacrimal bone

Mandible (include labels
    for the alveolar process
    and for the condylar
    process)

Maxillary bone

Nasal bone

Occipital bone (include
    a label for the foramen
    magnum)

Parietal bone

Sphenoid bone

Squamous suture

Temporal bone (include
    labels for the external
    auditory meatus, the
    mandibular fossa, the
    mastoid process, the
    styloid process, and the
    zygomatic process)

Zygomatic bone (include
    a label for the temporal
    process)

IV. *Using the list of terms provided, label the illustration below of the skull, inferior view, with the appropriate bone names and markings.*

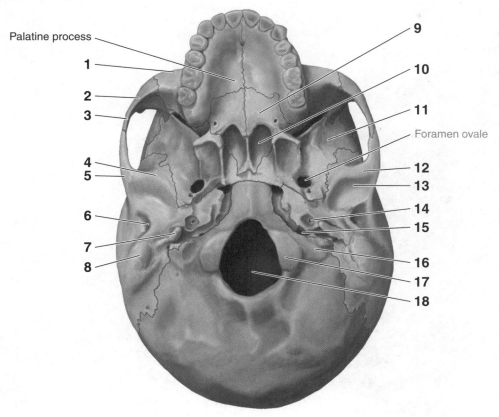

Palatine process

1. _____
2. _____
3. _____
4. _____
5. _____
6. _____
7. _____

8. _____
9. _____
10. _____
11. _____
12. _____
13. _____
14. _____

15. _____
16. _____
17. _____
18. _____

Maxilla

Occipital bone (include labels for the occipital condyle and for the foramen magnum)

Palatine bone

Sphenoid bone

Temporal bone (include labels for the carotid canal, the external auditory meatus, the jugular foramen, the mandibular fossa, the mastoid process, the styloid process, and the zygomatic process)

Vomer bone

Zygomatic bone (include a label for the temporal process)

V. *Using the list of terms provided, label the illustration below of the skull, sagittal section, with the appropriate bone names.*

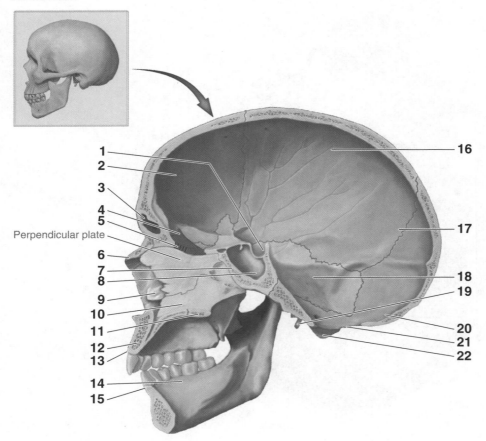

Perpendicular plate

1. _____
2. _____
3. _____
4. _____
5. _____
6. _____
7. _____
8. _____

9. _____
10. _____
11. _____
12. _____
13. _____
14. _____
15. _____
16. _____

17. _____
18. _____
19. _____
20. _____
21. _____
22. _____

Ethmoid bone (include labels for the cribriform plate [olfactory foramina], the crista galli, and the perpendicular plate)

Frontal bone (include a label for the frontal sinus)

Inferior nasal concha

Lambdoid suture

Mandible (include a label for the alveolar margin)

Maxilla (include a label for the alveolar margin)

Nasal bone

Occipital bone (include labels for the foramen magnum and for the occipital condyle)

Palatine bone

Parietal bone

Sphenoid bone (include labels for the sella turcica and for the sphenoidal sinuses)

Temporal bone (include a label for the styloid process)

Vomer bone

Hyoid Bone

Why is the hyoid bone unique?_____

_____

The hyoid bone is located in the _____ suspended from the styloid process of the temporal bone by ligaments and muscles. The hyoid bone supports the tongue.

Vertebral Column

The **vertebral column** extends from the base of the skull to the pelvis and is composed of bones called **vertebrae. Intervertebral discs**, made of _____ are situated between each vertebra. The vertebral column protects the spinal cord, which extends through the openings in the vertebrae called the _____.

How many vertebrae are found in the vertebral column?_____

When the sacrum and coccyx are considered as individual bones, the total number of bones in the vertebral column is _____ bones.

How many vertebrae are in each region of the spine?

- _____ **cervical vertebrae** (neck)
- _____ **thoracic vertebrae** (thorax)
- _____ **lumbar vertebrae** (lower trunk)
- _____ **sacral vertebrae** (fused to form the **sacrum**)
- _____ **coccygeal vertebrae** (fused to form the **coccyx**)

> **TIP!** Use this tip to remember how many vertebrae are found in the cervical, thoracic, and lumbar regions: 7, 12, and 5 are the times for breakfast, lunch and dinner. There are 7 cervical vertebrae, 12 thoracic vertebrae, and 5 lumbar vertebrae.

Curves of the vertebral column correspond to the regions of vertebrae.

- **Cervical curve** bends _____ (concave)
- **Thoracic curve** bends _____ (convex)
- **Lumbar curve** bends _____ (concave)
- **Sacral curve** bends _____ (convex)

What functions do these curves serve? _____

_____

What curve does a newborn have? _____

_____

When do the other curves develop?_____

_____

- Cervical curve develops when: _____
- Lumbar curve develops when: _____

A Typical Vertebra

- **Body** is the single, drum-shaped portion that is the weight-bearing part of the vertebra.
- **Vertebral arch** extends from the body and completes the bony circle around the opening.
- **Vertebral foramen** is an opening through which the _____ passes.
- **Pedicles** are two bridges attached to the body.

- **Laminae** are two plates that extend from the pedicles backward.
- **Spinous process** is a single posterior projection.
- **Transverse processes** are two lateral projects extending from the _____.
- **Superior** and **inferior articulating processes** are four upward and downward facing projections. These processes unite with vertebrae above and below.

As we discuss the parts of the vertebra, add labels to the illustration below. When you are done, you should be able to identify the parts of a typical vertebra listed below.

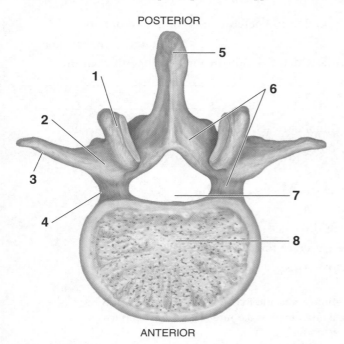

POSTERIOR

ANTERIOR

1. _____
2. _____
3. _____
4. _____
5. _____
6. _____
7. _____
8. _____

Body	Spinous process	Vertebral arch
Lamina	Superior articulating process	Vertebral foramen
Pedicle	Transverse process	

Cervical Vertebrae

Unique features of the cervical vertebrae:
- Cervical vertebrae are smaller and lighter in size than other vertebrae.
- Cervical vertebrae have a small hole in each transverse process, known as a **transverse foramen**, through which arteries travel to the brain.
- **Atlas**, C1, is the _____ cervical vertebra. It has _no_ body and has large superior articulating processes with cartilage-covered surfaces called **facets**. The joint of the atlas with the occipital condyles of the skull allow you to nod your head up and down (as if saying "yes").
- **Axis**, C2, is the _____ cervical vertebra. It has a body and an **odontoid process** (**dens**). The odontoid process projects up through the ring of the atlas and allows you to pivot your head (as if saying "no").

As we discuss the parts of the cervical vertebra, add labels to the illustration below. When you are done, you should be able to identify the parts of the cervical vertebra listed below.

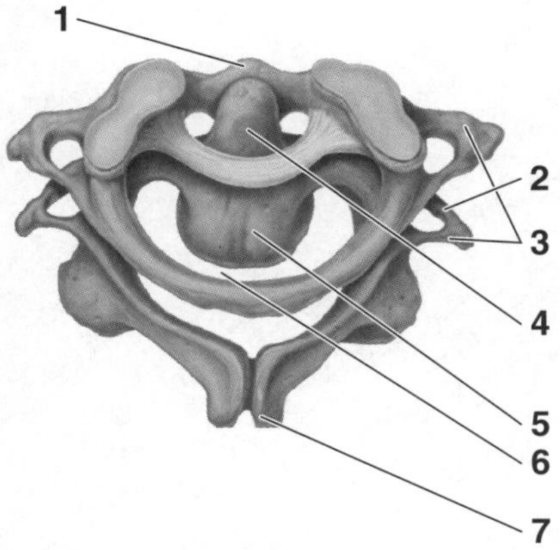

1. _____

2. _____

3. _____

4. _____

5. _____

6. _____

7. _____

Axis   Dens (odontoid process)   Vertebral foramen

Atlas   Spinous process

Body   Transverse process

Thoracic Vertebrae

How many thoracic vertebrae are in your vertebral column?_____

Unique features of the thoracic vertebrae:

- The thoracic vertebrae are the only members of the vertebral column to articulate with the

  _____.

- **Facets** are smooth articulating surfaces present on thoracic vertebrae on the sides of their bodies and on the transverse processes where ribs attach.

Lumbar Vertebrae

Unique features of the lumbar vertebrae:

- Lumbar vertebrae are larger and thicker than the cervical and thoracic vertebrae, particularly at the

  _____.

- Lumbar vertebrae handle more stress from the body weight they support.

Sacrum

How many vertebrae fuse to form the sacrum? _____

Where is the sacrum located? _____

- **Median sacral crest** is a remnant of the spinous processes of the five fused vertebrae.
- **Superior articular processes** are the two superior processes that articulate with the

  _____ lumbar vertebra.

- **Sacral canal** is the extension of the vertebral canal that continues from the lumbar region into the

  _____.

- **Sacral hiatus** is where the sacral canal opens at the opposite end of the sacrum.
- **Sacral foramina** are four pairs of openings alongside the median sacral crest; nerves and

  _____ travel through these openings.

As we discuss the parts of the sacrum, add labels to the illustration below. When you are done, you should be able to identify the parts of the sacrum listed below.

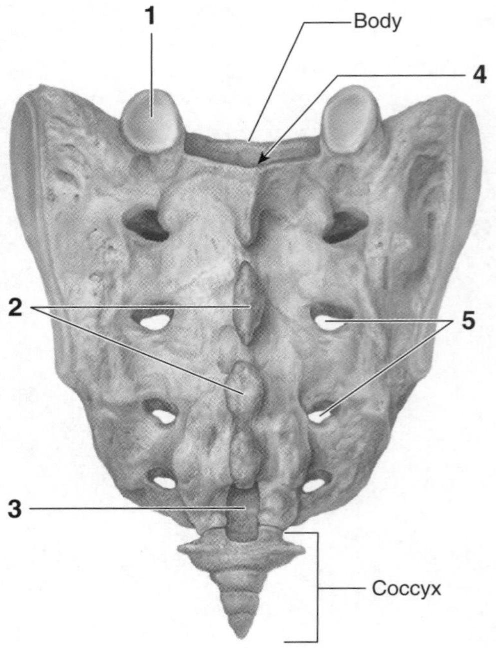

1. _____
2. _____
3. _____
4. _____
5. _____

Dorsal sacral foramina	Sacral canal	Superior articular process
Median sacral crest	Sacral hiatus	

Thoracic Cage

The thoracic cage is formed by the thoracic vertebrae, sternum, and ribs. It encloses the organs of the chest and supports the shoulder girdle and upper limbs.

Sternum

The **sternum**, or breastbone, is located along the midline of the chest. The sternum articulates with the two _____ at the superior end and with the ribs by cartilage along its lateral borders.

- **Manubrium** is the superior part.
- **Body** is the middle part.
- **Xiphoid process** is the inferior part.

Ribs

Each of the 12 pairs of ribs attaches to the thoracic vertebra and curves around the front toward the sternum.
- **True ribs** are directly connected to the sternum by **costal cartilage**. True ribs are the first seven pairs of ribs.
- **False ribs** are the last five pairs of ribs and have either an indirect connection to the _____ or no direct connection at all.
- **Floating ribs** are the last two or three pairs that lack _____ completely.

Features of a typical rib:
- **Shaft** curves around in a semicircle.
- **Head** is a proximal (or posterior) enlargement; articulates with the _____ of one or two thoracic vertebrae.

• **Tubercle** is a small projection near the head which articulates with the _____ process of the thoracic vertebra.

As we discuss the parts of the thoracic cage, add labels to the illustration below. When you are done, you should be able to identify the parts of the thoracic cage listed below.

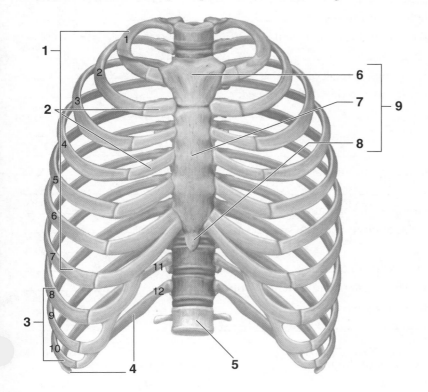

1. _____
2. _____
3. _____
4. _____
5. _____
6. _____
7. _____
8. _____
9. _____

Costal cartilages
False ribs (8 to 12)
Floating ribs (11, 12)
L1 vertebra

Sternum (include labels for the
   body, manubrium, and
   xiphoid process)
True ribs (1 to 7)

Review Time!

I.   Provide a brief answer for each of the following questions.

1. Name the two bones that articulate with the teeth.
   1. _____
   2. _____
2. List the bones that form the thoracic cage.
   1. _____
   2. _____
   3. _____
3. What bones are united by the coronal suture?
   1. _____
   2. _____

4. Name the bones, paired and individual, that form the cranium.

    1. _____   4. _____

    2. _____   5. _____

    3. _____   6. _____

5. Which bone is the only movable bone in the skull?_____

6. Name the only bone in the skeleton that does not articulate with another bone.

    _____

7. How many pairs of true ribs exist in the thoracic cage?_____

8. What is the name of the hole that forms the opening to the ear?_____

    _____

9. What is the role of costal cartilage?_____

    _____

10. List the numbers for cervical, thoracic, and lumbar vertebrae._____

    _____

11. Through what part of the vertebra does the spinal cord pass?_____

12. Through what opening in the occipital bone does the spinal cord pass?_____

    _____

13. What is the shape of the cervical curvature?_____

14. What gland is supported by the sella turcica of the sphenoid bone?_____

15. Identify the bones that house the sinuses.

    1. _____   3. _____

    2. _____

16. Name the two bones that form the roof of the mouth.

    1. _____

    2. _____

17. How many total rib pairs does a person normally have?_____

18. Name the three parts of the sternum.

    1. _____

    2. _____

    3. _____

19. Name the two bones, or parts, that form the nasal septum.

    1. _____

    2. _____

20. Name the two processes that form the zygomatic arch and create the prominence of the cheekbone.

    1. _____

    2. _____

CONCEPT 5

The Appendicular Skeleton

Concept: The appendicular skeleton includes the bones that lie outside of the central axis of the body. They include the bones of the pectoral girdle, upper limb, pelvic girdle, and lower limb.

LEARNING OBJECTIVE 15. Identify the bones of the appendicular skeleton.

LEARNING OBJECTIVE 16. Identify the prominent features of the appendicular bones.

List the bones of the appendicular skeleton.

1. _____ girdle includes the scapula and clavicle.
2. Upper limb bones include the: _____

   _____
3. Pelvic girdle includes two coxal bones and the sacrum.
4. Lower limb bones include the: _____

   _____

Pectoral Girdles

Each of the two pectoral girdles contains a clavicle (collarbone) and scapula (shoulder blade).

Clavicles

Clavicles are slender "S"-shaped bones. Each bone extends between the sternum and the scapula at the base of the neck.

The **acromioclavicular joint** is formed where the clavicle joins the scapula. Along with the glenohumeral joint (discussed below), the acromioclavicular joint is one of two in the shoulder. What is the function of this joint?_____

_____

Scapula

Each triangular **scapula** is lateral to the clavicle on the upper back.
- **Subscapular fossa** is the anterior surface.
- **Spine** is a _____ on the posterior surface that divides the scapula into two unequal portions.
- **Supraspinous fossa** is the portion of the scapula superior to the spine.
- **Infraspinous fossa** is the portion of the scapula inferior to the spine.
- **Acromion process** is at the lateral end of the scapula; it unites with the _____ (bone).
- **Coracoid process** is anterior to the acromion and curves laterally. It is an attachment site for muscles of the arm and chest.
- **Glenoid cavity** is an oval depression along the lateral edge that articulates with the head of the

  _____.
- **Glenohumeral joint** is created where the glenoid cavity of the scapula articulates with the head of the humerus. What is the other shoulder joint (previously discussed)? _____

As we discuss the parts of the scapula, add labels to the illustration below. When you are done, you should be able to identify the parts of the scapula listed below. You may use terms more than once.

1. _____
2. _____
3. _____
4. _____
5. _____
6. _____
7. _____
8. _____
9. _____
10. _____
11. _____

Acromion process   Infraspinous fossa   Subscapular fossa
Coracoid process   Spine   Supraspinous fossa
Glenoid cavity

Upper Limb

How many bones are found in the two upper limbs?_____

Each upper limb includes the:

- Humerus (arm)
- Radius and _____ (forearm)
- Metacarpals (wrist)
- Carpals (hand)
- _____ (fingers)

Humerus

The humerus is the long bone of the arm that extends from the shoulder to the elbow. The features, next, are presented from the proximal to the distal end.

- **Head** of the humerus articulates with the _____ cavity of the scapula. What joint is formed by this articulation? _____

- **Anatomical neck** is a narrow circular groove distal to the head that separates the head from two _____.

- **Greater tubercle** is a projection on the _____ side; it provides an attachment for muscles that move the arm at the shoulder.

- **Lesser tubercle** is a projection on the _____ side; it provides an attachment for muscles that move the arm at the shoulder.

- **Intertubercular groove** is a narrow channel that runs between the greater and lesser tubercles.

- **Surgical neck**, a region commonly fractured, is _____ to the tubercles.

- **Capitulum** is a smooth, round process on the distal end of the humerus that articulates with the _____.

- **Trochlea** is on the medial, distal side of the humerus that articulates with the _____.

- **Epicondyles** (medial and lateral) form the medial and lateral borders of the distal end of the humerus. They are attachment sites for muscles and ligaments of the _____.

- **Coronoid fossa** is a depression on the anterior side that receives a portion of the ulna.
- **Olecranon fossa** is a depression on the posterior side that receives a portion of the ulna when the
_____ is extended straight out at the elbow.

As we discuss the parts of the humerus, add labels to the anterior and posterior views below. When you are done, you should be able to identify the parts of the humerus listed below. You may use terms more than once.

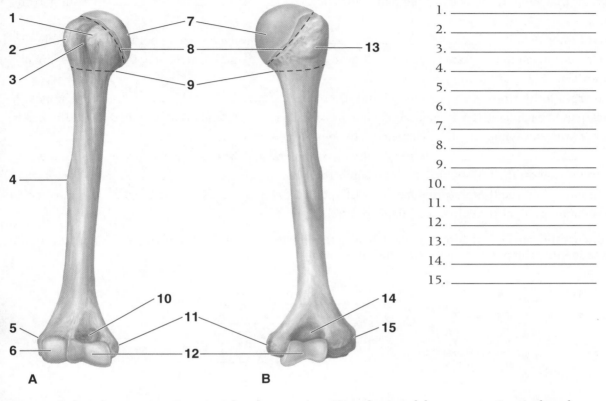

1. _____
2. _____
3. _____
4. _____
5. _____
6. _____
7. _____
8. _____
9. _____
10. _____
11. _____
12. _____
13. _____
14. _____
15. _____

Anatomical neck	Greater tubercle	Lateral epicondyle	Surgical neck
Capitulum	Head	Lesser tubercle	Trochlea
Coronoid fossa	Intertubercular groove	Medial epicondyle	
Deltoid tuberosity		Olecranon fossa	

Radius

The radius is the lateral bone of the forearm; it is the bone always in line with the thumb.

- **Head** is on the proximal end of the radius. It articulates with the capitulum of the
_____ and a notch on the ulna.
- **Radial tuberosity** is a roughened surface distal to the head which is an attachment for the
_____ muscle of the arm.
- **Styloid process** is at the distal end of the radius; it provides an attachment for ligaments of the
_____.

Ulna

The ulna is medial to the radius in the forearm.

- **Olecranon process** is a large projection at the proximal end that forms the bony tip of your elbow.
- **Coronoid process** is a projection distal to the olecranon process.
- **Trochlear (semilunar) notch** is a semicircular depression between the olecranon process and the coronoid process. It receives the trochlea of the _____.

- **Head** is at the distal end and is separated from the wrist by a _____ disc.
- **Styloid process** provides an attachment site for ligaments of the wrist.

Hand

The bones of the hand consist of the carpals that form the _____, the metacarpals that support the body of the hand, and the _____ that support the fingers.

- **Carpal bones** include _____ (*how many?*) small bones bound together by ligaments arranged in two transverse rows (four to a row). The carpals articulate with the radius, ulnar fibrocartilage disc, and the metacarpals.
- **Metacarpal bones** form the palm of the hand. There are _____ (*how many?*) metacarpals in each hand. Each metacarpal bone has a flat base, shaft, and distal, rounded head. The heads form the knuckles when the fist is clenched. The metacarpals articulate with the _____ bones on the proximal end and with the phalanges on the distal end.
- **Phalanges** support the fingers (digits) of the hand. There are _____ (*how many?*) in each hand: 2 in the thumb (proximal and distal) and _____ (*how many?*) in each remaining finger (proximal, middle, and distal).

As we discuss the parts of the forearm, add labels to the illustration below. When you are done, you should be able to identify the parts of the forearm listed below.

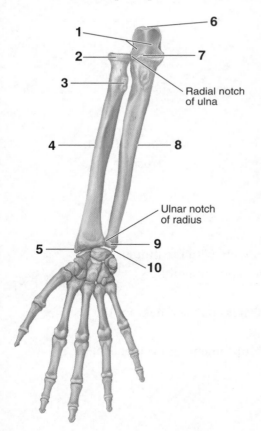

Radial notch of ulna

Ulnar notch of radius

1. _____
2. _____
3. _____
4. _____
5. _____
6. _____
7. _____
8. _____
9. _____
10. _____

Radius (include labels for the head of radius, radial tuberosity, and styloid process)

Ulna (include labels for the coronoid process, head of ulna, olecranon process, styloid process, and trochlear notch)

As we discuss the bones of the hand, add labels to the illustration below. When you are done, you should be able to identify the bones of the hand listed below.

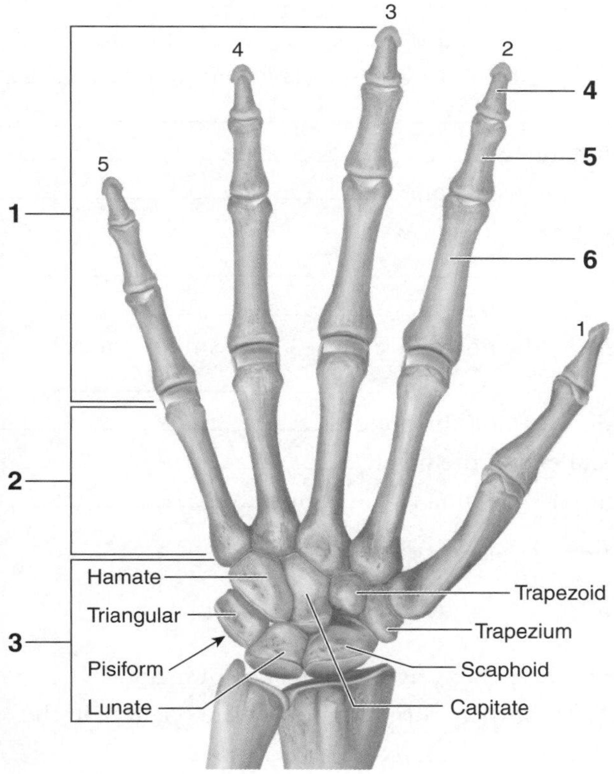

1. _____
2. _____
3. _____
4. _____
5. _____
6. _____

Hamate
Triangular
Pisiform
Lunate
Trapezoid
Trapezium
Scaphoid
Capitate

Carpals   Phalanges   Middle phalanx

Metacarpals   Proximal phalanx   Distal phalanx

Review Time!

I.   *Provide a brief answer for each of the following questions.*

     1. Name the two bones in the forearm.

        1. _____

        2. _____

     2. With what bone does the trochlea of the humerus articulate?_____

     3. With what bone does the capitulum of the humerus articulate?_____

     4. List the bones in the arm, forearm, and hand in anatomical order from superior to inferior.

        _____

        _____

        _____

        _____

        _____

     5. What part of the humerus articulates with the glenoid cavity of the scapula?_____

6. Name the two joints that form the shoulder joints.

   1. _____

   2. _____

7. Which forearm bone is situated on the thumb side?_____

8. What part of the scapula articulates with the clavicle to form the acromioclavicular joint?_____

   _____

9. How many carpal bones are there in total in each hand?_____

10. Which digit of the hand has only a proximal bone and distal bone?_____

11. List the bones of the pectoral girdle.

   _____

   _____

12. Which is situated closer to the head of the humerus—the anatomical neck *or* the surgical neck?

   _____

13. Is the head of the radius on the proximal *or* the distal end of the bone?_____

14. Is the head of the ulna on the proximal *or* the distal end of the bone?_____

15. In anatomical position, which forearm bone is lateral—the ulna *or* the radius?_____

Pelvic Girdle

The pelvic girdle is a frame that supports the lower limbs to carry the weight of the body. It includes the **coxal** (pelvic or hip) **bones** that unite with the **sacrum** posteriorly to form the pelvis. The opening in the center of the pelvis is known as the pelvic _____.

Functions: The pelvis provides support for the upper body parts, attachment to lower limbs, and protection for organs of the lower trunk. In females, it forms the skeletal part of the _____ canal. Male and female pelvises are structurally different.

Can you list at least three differences here?

	Male	Female
1.		
2.		
3.		

Coxal Bones

In a newborn, each coxal bone consists of three separate bones.

1. **Ilium**

2. _____

3. **Ischium**

As the child grows, the three bones fuse until they merge completely in the adult, where they become subdivisions of a single bone. The area of fusion is a cup-shaped depression called the **acetabulum**. The acetabulum serves as a socket for the head of the _____.

Let's discuss the markings on each of the three coxal bone subdivisions.

1. The **ilium** is the largest of the coxal bone's subdivisions; it forms the bony ridge of the hip.
   - **Iliac crest** is the superior bony ridge of the hip.
   - **Auricular surface** is the roughed surface along the posterior margin of the _____.
   - **Sacroiliac joint** is created when the auricular surface unites with the _____.
   - **Anterior superior iliac spine** is the most prominent spine and is anterior on each

     _____.

2. The **ischium** is the inferior and the posterior portion of the coxal bone with an "L" shape.
   - **Ischial spine** is a projection with the superior border near the _____.
   - **Ischial** _____ is a roughened, elevated surface at the angle of the "L" that supports your weight when sitting.
   - **Ramus** is a flat region that fuses with the _____.

3. The **pubis** is the inferior and the anterior part of the coxal bone.
   - **Symphysis pubis** is the joint created when the pubis bones of opposite _____ bones come together.
   - **Pubic arch** is the inferior angle formed by the two coxal bones in the pubic region.
   - _____ **foramen** is the opening formed by the curvatures of the pubis and _____. Parts of muscles, blood vessels, and nerves pass through this hole, the largest foramen in the body.

> **TIP!** Having trouble keeping the three portions of the coxal bone straight? Remember the "S" in ischium. The "S" reminds us the ischium bone is for sitting.

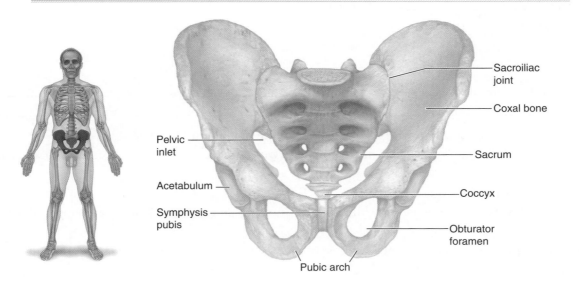

As we discuss the parts of the coxal bone, add labels to the illustration below. When you are done, you should be able to identify the parts of the coxal bone listed below.

1. _____
2. _____
3. _____
4. _____
5. _____
6. _____
7. _____
8. _____
9. _____
10. _____
11. _____

Acetabulum

Obturator foramen

Ilium (include labels for the anterior superior iliac spine, auricular surface, and iliac crest)

Ischium (include labels for the ischial spine, ischial tuberosity, and ramus)

Pubis

Lower Limb

How many bones are found in the two lower limbs?_____

Each lower limb includes the:

• Femur (thigh)

• _____ (kneecap)

• Tibia and _____ (leg)

• Tarsals and metatarsals (foot)

• Phalanges (toes)

Femur

What makes the femur a unique bone of the body?_____
_____

The femur extends from its union with the coxal bone at the hip joint to the knee.

• **Head** is ball shaped and projects medially to articulate with _____ of the coxal bone.

• **Neck** is the constricted area below the head.

• **Greater trochanter** is a large process by the base of the neck and is situated lateral and upper of the two trochanters.

• **Lesser trochanter** is the medial, lower process of the two trochanters. These trochanters provide attachment sites for muscles of the _____ and _____.

- **Linea aspera** is a line down the posterior side of the shaft of the _____; it, too serves as an attachment site for muscles.
- **Lateral condyle** and **medial condyle** are two rounded processes on the distal end of the femur that articulate with the tibia.
- **Intercondylar fossa** is a depression situated between the lateral and medial condyles.
- **Patellar surface** is a depression on the _____ side of the distal end of the femur.

As we discuss the parts of the femur, add labels to the anterior and posterior views below. When you are done, you should be able to identify the parts of the femur listed below.

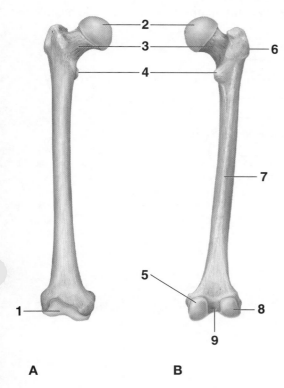

1. _____
2. _____
3. _____
4. _____
5. _____
6. _____
7. _____
8. _____
9. _____

A   **B**

Greater trochanter	Lateral condyle	Medial condyle
Head	Lesser trochanter	Neck
Intercondylar fossa	Linea aspera	Patellar surface

Patella

The **patella** (kneecap) is located within a large tendon (quadriceps tendon) that wraps over the anterior side of the knee.

Tibia

The **tibia** is the larger of the two bones of the leg; it is also medial and extends between the knee and ankle.

- **Lateral condyle** and **medial condyle** are situated on the proximal end and articulate with the condyles of the _____.
- **Tibial tuberosity** is a roughened surface on the anterior side of the tibia. It is an attachment site for the _____ ligament.
- **Medial malleolus** is on the distal end of the tibia which forms the medial side of the _____.

Fibula

The **fibula** is a thin bone located lateral to the tibia in the leg.
- **Head** of the fibula is at its proximal end; it articulates with the _____ of the tibia.
- **Lateral malleolus** is on the distal end that forms the lateral ankle. It articulates with the _____, a large bone in the foot.

> **TIP!** How can you tell the tibia from the fibula? The tibia bone has the shape of a big "T."

As we discuss the leg bones, add labels to the illustration below. When you are done, you should be able to identify the parts of the leg bones listed below.

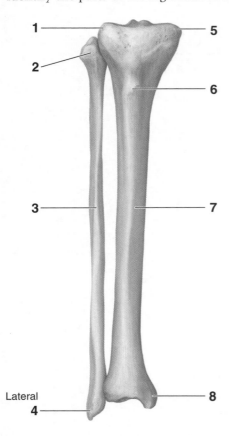

1. _____
2. _____
3. _____
4. _____
5. _____
6. _____
7. _____
8. _____

Tibia (include labels for the lateral condyle, medial condyle, medial malleolus, and tibial tuberosity)

Fibula (include labels for the head of the fibula and lateral malleolus)

Foot

The foot contains _____ (*how many?*) bones that comprise the ankle, foot, and toes.
- **Tarsal bones** (7) form the ankle. The two most prominent are **talus**, which is the only bone that articulates with the tibia and fibula, and _____, the heel bone that supports the weight of the body.
- **Metatarsal bones** (5) consist of a proximal base, a shaft, and a distal head (forms the ball of the foot). Between the calcaneus and the ball of the foot are the **arches**, which elevate the midsection of the foot.
- **Phalanges** (14) support the toes. Two phalanges are in the great (big) toe while there are _____ (*how many?*) in the other four toes.

As we discuss the bones of the foot, add labels to the illustration below. When you are done, you should be able to identify the bones of the foot listed below.

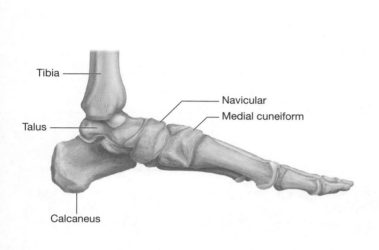

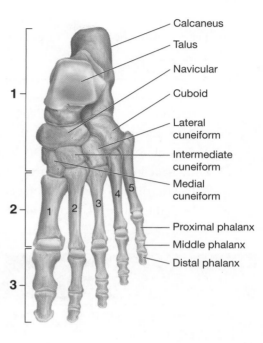

A

B

1. _____
2. _____
3. _____

Metatarsals
Phalanges
Tarsals

Review Time!

I.   Provide a brief answer for each of the following questions.

1. Name the two bones in the leg.

   1. _____
   2. _____

2. What part of the femur articulates with the acetabulum of the coxal bone? _____

3. How many metatarsal bones are in the instep of the foot? _____

4. Which leg bone is medial, the tibia *or* the fibula? _____

5. What parts of the tibia articulate with the condyles of the femur? _____
   _____

6. What two projections create the medial and lateral ankles? _____

7. List the bones that create the sacroiliac joint. _____
   _____
   _____

8. List the bones that create the pelvis. _____
_____
_____

9. List the three bones that fuse after birth to create the coxal bone.
    1. _____
    2. _____
    3. _____

10. Name the tarsal bone that serves as the heel bone. _____

11. What is the largest foramen in the body? _____

12. Is the pubic arch wider than 90 degrees in males *or* in females? _____

13. On what roughened part of the coxal bone do you sit? _____

14. Which portion of the coxal bone is the hip? _____

15. Why is the pelvic inlet wider in a female than in a male? _____
_____

CONCEPT 6

Joints

Concept: Joints are the junctions between bones. There are three types, which differ according to the nature of the material connecting the bones together and the degree of movement permitted.

LEARNING OBJECTIVE 17. **Distinguish between the three types of joints in the body and provide examples of each type.**

Joints, or **articulations**, are junctions between opposing bones. Joints may permit:
- No movement and be *immovable*
- Little movement and be *slightly movable*
- Unrestricted movement and be *freely movable*

Joints may be classified on the basis of their binding material and be:
- Fibrous
- Cartilaginous
- Synovial

Fibrous Joints

Fibrous joints consist of fibrous (dense) _____ tissue between articulating bones. Joints with little movement or no movement are called *synarthroses*.
- **An example of this type of joint is** _____
_____

Cartilaginous Joints

Cartilaginous joints bind opposing bones together with cartilage (hyaline or fibrocartilage). Cartilaginous joints are slightly movable. Slightly movable joints are known as *amphiarthroses*.
- **An example of this type of joint is** _____
_____

Synovial Joints

Synovial joints permit a greater range of motion than fibrous or cartilaginous joints and are freely movable. Freely movable joints are known as *diarthroses*.

* **Some examples of this type of joint are** _____
_____
_____

Parts of a Synovial Joint

Following are the parts of a typical synovial joint:

* **Synovial cavity** is the fluid-filled space between opposing bones.
* **Articular capsule** is a tubular capsule that encloses the _____ cavity.
* **Fibrous capsule** is the outer layer of the articular capsule and is continuous with the
_____ of the articulating bones and reinforced by ligaments.
* **Synovial membrane** is the inner layer of the articular capsule. It secretes a thick, clear fluid (**synovial fluid**) into the synovial cavity. The function of synovial fluid is _____
_____
* **Articular cartilage** constructed of hyaline cartilage covers the surfaces of the articulating bones that are exposed to the synovial cavity.

Accessory Structures of a Synovial Joint

These accessory structures improve movement in the synovial joint.

* **Menisci** are discs of fibrocartilage that subdivide the synovial cavity into two or more separate cavities. How do these discs serve the joint? _____
* **Ligaments** serve to stabilize joints by restricting the movement in the joint.
* **Bursae** are sacs lined with _____ membrane and contain synovial fluid. The bursae sacs are found _____
_____

* **Tendon sheaths** are elongated bursae that are wrapped about tendons in the hand and foot.

Types of Synovial Joints

LEARNING OBJECTIVE 18. Describe the six types of synovial joints.

How are synovial joints classified?_____
_____

Provide examples for the following six types of synovial joints:

1. **Pivot:** Movement is rotation about a central axis. Cylindrical surface of one bone rotates within a ring formed by another bone.
   * **An example of a pivot synovial joint is** _____
   _____

2. **Gliding:** Movement is back-and-forth sliding. Flat articulating surfaces create gliding joints.
   * **An example of a gliding synovial joint is** _____
   _____

3. **Condyloid:** Movement is back-and-forth and circular. A rounded condyle "knuckle" of one bone fits into a cavity of another bone.
   * **An example of a condyloid synovial joint is** _____
   _____

4. **Saddle:** Movement is back-and-forth, side-to-side, and some pivotal movements. Convex surface of one bone fits into the concave surface of another bone.
   - **An example of a saddle synovial joint is** _____
   _____

5. **Hinge:** Movement is back-and-forth (like a door). Convex surface of one bone fits into the concave surface of another bone.
   - **An example of a hinge synovial joint is** _____

6. **Ball and socket:** Movement is greater than any other joint type. Ball-shaped process of one bone fits into a cup-shaped socket of another bone.
   - **An example of a ball and socket synovial joint is** _____
   _____

Types of Movements at Synovial Joints

LEARNING OBJECTIVE   19. Define and describe the movements that are possible at synovial joints.

Contraction of skeletal muscles produces movement in synovial joints. Muscles are typically attached by tendons to two bones; one bone is held stationary while the other bone is pulled. The movement is called an **action**. Fourteen actions follow; provide an example where requested:

1. **Flexion** is a _____ in the angle between two bones.
   - **Dorsiflexion** occurs at the ankle when the top of the foot is moved toward the ankle.
   - **An example of flexion is** _____
   _____

2. **Extension** is an increase in the angle between two bones.
   - **Hyperextension** increases the angle beyond any normal anatomical position.
   - **Plantar flexion,** a special type of extension, occurs when you stand on your toes.
   - **An example of extension is** _____
   _____

3. **Abduction** is movement away from the vertical midline of the body.
   - **An example of abduction is** _____
   _____

4. **Adduction** is movement _____ the vertical midline of the body.

   > **TIP!** To perform "jumping jacks" you must move your arms and legs in alternating abduction and adduction movements.

   - **An example of adduction is** _____
   _____

5. **Circumduction** is movement of a limb such that its distal end forms a circular pattern.
   - **An example of circumduction is** _____
   _____

6. **Rotation** is movement of a part around a central axis.
   - **An example of rotation is** _____
   _____

7. **Pronation** occurs at the _____ when you turn your hand so that the palm is positioned inferiorly or posteriorly.

8. **Supination** occurs at the wrist and is opposite to _____. This movement occurs when you turn your hand so that the palm is positioned superiorly or anteriorly.

> **TIP!** When you carry a *soup* bowl with both hands, your hands are in a supine position.

9. **Eversion** occurs only with the foot at the _____, when the foot is turned to point the sole outward.

10. **Inversion** occurs with the foot at the ankle and is opposite to _____; the foot is turned to point the sole inward.

11. **Protraction** involves the movement of a body part straight outward from midline.
    - **An example of protraction is** _____
    _____

12. **Retraction** is the opposite of _____ and involves returning the body part straight back to the midline.
    - **An example of retraction is** _____
    _____

13. **Elevation** occurs when a body part is raised toward the head.
    - **An example of elevation is** _____
    _____

14. **Depression** is the opposite of _____.
    - **An example of depression is** _____
    _____

Review Time!

I. *Using the terms in the list below, write the appropriate type of joint in each blank. You may use a term more than once.*

Cartilaginous　　　　　Fibrous　　　　　Synovial

1. Joint consisting of dense connective tissue between articulating bones _____

2. Joint lubricated by synovial fluid _____

3. Elbow joint _____

4. Joint experiencing a wide range of motion _____

5. Symphysis pubis of the pelvic girdle _____

6. Knee joint _____

7. Diarthroses _____

8. Hyaline cartilage or fibrocartilage creates a firm but slightly movable joint _____

9. Skull sutures _____

10. Intervertebral discs of the vertebrae _____

II. *Using the terms in the list below, write the appropriate type of synovial joint in each blank. You may use a term more than once.*

Ball and socket   Condyloid   Gliding   Hinge

Pivot   Saddle

   1. Elbow joint   _____
   2. Joint that permits back-and-forth movement like a
      single-hinged door   _____
   3. Acromioclavicular joint   _____
   4. Joint between the radius and ulna   _____
   5. Joint created between the acetabulum of the coxal bone and
      the head of femur   _____
   6. Joint movement is limited to rotation around a central axis   _____
   7. Joint between axis and atlas of the vertebral column   _____
   8. Back-and-forth sliding motion between two nearly flat
      articulating surfaces   _____
   9. Glenohumeral joint   _____
  10. Joint between a carpal and the metacarpal of the thumb   _____

III. *Using the terms in the list below, write the appropriate type of synovial joint movement in each blank. You may use a term more than once.*

Abduction   Adduction   Extension   Flexion

Circumduction   Rotation   Pronation   Inversion

   1. Bending the elbow   _____
   2. Movement away from the vertical midline of the body   _____
   3. Movement opposite to supination   _____
   4. Movement of a limb so that its distal end forms a
      circular pattern   _____
   5. Occurs at the wrist   _____
   6. Turning your head left and right to say "no"   _____
   7. Straightening the leg at the knee   _____
   8. Occurs with the foot at the ankle   _____
   9. Movement opposite to eversion   _____
  10. Raising the arm horizontally from the side   _____

IV. *Provide a brief answer for each of the following questions.*
   1. Describe features of the synovial joint that act to absorb shock. _____

   2. Describe the type of movement that can occur in amphiarthroses. _____

   3. What type of joint experiences a free range of motion? Provide the name of this joint based on its
      binding material. _____

   4. Provide the name of joints that are freely movable. _____

5. Explain the contributions of bursae and tendon sheaths to a synovial joint.

_____

_____

_____

6. What function(s) does synovial fluid serve? _____

_____

_____

7. Describe how dorsiflexion and plantar flexion are opposite actions. _____

_____

_____

8. Describe the range of motion in synarthroses, amphiarthroses, and diarthroses. _____

_____

_____

_____

9. What type of synovial joint permits the greatest degree of movement? _____
   List two examples of this type of joint. _____

_____

_____

10. Do you recall from a previous chapter what type of tissue creates a synovial membrane?

_____

11. Using what you've learned in a previous chapter, why do you think torn menisci are difficult to
    heal?_____

_____

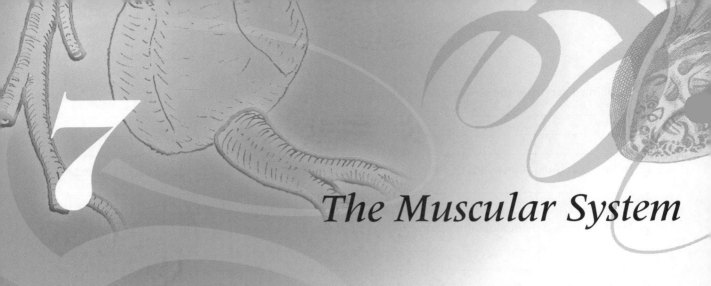

7 *The Muscular System*

Tips for Success as You Begin

Read Chapter 7 from your textbook before attending the class. Listen when you attend the lecture and fill in the blanks in this notebook. You may choose to complete the blanks before attending the class as a way to prepare for the day's topics. The same day you attend the lecture, read the material again, and complete the exercises after each section in this notebook. Start studying early and study this material often—you are now encountering some more complex physiology as well as numerous skeletal muscles you may have to learn.

Introduction

LEARNING OBJECTIVE   **1. Indicate the primary function of muscles.**

Recall from Chapter 4 the three types of muscle tissue:

1. Smooth muscle
2. Cardiac muscle
3. Skeletal muscle

Which of the three tissue types is the major component of the roughly 600 muscles in the human body?

_____

Skeletal muscle tissue contracts (shortens) to move the bones to which it is attached. The three major functions of the muscular system are:

1. _____: Movement relies on the integration of bones, nerves, joints, and nearby muscles to produce a movement.

2. _____: Rigid connections hold the body in an upright posture and strengthen the frame.

3. _____: Movement produces heat that helps to maintain body temperature.

CONCEPT 1

Muscle Structure

Concept: A muscle is an organ bound by several layers of connective tissue and mainly consists of skeletal muscle tissue. Each skeletal muscle cell is a long filamentous fiber containing contractile proteins in a highly ordered arrangement.

LEARNING OBJECTIVE 2. Describe the connective tissues associated with muscles.

Muscles usually extend from one bone to another. Muscles are a combination of skeletal muscle tissue, connective tissue, nerves, and a blood supply.

Connective Tissues of Muscle

The most abundant connective tissue associated with muscle is _____.

- **Superficial fascia** exists between skin and muscles or it may surround muscles.
- **Deep fascia** is part of the muscle, the organ. Deep fascia internally divides the muscle and is composed of connective tissue rich in _____ fibers.

Layers of Deep Fascia in Muscle

The following three layers are deep fascia. Each layer brings blood vessels and nerves to the deep compartments of muscle and provides support to the muscle.

1. **Epimysium** surrounds the entire muscle, covering it like a sheath.
2. **Perimysium** divides the muscle into compartments, known as **fascicles**. Fascicles are bundles of skeletal muscle cells.
3. **Endomysium** is the thinnest, innermost fascia that surrounds each individual muscle cell.

Connecting Muscle to Bone and Muscle to Muscle

- **Tendons** are narrow bands formed from the union of the three layers of deep fascia found in the muscle. Tendons attach the muscle to the bone. Do you recall the type of connective tissue that forms tendons?_____
- **Aponeuroses** are broad sheets of dense connective tissue that anchor muscles to bone or muscles to other muscles.

Other tissues associated with muscle include loose connective tissue (areolar tissue) and adipose tissue.

TIP! Build your own muscle, complete with connective tissue layers.

What you'll need: A handful of straws (with paper wrappers), one paper plate, several napkins, or paper towels.

How to build your muscle: Each straw is a muscle cell. The paper covering on the straw is deep fascia known as the endomysium. Take a bundle of straws in your hand. You now hold a fascicle (bundle) of muscle cells; each muscle cell is individually wrapped by its own endomysium. Use the napkin or paper towel to wrap this bundle. The napkin serves as the perimysium. Do the same to create more fascicles of straws with a paper towel perimysium. Finally, take the paper plate and wrap all of your bundles. The paper plate is the muscle's epimysium.

Microscopic Structure of Muscle

LEARNING OBJECTIVE 3. Identify and describe the microscopic components of skeletal muscle tissue.

Muscle cells are also known as muscle _____. Muscle cells are unique in that they are multinucleate.

- The plasma membrane of a muscle cell is called the _____ and the cytoplasm is termed _____.
- Muscle cells contract and return to their original strength. To accommodate this function, many mitochondria work to produce ATP for contractions.
- **Sarcoplasmic reticulum (SR)** is a membranous sac that stores _____ for muscle contractions.
- **Transverse (T) tubules** are tubes situated between the SR; they unite with the sarcolemma. T tubules form channels to enable the quick flow of _____ between the sarcoplasm and the SR.
- **Myofibrils** are cylindrical cords of protein deep to the SR that lay parallel to one another. Myofibrils have two kinds of proteins: **thick filaments** and **thin filaments.**
  1. What protein forms the thick filaments?_____
  2. What proteins form the thin filaments?_____
- The myosin filaments composing of the thick filaments have swellings known as **heads** (cross bridges) while actin, troponin, and tropomyosin form a thin filament.

Patterns of Filaments

Thick and thin filaments create a light–dark striation pattern that is identical in muscle fibers. The arrangement is discussed next.

- **A band:** A *dark* region where thick and thin filaments overlap. "A" comes from **a**nisotropic.
- **H zone:** A region within the A band where only _____ filaments are found.
- **I band:** A *light* region where only thin filaments are found. "I" comes from **i**sotropic.
- **Z lines:** A strand of proteins with a zig-zag appearance that intersects the thin filaments at regular intervals.
- **Sarcomere:** Distance between two adjacent _____. Each sarcomere contains half of two _____ bands on either side of an _____ band. The sarcomere is the primary structural and functional unit of a muscle fiber.

> **TIP!** Remember that the "I" in light bands reminds us that I bands are the light bands. Likewise, the "A" in dark bands reminds us that A bands are dark bands.

Review Time!

I.   *Using the terms in the list below, write the appropriate muscle anatomy in each blank. You may use a term more than once.*

| Myofibril | Sarcolemma | Sarcoplasm | Sarcoplasmic reticulum |
| Thick filaments | Thin filaments | Transverse (T) tubules | |

1. Type of protein filament composed of myosin   _____
2. Enables the flow of ions between the sarcoplasm and the sarcoplasmic reticulum   _____
3. Another name for the cytoplasm of a muscle fiber   _____

4. Stores calcium ions for muscle contractions _____

5. Type of protein filament composed of actin, troponin,
   and tropomyosin _____

6. Another name for the plasma membrane of the muscle fiber _____

7. Has swellings known as heads (cross bridges) _____

8. May be composed of thick or thin filaments _____

9. Connected to the sarcoplasmic reticulum and the sarcoplasm _____

10. Membranous sac similar to the endoplasmic reticulum in
    other cells _____

II. *Using the terms in the list below, write the appropriate part of the sarcomere in each blank. You may use a term more than once.*

   A band   *H zone*   *I band*   *Sarcomere*   *Z line*

1. Region where only thin filaments are found _____

2. Isotropic _____

3. Structural and functional unit of the muscle fiber _____

4. Zig-zag appearance to a strand of proteins _____

5. Light region _____

6. Segment between two adjacent Z lines _____

7. Protein strands that intersect the thin filaments at
   regular intervals _____

8. Dark region _____

9. Region within the A band where only thin filaments are found _____

10. Region where thin and thick filaments overlap _____

III. *Using the terms in the list below, label this sarcomere of skeletal muscle. You may use a term more than once.*

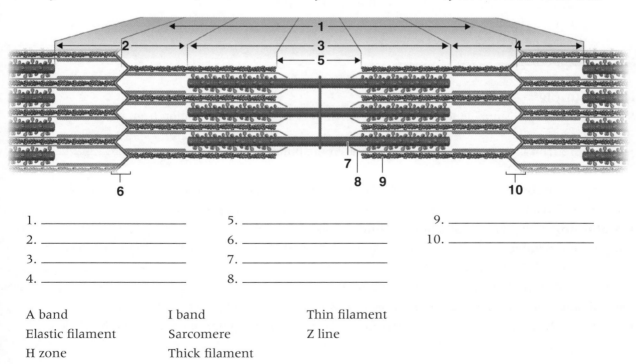

1. _____   5. _____   9. _____

2. _____   6. _____   10. _____

3. _____   7. _____

4. _____   8. _____

A band   I band   Thin filament

Elastic filament   Sarcomere   Z line

H zone   Thick filament

IV. Provide a brief answer for each of the following questions.

1. Place the following layers of fascia in order from superficial to deep: endomysium, epimysium, perimysium. _____

2. Under the microscope, you see alternating light and dark bands when viewing a section of skeletal muscle tissue. Explain what forms those light and dark bands. _____

3. Describe the function of the transverse (T) tubules. _____

4. What does the distance between two adjacent Z lines create? _____

5. Why does a muscle fiber need hundreds of mitochondria? _____

6. Complete this sentence with an appropriate directional term: The sarcolemma is _____ to the endomysium.

7. Describe the two types of filaments that form the myofibril. _____

8. Compare and contrast the function of tendons and aponeuroses. _____

9. Complete this sentence with an appropriate directional term: The sarcoplasm is _____ to the sarcolemma.

10. What is a fascicle? _____
    What type of fascia wraps fascicles? _____

Nerve Supply

Since a muscle fiber is unable to contract on its own, it must rely on stimulation from nerve impulses to contract.

- **Motor neuron** is the nerve cell that originates in the brain or _____ and travels to the muscle.
- **Synaptic knobs** (bulbs) are the branched distal ends of the motor neuron. The synaptic knobs are slightly enlarged. *Each* synaptic knob forms a junction with *one* muscle fiber.
- **Motor unit** is the functional unit consisting of a single motor neuron, its branches, and the numerous muscle fibers innervated by the neuron. An impulse carried by the single motor neuron will stimulate all the muscle cells in the motor unit to _____.
- **Motor end plate** is a highly folded region of the _____ (muscle cell's plasma membrane) that has many receptors embedded within the phospholipid bilayer.
- **Synaptic cleft** is a fluid-filled gap between the synaptic knob of a motor neuron and the _____ of a muscle fiber.

- **Neuromuscular junction** includes the synaptic knob of a motor neuron, the synaptic cleft, and the sarcolemma of a muscle fiber.
- **Synaptic vesicles** are located in the cytoplasm of the synaptic knob of a motor neuron. These vesicles contain a chemical called a **neurotransmitter**. Neurotransmitters transmit nerve signals from one neuron to a _____ or _____. The specific type of neurotransmitter housed in the vesicle is _____, or **ACh.**

Nerve Impulse Transmission

1. Nerve impulse arrives at the terminal end of a motor neuron. Acetylcholine (ACh) is stimulated to be released from synaptic vesicles.
2. Once released, ACh diffuses across the _____ and binds with receptors in the motor end plate of the muscle fiber.
3. Binding of ACh to receptors triggers muscle contraction (our next topic).

Review Time!

I. Provide a brief answer for each of the following questions.

1. Explain how the motor unit and neuromuscular junction differ._____

2. What is a neurotransmitter? What is its function?_____

3. Are the motor neuron and the motor unit the same? Explain._____

4. Where is the synaptic cleft located? Be specific._____

5. What chemical is housed within synaptic vesicles?_____
6. What is the function of ACh?_____

7. What chemical promotes the contraction of a muscle cell?_____
8. Where is the motor end plate located?_____
9. Can a skeletal muscle fiber contract on its own without stimulation? Explain.

10. To what type of cell—the nerve cell or the muscle cell—do synaptic knobs belong?

CONCEPT 2

Physiology of Muscle Contraction

Concept: Muscle contraction is achieved when the sarcomeres of muscle fibers shorten in length. This movement requires a stimulus, calcium ions, and energy in the form of ATP.

> **LEARNING OBJECTIVE** 4. Identify the parts of the neuromuscular junction.

> **LEARNING OBJECTIVE** 5. Explain the sliding filament mechanism of muscle contraction.

> **LEARNING OBJECTIVE** 6. Describe in their proper order of occurrence the events leading to muscle contraction.

In a motor unit, muscle fibers contract simultaneously to produce a smooth contraction. Upon stimulation, the contraction of a single muscle fiber is accomplished by the sliding action of the thin filaments inward toward the _____ zones, causing _____ to shorten. The shortening of myofibrils produces muscle contractions, a concept known as the **sliding filament mechanism**.

The Muscle Fiber at Rest

- Calcium ions are stored within the sarcoplasmic reticulum.
- ATP is bound to thick filaments made of the protein _____.
- Thin filaments are intact with all three proteins (actin, _____, and
  _____).

Role of the Stimulus

- ACh is released into the synaptic cleft. ACh provides the stimulus that is needed for muscle contraction to start.
- ACh binds to receptors on the motor end plate of the _____ fiber.
- An impulse is generated through the _____, down T tubule membranes, and to the sarcoplasmic reticulum.
- The SR releases calcium into the sarcoplasm. Calcium diffuses to the _____.

Muscle Contraction

- Calcium binds to troponin on the thin filaments. Troponin and actin undergo a shape change, revealing actin-binding sites on the _____ filaments.
- Once the actin-binding sites are exposed, myosin heads on the _____ filaments bind. The connection, or *coupling*, between thick and thin filaments occurs by a chemical bond.
- Coupling requires calcium ions from the SR, but does not need energy input.
- Calcium ions activate the breakdown of ATP that is bound to the _____ filaments.
- Myosin catalyzes the breakdown of ATP into ADP, a phosphate group, and energy. The energy is stored in the myosin head momentarily and then it is released. The release of the energy pivots the myosin head, producing a *power stroke*.
- The pivot of the myosin head causes the _____ filament to slide toward the center of the sarcomere. Once the pivot action is complete, another ATP molecule binds to the _____ head and is broken down to produce energy, causing the head to release from the thin filament.

- Since the binding site is now exposed, another myosin head can bind. What happens next?

  _____

  _____

- The process repeats: coupling, power stroke, detachment. The thin filaments slide toward the center of the sarcomere. Z lines move closer together and the _____ shortens. Sarcomere shortening also shortens the myofibril, leading to contraction of the muscle fiber.
- **Rigor mortis** occurs after death because no ATP is available for the release of myosin heads from the actin-binding sites. This condition of muscular rigidity is not permanent as muscle decomposition occurs.

Return to Rest

- Although ACh release stops once the nerve impulse no longer travels down the motor neuron, the stimulus does not end until all ACh is inactivated. What enzyme is responsible for the inactivation of ACh molecules? _____ (AChE)
- Calcium ions are returned to the _____ by enzymes through active transport (requires ATP).
- What happens to the actin-binding sites if calcium is no longer present?_____

  _____

- The lack of binding sites breaks attachments to myosin heads.
- Thin filaments slide back to their original position in the sarcomere.

Review Time!

I. *Place a number from 1 to 6 in the blank before each statement to indicate the correct order of the steps of muscle contraction.*

_____ Myosin heads bind to exposed actin-binding sites on the thin filaments.

_____ After the myosin head detaches from the actin-binding site, it can attach to a binding site on another thin filament closer to the sarcomere's center.

_____ The breakdown of a second ATP powers the release of the myosin head from the thin filament.

_____ Calcium binds to troponin molecules in the thin filaments causing a change in the shape of actin and troponin.

_____ The sarcomere shortens as Z lines are drawn together.

_____ The breakdown of a first ATP promotes a power stroke of a myosin head.

II. *Provide a brief answer for each of the following questions.*

1. Since the thick and thin filaments do not shorten during muscle contraction, how is muscle shortening accomplished?_____

   _____

   _____

2. Describe the events of the sliding filament mechanism of muscle contraction.

   _____

   _____

   _____

   _____

3. Explain the role of ACh in stimulating a muscle to contract. _____

   _____

4. List and discuss two events during muscle contraction and relaxation that require the use of ATP.

_____

1. _____

_____

2. _____

_____

5. How does the sarcomere shorten during muscle contraction?_____

_____

_____

6. What is the role of acetylcholinesterase in returning the muscle to rest?_____

_____

_____

7. Where is calcium stored when the muscle is not contracting?_____

8. Discuss two roles of calcium during muscle contraction. _____

1. _____

_____

2. _____

_____

9. Why does rigor mortis occur after death? Explain this condition. _____

_____

_____

10. What happens during "coupling"? Explain. _____

_____

_____

LEARNING OBJECTIVE 7. Indicate the roles of ATP in muscle contraction and how this energy is supplied.

LEARNING OBJECTIVE 8. Describe the oxygen debt and muscle fatigue.

Energy for Contraction

List three times during muscle contraction and relaxation when energy (ATP) is required.

1. _____

2. _____

3. _____

Discuss the three methods of producing ATP.

1. **Cellular respiration:** Energy is made available when ATP is broken down to yield

_____ + phosphate (PO_4^{2-}) + energy. Do you recall from Chapter 3 where

ATP is made in the cell? _____. ATP is made during cellular respiration

when sugar molecules are degraded to release energy. That energy is stored temporarily in ATP in

muscle fibers, but used up within seconds once muscle contractions begin.

2. **Creatine phosphate:** Once muscle contractions begin, ATP made by cellular respiration is used up

quickly, so another source of energy is necessary. Creatine phosphate (phosphocreatine) is a high-

energy molecule that includes a phosphate group (PO_4^{2-}) that can be transferred to ADP to form

_____. What are the advantages of creatine phosphate over ATP?

• Creatine phosphate can be stored for longer periods than ATP in muscle fibers.

• Creatine phosphate is four to six times more abundant than ATP in muscle.

3. **Other Sources:** Together, stored ATP and creatine phosphate only power muscle contractions for 15 seconds. Once ATP and creatine phosphate are depleted, free molecules of *glucose* are metabolized to make ATP, then *glycogen* is broken down into _____ and used to generate ATP. Finally, strenuous or prolonged exercise promotes the use of _____, which store the most energy.

Metabolism and Fitness

Cellular respiration is a form of catabolism that involves the breakdown of _____ molecules by mitochondria to form ATP.

- If oxygen is available during cellular respiration, the maximum number of ATP molecules can be generated (36) from each molecule of glucose. The process is called **aerobic cellular respiration.**
- If oxygen is *not* available during cellular respiration, glucose is only partially broken down through a process that yields only 2 ATP molecules and a byproduct called lactic acid. The process is less efficient than aerobic respiration and known as **anaerobic respiration** (fermentation).

Myoglobin is a protein in muscle tissue that binds to _____ and stores it until it is needed. After several minutes of strenuous exercise, myoglobin will become depleted and the respiratory and cardiovascular systems won't be able to bring in enough oxygen. Cells now enter _____ respiration and lactic acid will be produced until oxygen is restored. The individual with greater cardiovascular fitness will produce lactic acid at a rate about half that for untrained individuals during heavy exercise.

Oxygen debt is the amount of oxygen needed to _____
_____

Muscle fatigue is the inability of a muscle to contract that can be caused by unavailability of _____, and accumulation of lactic acid and a decrease in pH.

Cramps may follow muscle fatigue when a muscle contracts spasmodically without relaxing. What is typically the cause of cramping? _____
_____

Comparing Muscle Tissues

Cardiac Muscle Cells

Cardiac muscle cells have:
- A single _____
- A rectangular shape
- Branches that contact adjacent cells
- **Intercalated discs**—thickenings of the cell membrane where neighboring cells contact each other. What is the function of intercalated discs?_____
_____

- Thick and thin filaments arranged into sarcomeres that produce striations
- Large amounts of myoglobin and a large blood supply volume
- Autorhythmic contractions (no external stimulus needed to start contractions)

Cardiac muscle cells do not:
- Produce contractions as forceful as skeletal muscle
- Develop oxygen debt or muscle fatigue

Smooth Muscle Cells

Smooth muscle cells have:

- A single nucleus
- A small, spindle shape
- The greatest ability of all three muscle types to sustain _____

Smooth muscle cells do not:

- Have troponin fibers and have few actin fibers in the thin filaments
- Have sarcomeres
- Possess striations
- House many sarcoplasmic reticula
- Produce fast, forceful _____
- Develop oxygen debt or muscle fatigue

Review Time!

I.   Using the terms in the list below, write the correct method of ATP production in each blank. You may use a term more than once.

Aerobic cellular respiration   *Anaerobic cellular respiration*   *Creatine phosphate*

1. Produces the most ATP per glucose molecule   _____

2. Besides aerobic cellular respiration, ATP production
   that only lasts about 15 seconds   _____

3. Produces lactic acid   _____

4. Utilizes oxygen to generate ATP   _____

5. Upon depletion of myoglobin, this form of respiration is used   _____

6. Also known as fermentation   _____

7. Stored in the muscles   _____

8. Utilized during strenuous activity   _____

9. Yields only 2 ATP per glucose   _____

10. Form of cellular respiration in which no oxygen is used to
    make ATP   _____

II. Using the terms in the list below, write the correct type of muscle tissue in each blank. You may use a term more than once.

Cardiac muscle tissue   *Skeletal muscle tissue*   *Smooth muscle tissue*

1. Lacks striations   _____

2. Autorhythmic contractions   _____

3. Most forceful contractions of all three types   _____

4. Lacks sarcomeres   _____

5. Experiences oxygen debt and muscle fatigue   _____

6. Lacks troponin fibers   _____

7. Intercalated discs   _____

8. Spindle-shaped cells with a single nucleus   _____

9. Rectangular cells that have a single nucleus   _____

10. Cells are branched   _____

III. Provide a brief answer for each of the following questions.

1. Rank these energy sources in order of their use by the body to produce ATP: glycogen, lipids, glucose. _____
   _____
   _____

2. Identify the process that produces the most ATP from a single glucose molecule.
   _____
   _____

3. An hour into his first hike of the season, David complains of being "out of breath" and is breathing heavily. What is he experiencing? Why?_____
   _____
   _____

4. A day after starting a new exercise program, Keisha has sore muscles in her legs. Explain to her why her leg muscles are sore and why the soreness won't be as bad if she continues to exercise.
   _____
   _____
   _____

5. How long could you exercise if you relied solely on cellular respiration and creatine phosphate to provide your ATP? Explain. _____
   _____

6. List some causes of muscle fatigue._____
   _____
   _____

7. What role does myoglobin play in cellular respiration? What happens once it is depleted?
   _____
   _____
   _____
   _____

8. Why is ATP needed during muscle contraction? List three times when ATP is necessary.
   _____
   _____
   _____
   _____

9. Compare cardiac muscle cells to skeletal muscle cells. How are these tissues similar?
   _____
   _____
   _____
   _____

10. What unique features do cardiac muscle cells have that allow them to work collectively as a unit?
   _____
   _____

CONCEPT 3

Muscle Mechanics

Concept: A muscle fiber responds to a stimulus of sufficient strength by contracting. The nature of contraction of the muscle may vary according to the number of motor units responding, the frequency of stimuli received, and how tension is applied.

LEARNING OBJECTIVE 9. Define threshold stimulus, and relate it to the concept of the all-or-none response.

LEARNING OBJECTIVE 10. Compare twitch, tetanic, isotonic, and isometric contractions.

All-or-None Response

Threshold stimulus is the weakest stimulus that can initiate a muscle to contract to its complete capacity. How does the muscle respond if the stimulus is less than threshold?_____

_____

All-or-none response means the muscle will either contract all the way, or not at all.

Each motor neuron stimulates motor units with their own unique threshold stimulus. Contractions increase in force as the intensity of stimulation increases and more motor units are activated (called **recruitment**). The greater the number of motor units stimulated, the greater the strength of contraction.

Measuring Muscle Contraction

Twitch contraction is a rapid response to a single stimulus that is slightly over threshold and experienced by a single muscle fiber. The measurement of a twitch is known as a **myogram.**

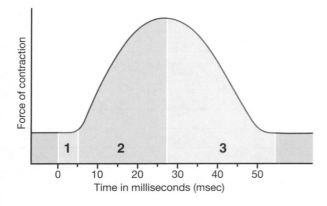

1. _____

2. _____

3. _____

As you consider the events of the twitch, label the myogram above with the following three periods.

• **Latent period:** Contraction is delayed after the stimulus. This is the time required for

_____ ions to be released, the activation of myosin, and cross bridge attachment to occur.

• **Period of contraction:** Tension increases in the muscle fiber as the sarcomere

_____.

- **Period of relaxation:** Muscle fiber returns to its original length. Calcium ions return to the SR and myosin heads detach from thin filaments.

Sustained Muscle Contraction

If a muscle fiber receives a series of stimuli, the muscle will respond as shown in the myogram below.

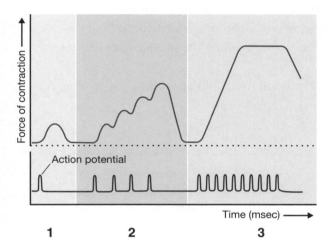

1. _____
2. _____
3. _____

As you study the myogram above, label the single twitch, summation, and complete tetanus.

- **Summation:** The time between stimuli is shortened to prevent the muscle fiber from _____. The twitches combine by summation. How is the force of contraction affected? _____
- **Tetanic contraction:** The time between stimuli is shortened further; this type of contraction will reach maximal force. **Complete tetanus** represents a fusion of twitches from many stimuli. The contraction is forceful and sustained. Your body movements, such as walking and moving your arms, are accomplished by muscles that reach complete tetanus. Complete tetanus also maintains **muscle tone**. What is muscle tone? _____ _____

Muscle tone keeps a muscle in a ready state so it can respond when a stimulus arrives. It helps with posture, for instance.

Isotonic and Isometric Contractions

Tension is the _____ exerted by muscle contraction. Isotonic and isometric contractions are two types of tetanic contractions.

- **Isotonic contractions** produce movement as a muscle pulls bone(s). Exercise through isotonic contractions increases _____ and _____.
- **Isometric contractions** produce muscle tension, but no shortening of the muscle, and no movement of the muscle. If you push against an immovable object, such as a wall, your muscles contract isometrically. Isometric contractions strengthen _____ and burn energy.

Review Time!

I. *Place a number from 1 to 5 in the blank before each statement to indicate the correct order of the periods of muscle contraction.*

_____ During the latent period, calcium ions must be released from the SR.

_____ The muscle fiber returns to its original length during the period of relaxation.

_____ The binding of myosin heads to thin filaments promotes cross bridge formation.

_____ The period of contraction occurs as the sarcomere shortens when the muscle fiber increases tension.

_____ Once the calcium ions are released from the SR, myosin heads can attach to actin-binding sites on thin filaments.

II. *Provide a brief answer for each of the following questions.*

1. Describe the all-or-none response. _____
   _____
   _____

2. A muscle fiber receives a subthreshold stimulus. How does the muscle respond? Explain.
   _____
   _____
   _____

3. Discuss the location of calcium ions during the latent period and during the period of relaxation.
   _____
   _____
   _____

4. April needs to move a 40 pound box. Explain how muscle recruitment will benefit her task.
   _____
   _____
   _____

5. What is the significance of muscle tone? Explain. _____
   _____
   _____

6. Why do you think we lose muscle tone after death? _____
   _____
   _____

7. Differentiate between summation of twitches and complete tetanus.
   _____
   _____
   _____

8. In gym class, Ken has run in place, completed a set of jumping jacks, and carried a weight in each hand from the storage room to the gymnasium. Which of these activities can be classified as isometric exercises? Explain your choice. _____
   _____
   _____

9. Do isometric or isotonic contractions bulk a muscle and increase its mass? Explain your choice.

_____

_____

_____

10. Chris wants to increase his endurance so that he can run a 10-kilometer race. Which type of exercise do you recommend to help him achieve his goal: isotonic or isometric exercises? _____. Discuss your choice. _____

_____

_____

CONCEPT 4

Production of Movement

Concept: Movement occurs when a muscle contracts, pulling a movable bone toward a more stationary bone. For most movements, many muscles are involved and each plays one of several possible roles.

LEARNING OBJECTIVE 11. Define origin and insertion, and describe the role of group actions in producing movement.

We will now explore the nature of muscle movement, including how the muscle is attached, the structure of the joint, and interactions of nearby muscles.

Origin and Insertion

Muscles produce movement by pulling on their attachments (tendons attached to bones). Most muscles cross a joint between two opposing bones. One end of the muscle is relatively _immovable_ while the other end of the muscle is _movable_. During contraction, the insertion is pulled toward the origin. In the muscles of the limbs, the origins are proximal and the insertions are _____.

- **Origin:** Point of attachment to the _more stationary_ bone
- **Insertion:** Point of attachment to the _more movable_ bone

Group Actions

Group action is the coordinated response of a group of muscles to bring about a body movement. Muscles within the group have specific roles:

- **Agonists** are prime movers because they cause the desired action by contracting.
- **Antagonists** _____ during the action.
- **Synergists** assist the _____ in performing the action.
- **Fixators** _____ the origin of the prime mover.

CONCEPT 5

Major Muscles of the Body

Concept: The muscles provide for movement of all movable bones of the body. Their names correspond to their appearance, location, action, or relationship to other structures.

LEARNING OBJECTIVE 12. Identify the primary muscles on the basis of their locations, origins, insertions, and actions.

For the remainder of this chapter, we cover the origin, insertion, and primary action of primary muscles.

Muscles of the Head and Neck, Muscles of Mastication, and Muscles Moving the Head

Complete the table below by supplying the primary action for each muscle listed.

Muscles of Facial Expression, Mastication, and Head Movement

Muscle	Origin	Insertion	Action
Frontalis	Occipital bone	Skin around the eye	
Occipitalis	Occipital bone	Skin around the eye	
Orbicularis oculi	Maxillary and frontal bones around the orbit	The eyelid	
Orbicularis oris	Muscles surrounding the mouth	Skin at the corner of the mouth	
Buccinator	Maxilla and mandible	Orbicularis oris	
Zygomaticus	Zygomatic bone	Skin and muscle at the corner of the mouth	
Masseter	Zygomatic process of the temporal bone and zygomatic arch	Mandible	
Temporalis	Temporal bone	Mandible	
Sternocleidomastoid	Manubrium of the sternum and the clavicle	Mastoid process of the temporal bone	

As we discuss the muscles of the head and neck, add labels to the illustration below. When you are done, you should be able to identify the muscles of the head and neck listed below.

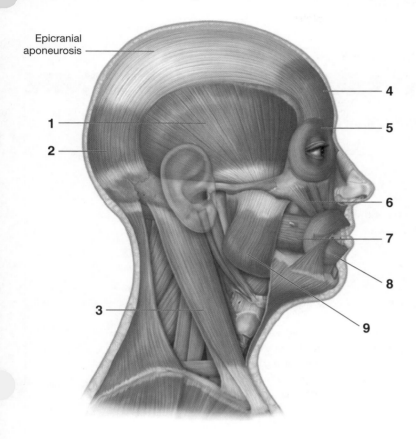

Epicranial
aponeurosis

1
2
3
4
5
6
7
8
9

1. _____

2. _____

3. _____

4. _____

5. _____

6. _____

7. _____

8. _____

9. _____

Buccinator	Occipitalis	Sternocleidomastoid
Frontalis	Orbicularis oculi	Temporalis
Masseter	Orbicularis oris	Zygomaticus

Muscles Moving the Pectoral Girdle and Trunk

Anterior Muscles of the Pectoral Girdle and Trunk

Complete the table below by supplying the primary action for each muscle listed.

Anterior Muscles of the Pectoral Girdle and Trunk

Muscle	Origin	Insertion	Action
Pectoralis major	Clavicle, sternum, and costal cartilages of the first 6 ribs	Greater tubercle of the humerus	
Pectoralis minor	Ribs 3–5	Coracoid process of the scapula	
Deltoid	Acromion and spine of the scapula, and the clavicle	Deltoid tuberosity of the humerus	
Serratus anterior	The first 8 ribs	Scapula	
Subscapularis	Anterior surface of the scapula	Lesser tubercle of the humerus	
Rectus abdominis	Pubic bone and symphysis pubis	Xiphoid process of the sternum and the costal cartilages of fifth to seventh rib	
External oblique	Lower 8 ribs	Iliac crest and the linea alba	
Internal oblique	A large aponeurosis of the lower back, the iliac crest, and the costal cartilages of the lower ribs	Linea alba and the pubic bone	
Transverse abdominis	A large aponeurosis of the lower back, the iliac crest, and the costal cartilages of the lower ribs	Linea alba and the pubic bone	
External intercostals	Ribs	Rib inferior to the rib of origin	
Internal intercostals	Ribs	Rib superior to the rib of origin	

As we discuss the muscles of the pectoral girdle and anterior trunk, add labels to the illustration below. When you are done, you should be able to identify the muscles of the pectoral girdle and anterior trunk listed below.

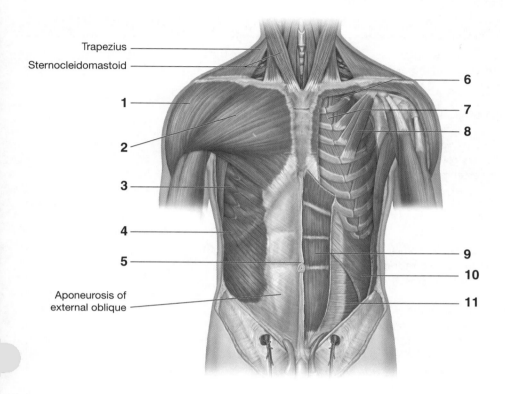

1. _____   5. _____   9. _____

2. _____   6. _____   10. _____

3. _____   7. _____   11. _____

4. _____   8. _____

Deltoid   Internal oblique   Rectus abdominis

External intercostals   Linea alba   Serratus anterior

External oblique   Pectoralis major   Transverse abdominis

Internal intercostals   Pectoralis minor

Posterior Muscles of the Pectoral Girdle and Trunk
Complete the table below by supplying the primary action for each muscle listed.

Posterior Muscles of the Pectoral Girdle and Trunk

Muscle	Origin	Insertion	Action
Trapezius	Occipital bone and spines of the cervical and thoracic vertebrae	Acromion and spine of the scapula	
Levator scapulae	First four cervical vertebrae	Scapula	
Rhomboids	Seventh cervical and first five thoracic vertebrae	Scapula	
Latissimus dorsi	Spines of lower six thoracic vertebrae, lumbar vertebrae, lower ribs, and iliac crest	Intertubercular groove of the humerus	
Supraspinatus	Posterior surface of the scapula superior to the spine	Greater tubercle of the humerus	
Infraspinatus	Posterior surface of the scapula inferior to the spine	Greater tubercle of the humerus	
Teres major	Scapula	Lesser tubercle of the humerus	
Teres minor	Scapula	Greater tubercle of the humerus	
Erector spinae	Vertebrae, pelvis	Superior vertebrae and ribs	

As we discuss the muscles of the pectoral girdle and posterior trunk, add labels to the illustration below. When you are done, you should be able to identify the muscles of the pectoral girdle and posterior trunk listed below. You may use one term more than once.

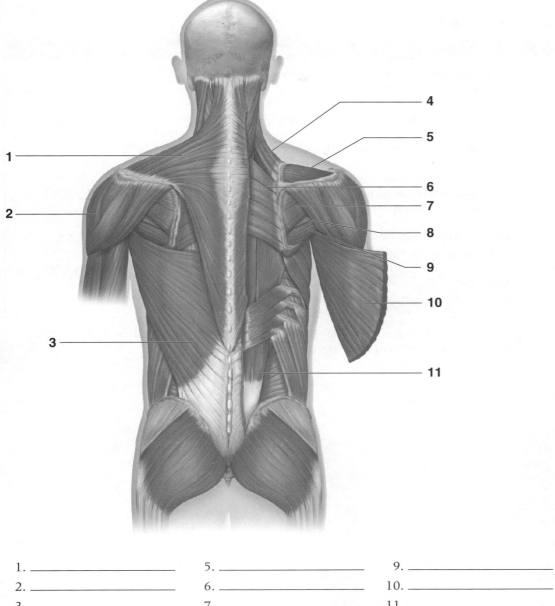

1. _____   5. _____   9. _____

2. _____   6. _____   10. _____

3. _____   7. _____   11. _____

4. _____   8. _____

Deltoid   Levator scapulae   Teres major

Erector spinae   Rhomboids   Teres minor

Infraspinatus   Supraspinatus   Trapezius

Latissimus dorsi

Muscles of the Upper Limb

Muscles that Move the Forearm

Complete the table below by supplying the primary action for each muscle listed.

Muscles that Move the Forearm

Muscle	Origin	Insertion	Action
Biceps brachii	Two heads of origin on the scapula	Radial tuberosity of the radius	
Brachialis	Shaft of the humerus	Coronoid process of the ulna	
Brachioradialis	Distal end of the humerus	Base of the styloid process of the radius	
Triceps brachii	Three heads of origin on the scapula and humerus	Olecranon process of the ulna	
Supinator	Distal end of the humerus and proximal end of the ulna	Proximal end of the radius	
Pronator teres	Distal end of the humerus and coronoid process of the ulna	Shaft of the radius	

As we discuss the muscles of the anterior arm, add labels to the illustration below. When you are done, you should be able to identify the muscles of the anterior arm listed below.

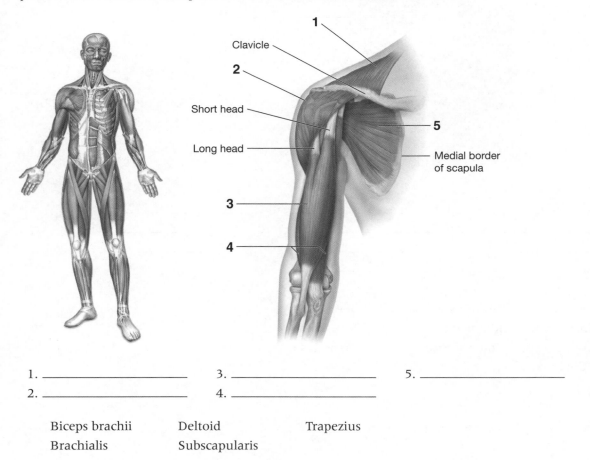

1. _____   3. _____   5. _____

2. _____   4. _____

    Biceps brachii   Deltoid   Trapezius

    Brachialis   Subscapularis

As we discuss the muscles of the posterior arm, add labels to the illustration below. When you are done, you should be able to identify the muscles of the posterior arm listed below.

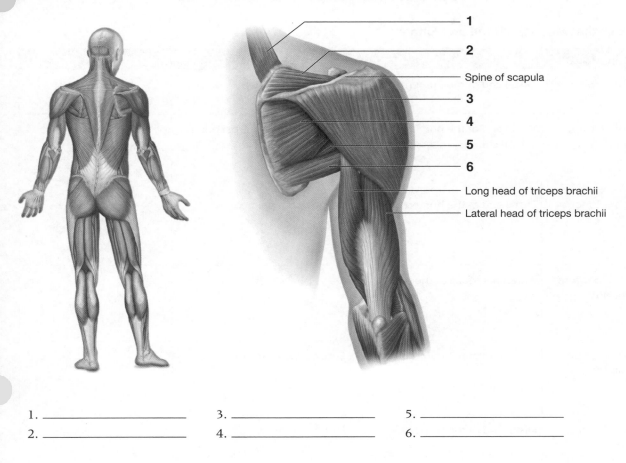

1 ———
2 ———
Spine of scapula
3 ———
4 ———
5 ———
6 ———
Long head of triceps brachii
Lateral head of triceps brachii

1. _____   3. _____   5. _____
2. _____   4. _____   6. _____

Deltoid   Levator scapulae   Teres major
Infraspinatus   Supraspinatus   Teres minor

Muscles that Move the Hand and Fingers

Complete the table below by supplying the primary action for each muscle listed.

Muscles that Move the Hand and Fingers

Muscle	Origin	Insertion	Action
Flexor carpi radialis	Distal end of the humerus	Second and third metacarpals	
Flexor carpi ulnaris	Distal end of the humerus and the olecranon process of the ulna	Carpal and metacarpal bones	
Palmaris longus	Distal end of the humerus	Fascia of the palm	
Flexor digitorum profundus	Anterior surface of the ulna	Distal phalanges of digits 2–5	
Extensor carpi radialis longus	Distal end of the humerus	Second metacarpal	
Extensor carpi ulnaris	Distal end of the humerus	Fifth metacarpal	
Extensor digitorum	Distal end of the humerus	Middle and distal phalanges in digits 2–5	

As we discuss the muscles of the anterior forearm, add labels to the illustration below. When you are done, you should be able to identify the muscles of the anterior forearm listed below.

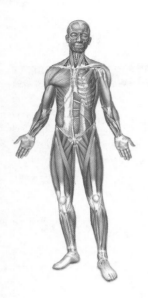 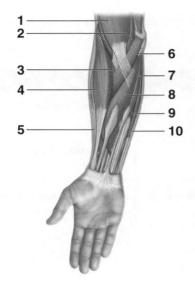 

1. _____
2. _____
3. _____
4. _____
5. _____
6. _____
7. _____
8. _____
9. _____
10. _____

Biceps brachii
Brachialis
Brachioradialis
Extensor carpi radialis longus

Flexor carpi radialis
Flexor carpi ulnaris
Flexor digitorum profundus
Palmaris longus

Pronator teres
Supinator

As we discuss the muscles of the posterior forearm, add labels to the illustration below. When you are done, you should be able to identify the muscles of the posterior forearm listed below.

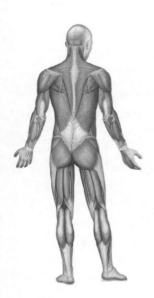 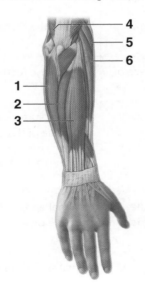

1. _____
2. _____
3. _____
4. _____
5. _____
6. _____

Brachioradialis
Extensor carpi radialis longus

Extensor carpi ulnaris
Extensor digitorum

Flexor carpi ulnaris
Triceps brachii

Muscles of the Lower Limbs

Muscles that Move the Leg

Complete the table below by supplying the primary action for each muscle listed.

Muscles that Move the Thigh and Leg

Muscle	Origin	Insertion	Action
Iliopsoas	Iliac fossa and lumbar vertebrae	Lesser trochanter of the femur	
Tensor fascia latae	Iliac crest of the ilium	Tibia by way of fascia of the thigh	
Adductor longus	Pubic bone and symphysis pubis	Posterior surface of the femur	
Adductor magnus	Ischial tuberosity	Posterior surface of the femur	
Gracilis	Pubic bone	Medial surface of the tibia	
Quadriceps femoris group:			
Rectus femoris	Ilium and margin of the acetabulum	Patella and tibial tuberosity by way of the quadriceps tendon	
Vastus lateralis	Greater trochanter and posterior surface of the femur	Same as the rectus femoris	
Vastus medialis	Medial surface of the femur	Same as the rectus femoris	
Vastus intermedius	Anterior and lateral surface of the femur	Same as the rectus femoris	
Gluteus maximus	Ilium, sacrum, and coccyx	Posterior surface of the femur and fascia of the thigh	
Gluteus medius	Ilium	Greater trochanter of the femur	
Biceps femoris	Two heads of origin: At the ischium and along the linea aspera of the femur	Proximal ends of the fibula and tibia by way of a common tendon	
Semitendinosus	Ischium	Medial surface of the tibia	
Semimembranosus	Ischium	Proximal end of the tibia	

As we discuss the muscles of the anterior thigh, add labels to the illustration below. When you are done, you should be able to identify the muscles of the anterior thigh listed below.

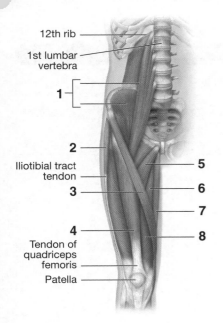

1. _____
2. _____
3. _____
4. _____
5. _____
6. _____
7. _____
8. _____

Adductor longus   Iliopsoas   Vastus lateralis

Adductor magnus   Rectus femoris   Vastus medialis

Gracilis   Tensor fasciae latae

As we discuss the muscles of the posterior thigh, add labels to the illustration below. When you are done, you should be able to identify the muscles of the posterior thigh listed below.

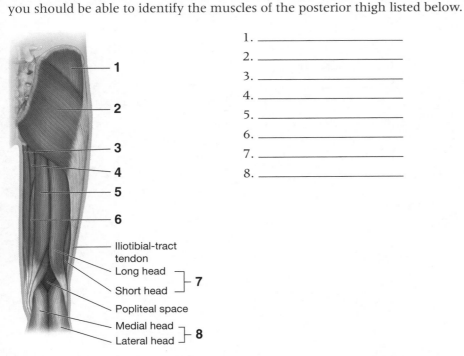

1. _____
2. _____
3. _____
4. _____
5. _____
6. _____
7. _____
8. _____

Adductor magnus   Gluteus maximus   Semimembranosus

Biceps femoris   Gluteus medius   Semitendinosus

Gastrocnemius   Gracilis

Muscles that Move the Foot and Toes

Complete the table below by supplying the primary action for each muscle listed.

Muscles that Move the Foot and Toes

Muscle	Origin	Insertion	Action
Tibialis anterior	Proximal two-thirds of the tibia	Tarsal bone (cuneiform) and the first metatarsal	
Extensor digitorum longus	Proximal end of the tibia, anterior surface of the fibula	Second and third phalanges of digits 2–5	
Gastrocnemius	Two heads, both at the distal end of the femur	Calcaneus by way of the calcaneal tendon	
Soleus	Proximal ends of the tibia and fibula	Calcaneus by way of the calcaneal tendon	
Peroneus longus	Proximal ends of the tibia and fibula	Tarsal and metatarsal bones	
Peroneus tertius	Distal surface of the fibula	Fifth metatarsal	

As we discuss the muscles of the anterior leg and foot, add labels to the illustration below. When you are done, you should be able to identify the muscles of the anterior leg and foot listed below.

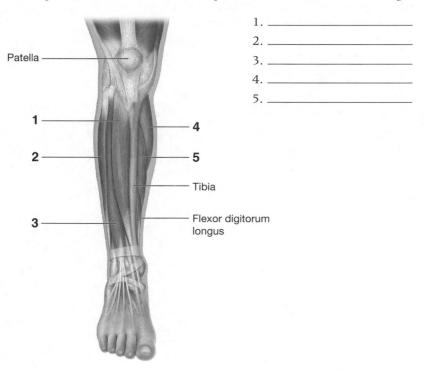

1. _____
2. _____
3. _____
4. _____
5. _____

Extensor digitorum longus   Peroneus longus   Tibialis anterior
Gastrocnemius   Soleus

As we discuss the muscles of the lateral and posterior leg and foot, add labels to the illustration below. When you are done, you should be able to identify the muscles of the laterial and posterior leg and foot listed below.

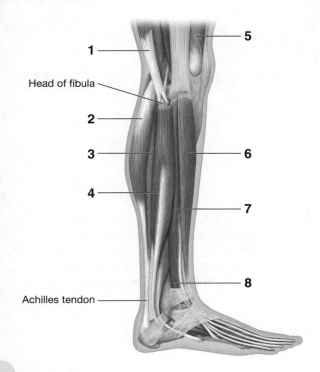

1. _____

2. _____

3. _____

4. _____

5. _____

6. _____

7. _____

8. _____

Biceps femoris

Extensor digitorum longus

Gastrocnemius

Peroneus longus

Peroneus tertius

Soleus

Tibialis anterior

Vastus lateralis

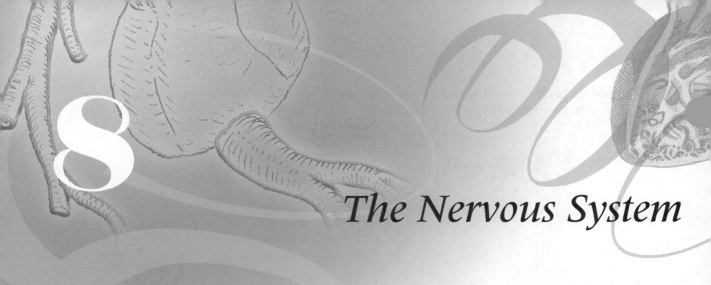

8 The Nervous System

Tips for Success as You Begin

Read Chapter 8 from your textbook before attending class. Listen when you attend lecture and fill in the blanks in this notebook. You may choose to complete the blanks before attending class as a way to prepare for the day's topics. The same day you attend lecture, read the material again and complete the exercises after each section in this notebook. Spend time every day with this chapter as it will help you make sense of the material. The nervous system is complex; you'll want to read and re-read the material in this chapter to gain a thorough understanding.

Introduction to the Nervous System

The nervous system has several functions. Provide a brief description of each.

1. Sensory function: _____
   _____

2. Integrative function: _____

3. Motor function: _____
   _____

The major organs of the nervous system are the brain, spinal cord, nerves, and sensory organs.

The primary responsibility of the nervous system is _____.

CONCEPT 1

Organization of the Nervous System

Concept: The nervous system consists of the central nervous system, which includes the brain and spinal cord, and the peripheral nervous system, containing the nerves, receptors, and ganglia.

LEARNING OBJECTIVE   1. Describe the divisions of the nervous system.

The two major categories of the nervous system are:

1. **Central nervous system (CNS)**
   • The major organs of the CNS are _____
   • The CNS receives all sensory nerve impulses and initiates all motor nerve impulses.

2. **Peripheral nervous system (PNS)**
   - The major organs of the PNS are _____
   - The PNS nerves communicate with the brain and the spinal cord.
   - The two subdivisions of the PNS are:
     a. _____ (SNS) is voluntary (under conscious brain control).
     b. _____ (ANS) is involuntary (under unconscious or automatic control).

CONCEPT 2

Nervous Tissue

Concept: The two types of cells in nervous tissue are neuroglia, which are supportive, and neurons, which conduct nerve impulses.

LEARNING OBJECTIVE 2. Distinguish both structurally and functionally between neurons and neuroglia.
3. Describe the structure of a neuron, and distinguish between myelinated and unmyelinated fibers.

Two types of cells in nervous tissue are:
1. **Neuroglia:** Support nervous tissue
2. **Neurons:** Conduct nerve impulses

Neuroglia

Neuroglia (or glial cells) form the majority (90%) of the brain and spinal cord and a small part of peripheral nerves. Although there are five types of neuroglia, we will only discuss the oligodendrocytes and Schwann cells in detail. Other types of neuroglia remove materials by phagocytosis or aid in the circulation of cerebrospinal fluid (CSF).

- *Oligodendrocytes* are neuroglia in the _____ that produce a fatty sheath around part of the neuron known as the _____. A disease known as *multiple sclerosis* (MS) is caused by the gradual deterioration of the oligodendrocytes. How are MS patients affected?

  _____

- *Schwann cells* are neuroglia that produce a fatty sheath around cells outside the brain known as the _____ sheath.

Neurons

Neurons are considered the primary functional unit of nervous tissue. The functions of neurons are to:
- Sense changes in the _____
- Integrate information
- Carry out a _____ response

Neuron Structure

As we discuss the three parts of a neuron (cell body, dendrites, and axon), add labels to the illustration below. When you are done, you should be able to identify the parts of a neuron listed below.

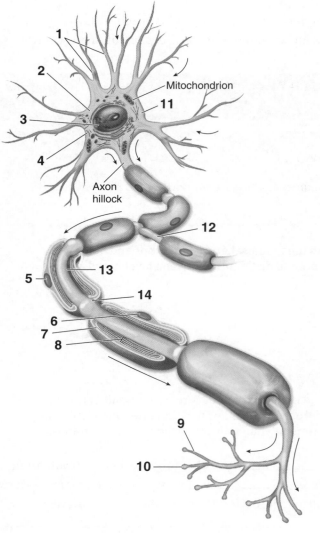

1. _____
2. _____
3. _____
4. _____
5. _____
6. _____
7. _____
8. _____
9. _____
10. _____
11. _____
12. _____
13. _____
14. _____

Axon   Dendrites   Nucleus of Schwann cell
Axon collateral   Neurofibril   Schwann cell—cytoplasm,
Axon terminal   Node of Ranvier   neurilemma, and myelin sheath
Cell body   Nucleus   Synaptic end bulb
Cytoplasm

Cell Body

The **cell body** consists of cytoplasm enclosed by a cell membrane, with a nucleus (and nucleolus) and organelles.

- What is missing from a mature neuron? _____
- What is a mature neuron not capable of performing? _____

Nissl bodies, which are a form of a rough endoplasmic reticulum, are unique to neurons. Ribosomes, present on Nissl bodies, indicate that _____ synthesis is taking place.

Neurofibrils, similar to microtubules, are also characteristic of neurons. An abnormal accumulation of neurofibrils occurs in *Alzheimer disease,* in which progressive mental confusion and short-term memory loss occurs.

Dendrites

Dendrites are thin, branching extensions originating from the cell body. Each dendrite is enveloped by the cell membrane. In most neurons, dendrites are short in length, highly branched, and quite numerous. Dendrites have receptors for receiving impulses from adjacent neurons. Do dendrites send nerve impulses *toward* or *away from* the cell body? _____

Axon

The **axon** is a part of the neuron that conducts impulses *away from* the cell body.

> **TIP!** Remember "a" for axon and "a" for away from the cell body.

Another name sometimes given to the axon is _____ **fiber**. An axon is surrounded by the cell membrane and reinforced by neurofibrils. How many axons are present in every neuron? _____. Side branches of an axon are called **collaterals**. The many small branches at the terminal end of an axon are called **synaptic end bulbs**. Some axons are as long as 1 meter and are partially enclosed with sheaths composed of **Schwann cells**. *Myelination* results when _____. Wrappings of Schwann cells form **myelin sheaths** and are rich in lipids. What is the function of the myelin sheath? _____, _____, and _____, for the axon. The cytoplasm and nuclei of the Schwann cells stay on the outer layer of the myelin sheath, forming the _____. Gaps between the Schwann cells where the myelin sheath is absent are known as **nodes of Ranvier**.

> **TIP!** Think of the myelin sheath as a roll of toilet paper—the tube in the center is like the axon while the toilet paper wrapped around the tube is like the Schwann cells that form the myelin sheath.

White Matter and Gray Matter

Unmyelinated fibers may be enclosed by _____ cells but lack the thick, multiple-layered myelin sheath. Groups of unmyelinated fibers, neuron cell bodies, and dendrites appear as _____ matter. Myelinated fibers have a thick myelin sheath (produced either by Schwann cells or oligodendrocytes) and appear white due to its presence. They are called _____ matter.

> **TIP!** Think of the neuron's structure like a tree. The tree branches are the dendrites while the trunk is the axon. The roots are the axon terminals.

Review Time!

I. *Using the terms in the list below, write the appropriate part of the neuron in each blank. You may use a term more than once.*

Axon   Cell body   Dendrite

1. Conducts nerve impulses toward the cell body   _____
2. Houses organelles and the nucleus   _____
3. May be myelinated by Schwann cells   _____
4. Numerous branches extending from the cell body   _____
5. One extension traveling from cell body   _____
6. Conducts nerve impulses away from the cell body   _____
7. Branches are known as collaterals   _____
8. Houses Nissl bodies   _____
9. May be wrapped by oligodendrocytes in the brain   _____
10. Terminal ends are called synaptic end bulbs   _____

II. *Provide a brief answer for each of the following questions about the nervous system organization and nervous tissue.*

1. List the two divisions of the nervous system and their functions.
    1. _____
    2. _____
2. List and describe the three functions of the nervous system.
    1. _____
    2. _____
    3. _____
3. What are the two types of cells in nervous tissue? How are they functionally different?
    1. _____
    2. _____
4. List the pathway of the nerve impulse along the neuron. _____
    _____
5. Name the two subdivisions of the PNS. _____
    1. _____
    2. _____
6. Describe the structure of the myelin sheath. _____
    _____
7. Differentiate between white matter and gray matter. _____
    _____
    _____
8. Compare and contrast the functions of oligodendrocytes and Schwann cells. _____
    _____
9. How are neurons functionally different from neuroglia? _____
    _____
10. Are mature neurons capable of mitosis? Explain. _____
    _____
    _____

Classifying Neurons

The following neurons are classified on the basis of *structural* differences. There are three major types of neurons.

1. **Multipolar neurons** have _____ dendrites arising from the cell body, and _____ axon. The neurons that carry impulses from the CNS to skeletal muscles are multipolar neurons.

2. **Bipolar neurons** have _____ dendrite and _____ axon arising from the cell body. Bipolar neurons are found _____.
   _____

3. **Unipolar neurons** contain a single nerve fiber extending from the cell body. The fiber splits into two branches: One branch extends to the spinal cord or brain and serves as the _____, the other branch extends to the peripheral part of the body and serves as the _____.
   • **An example of a unipolar neuron is** _____
   _____

The following neurons are classified on the basis of *functional* differences. There are also three major types of neurons.

1. **Sensory neurons** (afferent neurons), often unipolar in structure, carry nerve impulses from a peripheral part of the body _____ the CNS.

2. **Association neurons** (interneurons), often multipolar in structure, are located within the CNS and form links between _____. They relay impulses from one region of the brain or spinal cord to another.

3. **Motor neurons** (efferent neurons), often multipolar in structure, carry nerve impulses _____ the CNS to **effectors** that respond to stimuli such as muscles or glands.

Review Time!

I. *Using the terms in the list below, write the appropriate type of structural neuron in each blank. You may use a term more than once.*

Bipolar neuron   *Multipolar neuron*   *Unipolar neuron*

1. Often function as motor neurons   _____
2. A single dendrite and a single axon arise from the cell body   _____
3. Carry impulses from skin receptors to the spinal cord   _____
4. Often function as sensory neurons   _____
5. Many dendrites arise from the cell body   _____
6. Single nerve fiber extends from the cell body   _____
7. Found in special sensory areas such as the eye, ear, and nose   _____
8. Carry nerve impulses from the CNS to skeletal muscles   _____
9. Carry nerve impulses to the CNS from peripheral parts of the body   _____
10. Often function as association neurons (interneurons)   _____

II.   *Using the terms in the list below, write the appropriate type of functional neuron in each blank. You may use a term more than once.*

Sensory neuron   *Association neuron*   *Motor neuron*

1. Carries nerve impulses to the CNS   _____

2. Carry nerve impulses to effectors   _____

3. Located within the CNS   _____

4. Interneurons   _____

5. Form links between neurons   _____

6. Carry nerve impulses from the CNS to muscles
    or glands   _____

7. Efferent neurons   _____

8. Often unipolar in structure   _____

9. Relay impulses from one region of the brain
    to another   _____

10. Afferent neurons   _____

III. *Provide a brief answer for each of the following questions about the different types of neurons.*

1. Contrast the function of sensory and motor neurons. _____

_____

_____

2. Which neuron, based on functional classification, is only found in the CNS?

_____

_____

3. On what bases are neurons classified?

    1. _____

    2. _____

4. What structure do association neurons and motor neurons share in common?

_____

_____

_____

5. Describe the role of association neurons in the CNS._____

_____

_____

_____

CONCEPT 3

Neuron Physiology

Concept: Neurons communicate by the production of action potentials, which are conducted along axons and transmitted to other neurons across synaptic junctions.

LEARNING OBJECTIVE 4. Describe the events involved in maintaining a resting potential and producing an action potential.

The primary function of a neuron is _____.
Resting potential, action potential, and transmission of the nerve impulse from cell to cell are covered next.

The Resting Membrane Potential

Potential difference occurs when there is a separation of _____ between
two points. The cell membrane separates an unequal distribution of ions, or charges, present in the
extracellular and intracellular environments. The difference in ions creates a *polarized* area, measured
in terms of voltage. The ions having the greatest influence on membrane potential in most cells are
_____ (Na$^+$) and _____ (K$^+$). **Resting membrane potential**
is the difference resulting from an uneven distribution of ions in a resting neuron in a *polarized* state.

- At rest, where are sodium ions?_____
- At rest, where are potassium ions?_____

The **sodium–potassium pump** uses _____ to pump _____
ions out of the cell and _____ ions into the cell.

- Why is the outside of the cell membrane positively charged? _____

  _____

- Why is the inside of the cell membrane negatively charged? _____

  _____

Since the uneven distribution of ions results in a *polarized* state, measured in terms of voltage, what is the
charge on the inside of a polarized membrane?_____ millivolts (mV).

> **TIP!** To keep straight the locations of ions, remember SOPI: **s**odium is **o**utside the neuron while
> **p**otassium is **i**nside during resting potential.

The Action Potential

The action potential is also known as a nerve impulse and includes depolarization, repolarization, and
hyperpolarization. Only neurons and muscle cells are capable of producing action potentials.

Depolarization

Excitability is the ability of neurons and muscle cells to respond to a change in the environment. When a cell
becomes excited and the permeability changes, _____ ions flow into the cell and
the cell becomes *depolarized*. **Depolarization** is the first step in an action potential. The entry of sodium
ions into the cell changes the voltage from −70 millivolts to _____ millivolts,
from a negative to a positive value. The charge outside the membrane changes from positive to negative.

Repolarization

Two problems must be solved during repolarization: (1) Restoration of the charge on the inside of the cell membrane of the neuron, and (2) restoration of ions back to resting potential locations.

1. Soon after depolarization has occurred, resting membrane potential becomes restored or
   _____. **Repolarization** involves the diffusion of _____
   ions through newly opened potassium-gated channels. *The charges are now restored.*

2. For a brief moment, there is an excess of sodium ions outside of the membrane before resting potential
   is restored. **Hyperpolarization** is a brief period when the sodium–potassium pump is restoring
   the membrane to resting potential by pumping sodium ions _____ and
   potassium ions _____.

Conduction of the Action Potential

The action potential starts at a localized region of the membrane where the stimulus caused the inside of the cell to become more positive than the outside during depolarization. The electrical gradient and current increase membrane permeability to nearby _____ ions. This current causes a reversal of ion distribution (_____ polarization), followed by _____ polarization and _____ polarization.

TIP! Think of the conduction of the action potential as the "wave" seen in a football stadium. Sometimes it takes a while for the wave to catch on. Once the threshold stimulus (Chapter 7) has been reached, the wave (action potential) has caught on and the action potential is conducted down the length of the axon. As you fling your arms in the air to pass along the wave, you are demonstrating action potential. Once seated, you have returned to resting potential and are ready to conduct the wave (action potential) again.

Saltatory Conduction

In myelinated fibers, nerve impulse conduction is faster than in unmyelinated fibers. Nerve impulses jump across the myelin sheath from one node of _____ to the next node in a process known as **saltatory conduction.** How does saltatory conduction benefit homeostasis? _____

Transmission of Impulses from Cell to Cell

LEARNING OBJECTIVE   5. Describe the structure of a synapse and explain how an impulse is transmitted from cell to cell.

A **synapse** is the junction between adjacent neurons. The impulse crosses this junction to pass from the **presynaptic neuron** to the **postsynaptic neuron.** The axon of the presynaptic neuron branches and terminates at a synaptic end bulb that contains **synaptic vesicles.** Synaptic vesicles contain _____ that carry the impulse across the synapse to contact the postsynaptic membrane. The postsynaptic membrane has an indented (concave) surface that forms a fluid-filled gap called the _____ **cleft.**

The process of nerve impulse transmission across a synapse follows these steps.

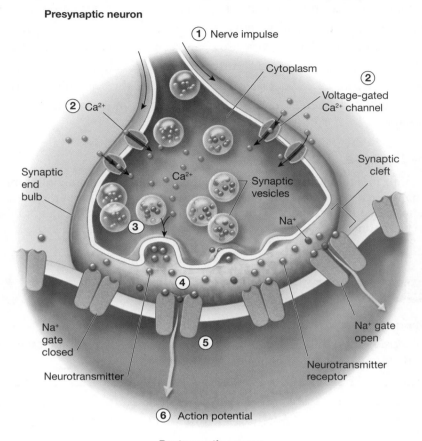

1. An action potential arrives at the synaptic end bulb of a presynaptic neuron.

2. _____
   _____

3. _____
   _____

4. _____
   _____

5. _____
   _____

6. Sodium ions flow into the postsynaptic membrane, promoting depolarization and action potential.

Excitatory and Inhibitory Transmission

Neurotransmitters can either increase membrane permeability to sodium ions, causing an action potential, or increase the membrane permeability to potassium ions, causing hyperpolarization.

1. **Excitatory transmission** increases postsynaptic membrane permeability to sodium ions.
   Neurotransmitters, such as _____ and _____, are required to cause the action potential.
   Facilitation is the accumulative effect of stimuli to produce an action potential.

2. **Inhibitory transmission** increases postsynaptic membrane permeability to potassium ions, decreasing the chance of an action potential being transferred across a synapse. The neurotransmitter contacts a receptor in the postsynaptic membrane and triggers _____-gated channels to open. Chloride ion channels are also opened and chloride ions enter the cell. What ions are not affected? _____

Positive ions collect _____ the cell while negative ions provide a negative charge along the _____ of the cell membrane, resulting in a hyperpolarized state.

Processing at the Synapse

Because the postsynaptic membrane may receive thousands of presynaptic end bulbs originating from thousands of presynaptic neurons, it is the overall effect of excitatory and inhibitory neurotransmitters on the postsynaptic membrane that determines whether an action potential will result or not. Homeostasis requires impulses to be channeled to specific areas of the body. *Plasticity* is _____

_____.

Review Time!

I.   *Provide a brief answer for each of the following questions about the action potential.*

1. How is a *polarized* neuron different from a *depolarized* neuron? Explain the establishment of a charge and the locations of ions involved in the creation of each state. _____

_____

_____

2. Explain how *hyperpolarization* helps return a neuron to its resting state. _____

_____

_____

3. What is the role of the sodium–potassium pump in maintaining resting potential?

_____

_____

_____

4. Discuss the role of potassium in depolarizing a cell and promoting an action potential.

_____

_____

_____

5. Contrast *excitation* of a neuron with *hyperpolarization*. _____

_____

_____

6. Discuss the role of chlorine and potassium ions in inhibitory transmission.

_____

_____

_____

7. Explain how myelination helps to speed a nerve impulse (action potential).

_____

_____

_____

8. Explain how a nerve impulse travels from a presynaptic neuron to a postsynaptic neuron.

_____

_____

_____

9. Discuss how calcium plays a critical role in transmission of a nerve impulse from one cell to another. _____

_____

10. Describe the difference between an excitatory transmission and an inhibitory transmission.

_____

_____

_____

11. If facilitation does not occur, do you think an action potential can be produced? Discuss.

_____

_____

12. A neuron receives a few inhibitory transmissions but many excitatory transmissions. Predict how you think the neuron will respond. _____

_____

_____

13. Explain how the lack of calcium can prevent the release of a neurotransmitter at the synapse.

_____

_____

14. Discuss how a cell maintains resting potential with a −70 millivolt charge on the inside of the cell membrane. _____

_____

_____

15. Discuss the role of sodium ions in conduction of an action potential. _____

_____

_____

CONCEPT 4

The Central Nervous System

Concept: The spinal cord and brain are the primary organs of the central nervous system (CNS). They are both protected by bone and membranes. The spinal cord carries nerve impulses to and from the brain, while the brain is the integrative center of the nervous system.

LEARNING OBJECTIVE   6. Identify the protective covering of the spinal cord and brain.

The organs of the CNS include the _____ and spinal cord.

The Spinal Cord

- **Overall structure:** The spinal cord is 42 centimeters (17 inches) from its exit from the brain through the foramen magnum to its end between lumbar segments L1 and L2. The spinal cord travels inferiorly within the vertebral canal.
- **Function:** The spinal cord serves as a two-way connection between the _____ and peripheral nerves.

Protective Coverings

The three protective coverings on the spinal cord are:

  1. _____

  2. _____

  3. _____ (membranes): All three meninges cover the brain and extend as a unit beyond the inferior end of the spinal cord.

    - **Dura mater** is a thick, tough outer sheath that is not attached to the vertebral column but instead borders a fat-filled space called the _____.
    - **Arachnoid** is the middle membrane with _____ fibers forming a cobweb network. The **subarachnoid space** is between the arachnoid and pia mater and filled with circulating **CSF.** CSF circulates around and through the spinal cord and brain. What is the function of CSF?_____
    _____
    _____

    - **Pia mater** is the delicate, thin, inner membrane attached to the _____ surface of the spinal cord surface.

Review Time!

I.   *Using the terms in the list below, write the appropriate spinal cord protection in each blank. You may use a term more than once.*

Arachnoid   *Cerebrospinal fluid*   *Dura mater*

Pia mater   *Vertebral column*

1. Bony protection for the spinal cord   _____

2. Layer through which CSF circulates   _____

3. Tough membrane layer   _____

4. Membrane layer that fills the epidural space   _____

5. Thin, delicate membrane layer   _____

6. Layer situated between dura mater and pia mater   _____

7. Deepest of the three membrane coverings   _____

8. Liquid cushion for the spinal cord   _____

9. Most superficial of the three membrane coverings   _____

10. Layer that has a cobweb appearance   _____

Spinal Cord Structure

LEARNING OBJECTIVE   7. Describe the structure of the spinal cord and distinguish between white and gray matter.

First, we'll discuss the linear, vertical structure of the spinal cord.

- The spinal cord has 31 segments. Each segment gives rise to a pair of **spinal nerves** by way of **spinal roots**. The function of the spinal nerves is _____

  _____

- Two areas of the spinal cord are thickened due to the many spinal nerves serving the appendages. They are:

  1. **Cervical enlargement** in the _____ region, which supplies the upper appendages.

  2. **Lumbar enlargement** in the _____ back region, which supplies the lower appendages.

- **Conus medullaris** is the tapered end of the spinal cord.

- _____ is the "horse tail" that extends beyond the conus medullaris and through the vertebral canal.

- **Filum terminale** is an extension of the pia mater that continues beyond the spinal cord to the back of the _____.

Now, we explore the spinal cord in its horizontal plane (cross section):

- Two **grooves** mark the surface.

  1. Anterior median fissure: _____ groove that divides the spinal cord into right and left portions.

  2. **Posterior median sulcus:** _____ groove that divides the spinal cord into right and left portions.

- **Gray matter** is composed of _____ fibers, cell bodies, and dendrites as well as neuroglia. Gray matter forms an H pattern in the center of the spinal cord.

1. **Posterior horns:** Two upper parts of the "H" of the gray matter. Terminal endings of _____ neurons are housed here. Sensory neurons originate in the skin, muscles, and visceral organs and their cell bodies lie outside the spinal cord in clusters known as **dorsal root** _____.

2. **Lateral horns:** Small projection between the anterior and posterior horns. Certain motor neurons of the _____ nervous system are housed here.

3. **Anterior horns:** Two lower parts of the "H" of the gray matter. Motor neurons that extend to _____ muscles originate here.

4. **Gray commissure** is a horizontal bar of matter that connects the right and left sides of the "H" together. A hole, the _____, in the center of the gray commissure carries CSF.

- **White matter** is composed of _____ fibers that surround the gray matter. The three regions, listed next, consist of bundles of myelinated fibers that represent nerve pathways up and down the spinal cord called **nerve** _____.

  1. **Posterior columns**
  2. **Lateral columns**
  3. **Anterior columns**

Spinal Cord Functions

LEARNING OBJECTIVE   8. Describe the conduction pathways of the spinal cord and the reflex arc.

The two main functions of the spinal cord are:

1. _____
2. _____

Nerve tracts carry information up to the brain and down away from the brain. By way of these tracts, the spinal cord ties together information received from sensory neurons, the integration power of the brain, and responding capabilities of motor neurons.

1. **Ascending tracts:** Carry _____ information to the brain.
2. **Descending tracts:** Carry _____ information away from the brain.

A **reflex** is a rapid response for emergencies that involves a minimal number of neurons. Why is a reflex so fast?_____

The **reflex arc** is a pathway for a reflex action.

1. _Sensory_ _____ at the end of a sensory neuron generates an action potential.
2. _Sensory_ _____ carries the nerve impulse to the CNS, such as the spinal cord.
3. _Association neurons_ receive the nerve impulse from the _____. The association neurons make up the _reflex center_ that processes the information and routes it to the appropriate _motor neuron._
4. _Motor neurons_ conduct impulses from the CNS to effectors.
5. _Effectors_ bring about a response.

Types of Reflexes

1. **Somatic reflexes:** Effectors are _____ muscles.
   - **Withdrawal reflex:** Withdrawal of a body part from potential injury, such as a hot stove, so as to minimize the extent of the injury.
   - **Patellar reflex:** Knee jerk reflex that involves only a sensory and a motor neuron.

2. **Visceral reflexes:** Effectors are _____ and _____ muscles. These reflexes cause automatic responses such as heart rate, breathing, vomiting, sneezing, and coughing.

Review Time!

I. *Using the terms in the list below, label the spinal cord illustration and horizontal cross-section.*

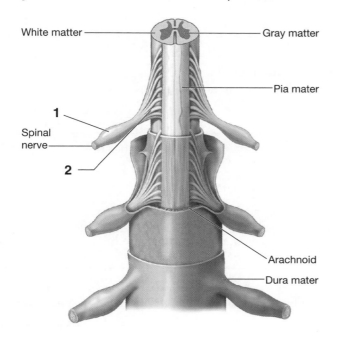

White matter — Gray matter

Pia mater

1

Spinal nerve

2

Arachnoid

Dura mater

1. _____
2. _____
3. _____
4. _____
5. _____
6. _____
7. _____
8. _____
9. _____
10. _____
11. _____
12. _____
13. _____

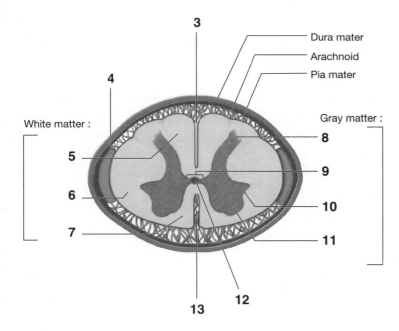

3

Dura mater
Arachnoid
Pia mater

4

White matter :

Gray matter :

5

8

6

9

7

10

11

12

13

Anterior column
Anterior horn
Anterior median fissure
Central canal
Dorsal root ganglion

Lateral column
Lateral horn
Gray commissure
Posterior column
Posterior horn

Posterior median sulcus
Subarachnoid space
Ventral root

II.   *Provide a brief answer for each of the following questions about spinal cord structure.*

1. At what point does the spinal cord end?_____
   What is the name of the tapered end below the spinal cord ending?

2. What are the functions of the horns of gray matter?_____
   _____
   _____

3. Which one of the three membranes forms the filum terminale?_____

4. Name the two enlargements of the spinal cord where many spinal nerves emerge.
   1. _____
   2. _____

5. What is the name of the horizontal bar of gray matter that forms the bar of the "H"?
   _____

6. Are nerve tracts part of white matter or part of gray matter? Explain _____
   _____

7. How many segments form the spinal cord?_____

8. Name the two grooves seen in a horizontal section of the spinal cord.
   1. _____
   2. _____

9. What type of neuron cell bodies are housed in the dorsal root ganglia outside the spinal cord?
   _____

10. What fluid circulates through the central canal of the spinal cord?_____
    _____

III. *Place a number from 1 to 6 in the blank before each statement to indicate the correct order of the steps of a withdrawal reflex.*

_____ Myosin heads bind to exposed actin-binding sites on the thin filaments.

_____ Nerve impulse is generated from the pain receptor along a sensory neuron to the CNS.

_____ Motor neurons conduct impulses from association neurons to the skeletal muscles in your arm to bring about a response.

_____ A sudden change stimulates a sensory receptor.

_____ Association neurons within the CNS make connections with other parts of the nervous system.

_____ Pain receptor is stimulated by a burn injury at the end of your finger.

IV.   *Provide a brief answer for each of the following questions about spinal cord function.*

1. What are the effectors of somatic reflexes?_____

2. Classify the patellar reflex as either somatic or visceral._____

3. What type of reflex causes an automatic response? _____

4. What type of information is carried by ascending tracts?_____

5. Do ascending tracts carry information *to* or *from* the brain?_____

6. What type of information is carried by descending tracts?_____

7. Is the information carried by descending tracts *motor* or *sensory*?_____

8. How does a withdrawal reflex promote homeostasis?_____
   _____

9. What part of the nervous system is bypassed in a reflex arc?_____

10. List the two functions of the spinal cord.

1. _____

2. _____

The Brain

The brain is housed within the _____ cavity. The parts of the brain are:

1. Cerebrum
2. Diencephalon (_____ and hypothalamus)
3. Cerebellum
4. Brain stem (midbrain, _____, and medulla oblongata)

Protective Coverings

The brain is protected by the cranium, _____ fluid, and three membranes. As a way of review, list the three meninges from superficial to deep:

1. _____

2. _____

3. _____

Cerebrospinal Fluid and Ventricles of the Brain

LEARNING OBJECTIVE   9. Identify the ventricles of the brain and explain how cerebrospinal fluid is produced, circulated, and drained.

CSF is a clear, colorless fluid that circulates within and around the spinal cord and brain. List the functions of CSF. _____

_____

_____

CSF circulates within the four ventricles of the brain:

1. The two **lateral ventricles** are located in each side of the cerebrum.
   - The **interventricular foramen** is a canal that connects each lateral ventricle to the third ventricle.
2. The **third ventricle** is located in the center of the diencephalon.
3. The **fourth ventricle** is located between the cerebellum and the medulla oblongata.
   - The **cerebral aqueduct** is a channel that connects the third with the fourth ventricle

CSF formation occurs at the _____ plexus in the ventricles. Choroid plexuses are networks of capillaries. *Hydrostatic pressure* pushes CSF through the brain and spinal cord. Between the walls of the capillaries and neuroglia (known as *ependymal cells*), the **blood–brain barrier** is formed.

- What substances are permitted to travel across the blood–brain barrier? _____

_____

- CSF is similar to blood plasma, but lacking in _____

_____.

- CSF is reabsorbed back into the blood stream across _____

_____

CSF Flow

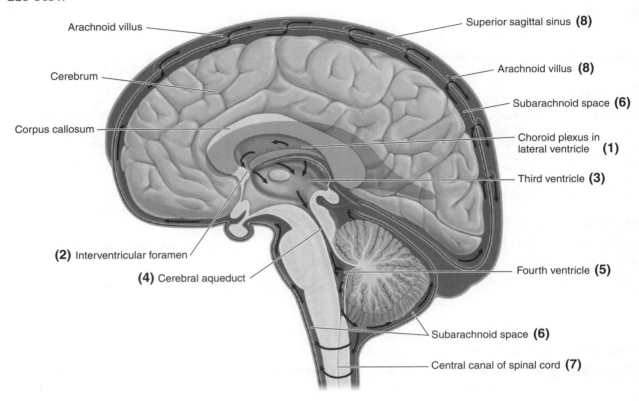

1. **Formed** by choroid plexus in lateral ventricles
2. _____ foramen
3. Third ventricle
4. Cerebral _____
5. Fourth ventricle
6. Subarachnoid space of the spinal cord, then cranium
7. Circulation also occurs in the central canal of spinal cord
8. **Reabsorbed** into the superior sagittal sinus

Cerebrum

LEARNING OBJECTIVE 10. Distinguish between the parts of the brain on the basis of structural and functional differences.

The cerebrum is the largest structure of the brain. It occupies most of the _____ cavity. The cerebrum is divided into right and left portions known as **cerebral hemispheres.**
Convolutions are wrinkles or folds on the cerebrum and include:

• _____ (upward projections)
• _____ (downward groove)
• **Fissures** (deep grooves)
   1. _____ **fissure** is a groove dividing the right and left cerebral hemispheres.
   2. _____ **fissure** is a groove dividing the cerebrum and the cerebellum.

TIP! To keep straight that gyri are upward projections while sulci are downward grooves, remember gyri are grand and sulci are shallow. Another way to remember: Sulcus is a downward groove, as to sulk (be "down in the dumps").

Lobes are surface features of the cerebrum and present on each cerebral hemisphere. The four lobes correspond to the cranial bones that lie above them. They are:

1. **Frontal lobe:** The frontal lobe is separated from the parietal lobe by a groove known as the _____ sulcus. The frontal and temporal lobes are separated by a groove known as the _____ sulcus.

2. **Parietal lobe**

3. _____ **lobe**

4. **Temporal lobe**

Once sectioned, the cerebrum reveals its internal features.

Gray matter (external) includes the cerebral cortex and three functional areas.

• **Cerebral cortex** is the external surface composed of _____ matter where cell bodies, synapses, and cerebral integration function are housed. The cerebral cortex includes three functional areas.

1. **Sensory areas** receive and interpret impulses from _____ receptors.

2. _____ **areas** initiate motor impulses.

3. **Association areas** integrate complex information and include conscious thought.

White matter (internal) is deep to the cerebral cortex and includes three major sets of myelinated fibers.

• **Commissural fibers** extend from hemisphere to hemisphere. The **corpus callosum** bridges the right and left cerebral hemispheres.

• _____ **fibers** extend from one region of a hemisphere to another within the same hemisphere.

• **Projection fibers** extend from one hemisphere downward to other parts of the brain.

Deep gray matter is embedded within each hemisphere. These masses of gray matter are known as **basal ganglia** or **basal** _____. The function of the basal nuclei is _____

_____

• What disease results from a degenerative lesion in one part of the basal ganglia?

_____

• What are the symptoms of this disease?_____

_____

Review Time!

I.   Provide a brief answer for each of the following questions about the cerebrum.

1. Where is CSF formed? _____

2. Where is CSF reabsorbed into the blood stream? _____

_____

3. List the four lobes found associated with the cerebral cortex. _____

_____

4. What is the function of the basal nuclei? _____

_____

5. Deep grooves associated with the cerebrum are known as _____

6. What is the function of the association areas of the cerebral cortex? _____
   _____

7. What lobes are divided by the central sulcus? _____
   _____

8. What type of myelinated fiber creates the corpus callosum? _____

9. What parts of the brain are divided by the longitudinal fissure? _____
   _____

10. Complete this sentence with a directional term: The basal nuclei, formed from gray matter, are
    _____ to the white matter of the cerebrum.

Diencephalon

The diencephalon is inferior to the corpus _____ of the cerebrum. The diencephalon is mostly gray matter and organized into two structures: thalamus and hypothalamus. It is also associated with two endocrine glands: _____ gland and _____ gland.

Thalamus

• **Structure:** Largest part of the diencephalon, surrounds the third ventricle beneath the corpus callosum, consists of two masses of gray matter surrounded by white matter.

• **Function:** Relay station for sensory nerve impulses on the way to the cerebral cortex and involuntary _____ impulses.

Hypothalamus

• **Structure:** Sits below the thalamus, partially in the sella turcica of the _____ bone. The **pituitary gland** is attached by a short stalk.

• **Function:** If you remember only one word for the hypothalamus, remember *homeostasis*.
  1. Regulates visceral activities for the _____ nervous system (digestion, respiration, blood pressure, heart rate).
  2. Regulates the _____ gland and serves as an intermediary between endocrine and nervous systems.
  3. Regulates body temperatures, food and water intake, waking and sleeping patterns, and sex drive.
  4. Manages physiological symptoms of _____.
  5. Plays a role in the development of _____ (tied to thalamus, cerebral cortex, basal ganglia, and other nuclei that form the **limbic system**).

Brain Stem

The brain stem includes the midbrain, pons, and medulla oblongata.

Midbrain

• **Structure:** Located between the diencephalon and the pons. Consists of an anterior portion, the cerebral peduncles, and a posterior portion, the _____.

• **Function:** The **cerebral peduncles** consist of bundles of myelinated fibers that connect motor pathways between cerebrum and _____. The **colliculi** serve as reflex centers for rapid eye, head, and trunk movements.

Pons

- **Structure:** Sits inferior to the midbrain as a rounded bulge of _____ matter.
- **Function:** Communicates with the medulla oblongata in regulation of breathing rhythm and relays sensory impulses from peripheral nerves to the _____.

Medulla Oblongata

- **Structure:** The most inferior part of the brain stem; unites with the spinal cord. White matter surrounds _____ matter. White matter consists of ascending (sensory) nerve fibers while the gray matter consists of descending (motor) nerve fibers. **Pyramids** result from descending fibers that cross to opposite sides to activate muscles. Fibers originating on the _left_ side activate muscles on the _____ side.
- **Function:** Gray matter consists of reflex centers for visceral reflexes, consciousness, and arousal. Visceral reflexes include:
  1. **Cardiac center** for the regulation of _____ rate.
  2. **Vasomotor center** for the regulation of _____.
  3. **Respiratory center** for the regulation of depth and rhythm of _____.

Cerebellum

- **Structure:** Located in the posterior and the inferior part of the _____. Like the larger cerebrum, it is divided into two hemispheres that are connected by the vermis and gray matter (cerebellar cortex) surrounds white matter (arbor vitae). Convolutions are known as _____ (upward folds) and _____ (shallow downfolds). The _____ fissure separates the cerebellum from the cerebrum.
- **Function:** Three bundled pairs of myelinated fibers, **cerebellar peduncles**, connect the cerebellum to other parts of the brain. The fibers carry the following:
  1. Sensory information is carried from muscles, joints, and the inner ear to inform the _____ about voluntary motor activities, equilibrium, and balance.
  2. Motor impulses that coordinate and provide precision to _____ muscle contraction, so that the cerebellum acts as an automatic pilot for motor responses (smooth response and posture maintenance).
  3. Sensory information from inner ear to provide a sense of _____.

Review Time!

I. _Using the terms in the list below, write the appropriate region or part of the brain in each blank. You may use a term more than once._

Cerebellum   Hypothalamus   Medulla oblongata

Pons   Thalamus   Midbrain

  1. Connected to the pituitary gland by a short stalk   _____
  2. Diencephalon part that serves as a relay station for sensory impulses on the way to the cerebral cortex   _____
  3. Houses the arbor vitae   _____
  4. Part of the limbic system   _____
  5. Houses the cardiac center, vasomotor center, and respiratory center   _____
  6. Consists of ascending and descending tracts that extend between brain and spinal cord   _____

7. Communicates with the medulla oblongata in regulating
   breathing rhythm   _____

8. The vermis connects the two hemispheres   _____

9. Attached to the pineal gland   _____

10. Regulates body temperature, food and water intake, and
    sex drive   _____

11. Houses cerebral peduncles and colliculi   _____

12. With the hypothalamus, forms the diencephalon   _____

13. Conveys motor impulses to coordinate and provide
    precision to skeletal muscle movement   _____

14. Regulates involuntary activities which have a direct
    effect on homeostasis   _____

15. Serves as reflex centers for rapid eye, head, and
    trunk movements   _____

II. *Provide a brief answer for each of the following questions about the regions of the brain*

1. List the two parts of the diencephalon.

   1. _____

   2. _____

2. What region of the brain serves as an automatic pilot for motor responses? _____

3. List the three parts of the brain stem.

   1. _____

   2. _____

   3. _____

4. Describe two functions of the thalamus.

   1. _____

   2. _____

5. Explain three roles the cerebellar peduncles play. _____

   _____

   _____

   _____

6. What three visceral reflex centers are housed in the medulla oblongata?

   1. _____

   2. _____

   3. _____

7. A stroke to the brain stem has left a patient unable to control the left side of his body. What
   specific part of the brain stem suffered damage? Explain. _____

   _____

   _____

8. Why do you think an overwhelming amount of stress can lead to problems with the endocrine
   system, limbic system, and maintaining homeostasis? Determine what part of the brain has been
   affected. _____

   _____

   _____

9. A brain injury to the posterior side of the cranium has left a patient with balance and equilibrium problems. Which part of the brain may have experienced damage? Explain. _____
_____
_____

10. Which part of the brain is to blame for imbalances with water intake? _____
_____

11. While walking down the street, you catch a whiff of perfume lingering in the air from a passerby. The woman's perfume was the same your dearly loved grandmother used to wear and the odor brought back a warm memory of her. What part of the diencephalon was involved in this emotional response?_____

12. Correct the false information in this statement: *Located between the cerebral cortex and midbrain, the thalamus regulates breathing rhythm along with the medulla oblongata.* _____
_____
_____

CONCEPT 5

The Peripheral Nervous System

Concept: The peripheral nervous system (PNS) consists of nerves, ganglia, and receptors that carry impulses between body organs and the CNS. It includes a somatic component managing voluntary functions and an autonomic component managing involuntary functions.

LEARNING OBJECTIVE   11. Identify the organs of the peripheral nervous system (PNS).

Organs of the PNS

The PNS includes organs such as nerves, ganglia, and sensory receptors.

Nerves

Nerves are true organs because they are composed of more than one type of _____ and perform a general function. The term "nerve" means something different from "nerve fiber." Each nerve consists of parallel bundles of nerve fibers (axons), which may be myelinated and are enclosed by wrappings of connective tissue.

• _____**neurium:** Tough, outer covering around the whole nerve.
• _____**neurium:** Thin wrapping around bundles of nerve fibers.
• _____**neurium:** Very thin, deep layer surrounding each individual nerve fiber.

Ganglia

Ganglia are clusters of neuron cell bodies located *outside* the CNS. Ganglia are enclosed by wrappings of _____ and contain blood vessels.

Sensory Receptors

Sensory receptors respond to stimuli, or changes in the environment. Many sensory receptors are the endings of _____ from sensory neurons.

- Many dendrites may be *free* within a body tissue where they pick up pain, pressure, or _____.
- Some dendrites are enclosed within a connective tissue capsule, such as fine touch or _____ receptors in the dermis of the skin.
- Some sensory receptors may be complex, such as the **special sensory organs** that include the _____, _____, _____ (tongue), and _____ organs (nose).

Cranial Nerves

LEARNING OBJECTIVE 12. Distinguish between cranial nerves and spinal nerves, and describe how spinal nerves branch.

Each of the _____ (*how many?*) pairs of cranial nerve has its own name and Roman numeral and is attached directly to the brain. The Roman numeral corresponds to the point of attachment to the brain (from anterior to posterior).

Three pairs of cranial nerves are strictly sensory and carry information to the CNS. List these pairs by name and Roman numeral.

1. _____
2. _____
3. _____

Five pairs of cranial nerves are strictly motor and carry information away from the CNS. List these pairs by name and Roman numeral.

1. _____
2. _____
3. _____
4. _____
5. _____

Four pairs contain both sensory and motor fibers and are considered _____ nerves. List these pairs by name and Roman numeral.

1. _____
2. _____
3. _____
4. _____

TIP! To keep the cranial nerves in correct numerical order, remember this mnemonic device:

Oh Oh Oh To Touch and Feel Very Green Vegetables AH

I	Oh = Olfactory	VII	Feel = Facial
II	Oh = Optic	VIII	Very =Vestibulocochlear
III	Oh = Oculomotor	IX	Green = Glossopharyngeal
IV	To = Trochlear	X	Vegetables = Vagus
V	Touch = Trigeminal	XI	A = Accessory
VI	And = Accessory	XII	H = Hypoglossal

Review Time!

I.   Using the terms in the list below, label the cranial nerves on this inferior view of the brain.

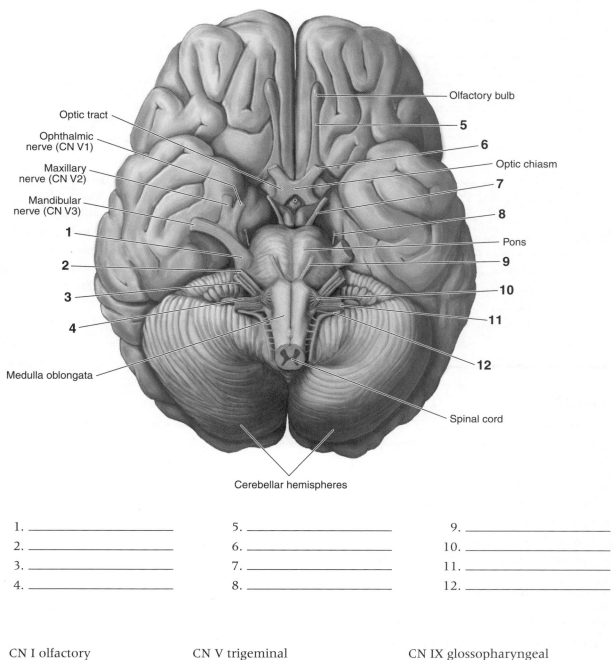

1. _____   5. _____   9. _____
2. _____   6. _____   10. _____
3. _____   7. _____   11. _____
4. _____   8. _____   12. _____

CN I olfactory   CN V trigeminal   CN IX glossopharyngeal

CN II optic   CN VI abducens   CN X vagus

CN III oculomotor   CN VII facial   CN XI accessory

CN IV trochlear   CN VIII vestibulocochlear   CN XII hypoglossal

II. *For each question below, provide the name and Roman numeral of the cranial nerve. You may want to have Table 8.2 from your book nearby as you practice this information.*

Name	Roman Numeral	Function
_____	_____	1. Sense of smell
_____	_____	2. Moves the tongue
_____	_____	3. Movement of the eye (name 3)
_____		
_____		
_____	_____	4. Sense of vision
_____	_____	5. Movement of the jaw for chewing
_____	_____	6. Sense of taste (name 2)
_____		
_____	_____	7. Sensations of visceral organs
_____	_____	8. Movement of the shoulders and head
_____	_____	9. Senses of hearing and equilibrium
_____	_____	10. Innervates the cells in the retina of each eye
_____	_____	11. Motor fibers innervate the heart
_____	_____	12. Controls the amount of light entering the eye
_____	_____	13. Innervates tear glands (name 2)
_____		
_____	_____	14. Movements of speech and swallowing
_____	_____	15. Innervates the inner ear

Spinal Nerves

Each of the _____ (*how many?*) pairs of spinal nerves is attached to the spinal cord and all are mixed in terms of function. Mixed nerves have both _____ and _____ nerve fibers. The spinal nerve pairs are:

- 8 pairs of cervical spinal nerves (C1 to C8)
- 12 pairs of thoracic spinal nerves (T1 to T12)
- 5 pairs of lumbar spinal nerves (L1 to L5)
- 5 pairs of sacral spinal nerves (S1 to S5)
- 1 pair of coccygeal spinal nerves (C0)

Roots of Spinal Nerves

Roots are nerve fibers extending from the horns of the spinal cord. At the intervertebral foramen, the roots combine to form a spinal nerve that is mixed in function.

- **Dorsal roots** unite with the posterior (dorsal) horns of the spinal cord are _____ in function. Collections of sensory neuron cell bodies form the **dorsal root ganglion.**
- **Ventral roots** unite with the _____ (ventral) horns of the spinal cord and are _____ in function.

Branches of Spinal Nerves

Once a spinal nerve emerges from the vertebral column, it splits into branches of mixed nerves.

Dorsal Ramus

Dorsal ramus is the small branch that extends to the _____ to supply muscles and skin.

Ventral Ramus

Ventral ramus is the larger branch that travels to the anterior body wall.

- In the trunk (T2 to T12), ventral rami directly supply body parts.
- **Plexuses** (other than in the trunk) are formed from ventral rami that branch and recombine to form complex networks. Due to the branching, individual body parts receive nerve impulses from more than one spinal nerve root. What is the advantage of the nature of the plexus?

  _____
  _____

- Three major plexuses are:
  1. **Cervical plexus** is formed by the branching of spinal nerves C1 to _____.
     The plexus is located beneath the _____ muscle in the anterior neck region.
     The _phrenic nerves_ innervate the diaphragm and send motor impulses to breathe.
  2. **Brachial plexus** is formed by the branching of spinal nerves C5 to _____.
     The plexus is located between the vertebral column and the axilla and supplies the skin and muscles of the upper limbs. Major branches include the _musculocutaneous, ulnar, median, radial,_ and _axillary nerves._
  3. **Lumbosacral plexus** is formed by L1 to _____ and S1 to _____.
     The plexus serves the skin and muscles of the abdominal wall, pelvic wall, thighs, legs, and feet. Major branches include the _femoral, obturator,_ and _sciatic nerves._

Review Time!

I. _Provide a brief answer for each of the following questions._
  1. Compare the number of spinal nerves to the number of vertebrae in each region of the vertebral column. Are the numbers the same or different?_____

  2. What does the dorsal ramus of a spinal nerve serve?_____

  3. Spinal nerves are known as mixed nerves. Explain the meaning behind the term _mixed_ nerve.

  4. Which plexus includes the phrenic nerves? Why are the phrenic nerves important?

  5. Contrast the type of impulse carried along the ventral root with that carried along the dorsal root.

6. What regions of the body are served by the lumbosacral plexus?_____
_____

7. What is the advantage of a nerve plexus?_____
_____
_____

8. Describe why damage to the cervical plexus could interrupt the process of breathing.
_____
_____

9. Why is a ramus considered a mixed nerve, yet the roots of a spinal nerve are not?
_____
_____

10. How are ventral rami and plexuses related?_____
_____
_____

Functional Divisions of the PNS

LEARNING OBJECTIVE   13. Distinguish between the somatic and autonomic nervous systems on the basis of their effectors and pathways.

The PNS has two divisions:
1. **Somatic:** Voluntary, under conscious control by the brain
2. **Autonomic:** Involuntary

Somatic Nervous System

The somatic nervous system is the part of the PNS that conveys information about *voluntary* activities such as
_____.

- **Sensory component:** Sensory receptors in skin, visceral organs, and special sensory organs; sensory nerves send impulses to the _____ nervous system. There is/are _____ (*how many?*) sensory neuron(s) between the sensory receptor and the CNS.
- **Motor component:** Motor nerves terminate in effectors, which are *always* _____ muscles. Which neurotransmitter is released at synapses with skeletal muscles to produce excitatory transmissions only? _____ (ACh). There is/are _____ (*how many?*) motor neuron(s) with a myelinated axon originating in the anterior gray horn of the spinal cord (CNS) and the effector.

Autonomic Nervous System

LEARNING OBJECTIVE   14. Distinguish between the sympathetic and parasympathetic autonomic divisions.

The autonomic nervous system is the part of the PNS that conveys information about *involuntary* activities such as _____. Reflex centers in the brain such as _____ and _____ regulate these functions.

- **Sensory component:** Sensory neurons transmit information from receptors in skin and visceral organs to centers in the _____, brain stem, or spinal cord.
- **Motor component:** Centers in the CNS route a motor response to promote or inhibit contractions of _____ or _____ muscles, or secretions from glands.

- **Two routes: Sympathetic** and _____ **divisions** are *antagonistic,* meaning the effect of an impulse from one division counteracts the effect of an impulse from the other division. Many visceral organs receive innervations from both divisions, known as *dual innervations.*

Autonomic Motor Pathways

For the sake of comparison, the somatic nervous system has a single neuron between the spinal cord and the skeletal muscle. The autonomic nervous system is a two-neuron pathway.

- A **preganglionic neuron** has its cell body situated in the _____ or spinal cord. The axon is *myelinated,* and it exits the CNS by way of a cranial or spinal nerve. It separates from the nerve and terminates at an autonomic ganglion.
- The **ganglion** is the site of _____ between the preganglionic and postganglionic neurons.
- A **postganglionic neuron** has its cell body situated in the ganglion and its axon is *unmyelinated.* This neuron extends to a _____ (smooth or cardiac muscle, or gland).

In summary, the pathway extends from preganglionic neuron, ganglion, to postganglionic neuron.

Sympathetic Division

- Preganglionic neurons originate from the _____ horn of spinal cord.
- Preganglionic neurons arise from spinal nerves T1 to _____ and L1 to L2 (or L3).
- The neurons take one of several pathways, such as the **sympathetic trunk ganglia** that lie along the vertebral column. (1) The preganglionic neuron may terminate at the first ganglion, or (2) it may travel and terminate at another ganglion. The postganglionic neuron travels with a _____ until it reaches a visceral effector. (3) The preganglionic neuron continues past the sympathetic trunk ganglia into the ventral body cavity and synapses with a postganglionic neuron. The postganglionic axon travels through a _____ before terminating at a visceral effector.

Parasympathetic Division

- Preganglionic neurons originate from the brain stem and the _____ region of the spinal cord (S2 to S4).
- The axons of preganglionic neurons emerge as part of a cranial nerve or the ventral root of a _____ nerve to end at **terminal ganglia** situated within or near visceral effectors.
- Postganglionic neurons travel a short distance to visceral effectors.

Autonomic Function

Autonomic impulses can either stimulate or inhibit the activities of smooth muscle, cardiac muscle, and glands. The dual function comes from the two different types of _____ released by the parasympathetic and sympathetic divisions of the autonomic nervous system.

- **Adrenergic fibers** include most sympathetic postganglionic fibers; they release _____ (noradrenalin).
- **Cholinergic fibers** include parasympathetic postganglionic fibers; they release _____.

The sympathetic and parasympathetic divisions either promote energy usage or conserve energy.

Sympathetic division is known as the "fight or flight divisions" because of its involvement in processes that use energy to prepare the body for quick thinking or physical reaction. Adrenergic fibers promote the following:

- *Increased* _____
- *Increased* blood _____ levels
- *Increased* _____ to skeletal muscles, lungs, heart
- *Increased* blood flow away from _____
- *Inhibit* _____.

Parasympathetic divisions are known as the "rest–digest" division because of the energy conservation efforts by _____ fibers, such as:

- *Stimulation* of smooth muscles in digestive organs and glands
- *Promotion* of digestion
- *Inhibits* heart rate

Review Time!

I.   *Provide a brief answer for each of the following questions about the divisions of the PNS.*

1. Why do you think different divisions of the autonomic nervous system use different neurotransmitters?_____
_____
_____

2. Which PNS division is responsible for motor control of skeletal muscle?
_____
_____

3. Compare the pathways for motor information for the autonomic and somatic pathways.
_____
_____
_____

4. Compare the pathways for motor information for the sympathetic and parasympathetic divisions.
_____
_____
_____

5. Provide two reasons the somatic nervous system is faster than the autonomic nervous system.
_____
_____

6. What neurotransmitter is released by adrenergic fibers? By cholinergic fibers?
_____
_____

7. Explain how the sympathetic and parasympathetic divisions are antagonistic.
_____
_____

8. Where do somatic motor neurons originate?_____
9. Where do preganglionic motor neurons of the autonomic nervous system originate?
_____
_____

10. Where do postganglionic motor neurons originate? _____
_____

11. In what organ(s) does the single neuron of the somatic nervous system terminate?
_____
_____

12. In what organ(s) does the postganglionic neuron of the autonomic nervous system terminate?
_____

13. Sanmitra was so nervous about giving her last speech for a class, she found her hands sweaty and her heart racing. Which division of the autonomic system is producing her experience? Explain.

_____

_____

_____

14. You may have been told to avoid swimming soon after a large meal. Which division of the autonomic nervous system favors digestive activities? Why do you think swimming should be avoided?

_____

_____

_____

_____

15. An 18-wheeler just nearly missed hitting Juan head-on while Juan was driving. Exasperated, he pulls over to the side of the road. Which autonomic nervous system division is in control? What symptoms do you think he's experiencing?_____

_____

_____

_____

16. You consciously decide to pick up your pen to write an answer to this question. Map the pathway from the spinal cord to the skeletal muscle. _____

_____

_____

17. For which nervous system division does acetylcholine produce skeletal muscle contractions?

_____

_____

18. Name two types of muscle tissue that bear receptors for norepinephrine (noradrenalin).

_____

_____

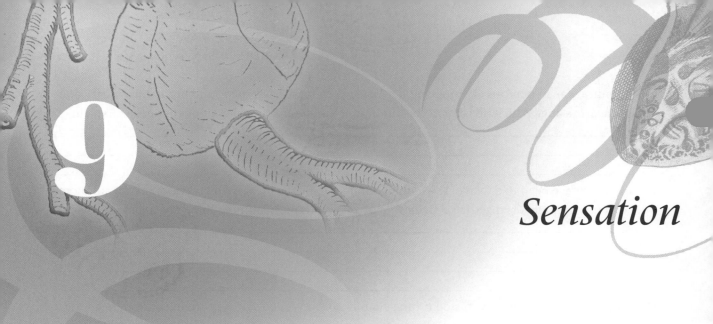

9

Sensation

Tips for Success as You Begin

Read Chapter 9 from your textbook before attending class. Listen when you attend lecture and fill in the blanks in this notebook. You may choose to complete the blanks before attending class as a way to prepare for the day's topics. The same day you attend lecture, read the material again and complete the exercises after each section in this notebook. Spend time every day with this chapter as it will help you make sense of the material. You'll want to practice linking together related structures so you can appreciate the pathway of various senses into the brain.

CONCEPT 1

Comparing Sensory and Motor Functions

Concept: Sensory functions provide the brain with information on conditions outside and inside the body in order to maintain homeostasis. Motor functions provide a means for responding to changes in the environment, with pathways arising from integration centers in the central nervous system (CNS).

LEARNING OBJECTIVE 1. Distinguish between the terms *sensory* and *motor*.

LEARNING OBJECTIVE 2. Describe the component in sensory and motor pathways.

What do sensory functions provide the brain with?_____

_____

What do motor functions enable the CNS to do?_____

_____

Sensory Functions

Sensations are a state of awareness of the external or internal conditions of the body and are needed for maintenance of homeostasis. Sensations are grouped into two categories:

1. **General senses** are detected by simple sensory receptors that include **somatic senses** and **visceral senses.**

- **Somatic senses** tell the brain about touch, pressure, temperature, _____,
  and body position.
- **Visceral senses** provide information about _____.

2. **Special senses** include the following:
   - _____ epithelium (smell)
   - Papillae of tongue (taste)
   - Eye (sight)
   - Ears (hearing and _____)

A **stimulus** is a change in the environment that is great enough to initiate a nerve impulse by a **sensory receptor.** The impulse is taken to the _____ nervous system.

Sensory Receptors

A sensory receptor originates sensation because it is capable of generating an action potential when a stimulus is received (known as _____). Threshold levels for receptors vary; receptors are sensitive to a particular stimulus but insensitive to others (known as *stimulus-specific*). The following receptors are classified by stimulus.

- _____ detect a mechanical or physical change such as touch, pressure, muscle tension, hearing, equilibrium, and blood pressure.
- **Thermoreceptors** detect _____ changes.
- **Nociceptors** detect pain.
- **Photoreceptors** detect changes in the amount of light and are present only in the _____ of the eye.
- _____ detect chemicals dissolved in fluid (taste and smell) and provide detection of oxygen and carbon dioxide levels in blood.

Sensory adaptation occurs when threshold level rises as a stimulus continues to be present. Do we continue to perceive the sensation as sensory adaptation occurs?_____

Sensory Pathways

There are two sensory conduction pathways.

1. **General sensory pathway** carries impulses from a *simple* receptor to the _____. Simple receptors are found in skin, visceral organs, and muscles. From the receptor, the impulse is sent along three neurons before reaching the brain.
   - First-order neuron is a sensory neuron that connects the sensory receptor to the
     _____.
   - Second-order neuron carries the impulse to the _____.
   - Third-order neuron conducts impulses to the cerebral _____ for processing.

2. **Special sensory pathway** carries impulses from a *complex* receptor such as the _____ and _____. The pathway is variable, but includes at least _____ neurons that connect the receptor to the cerebral cortex along a cranial nerve. In most cases the impulse is routed through the _____ before continuing to the cerebral cortex.

Review Time!

I.   *Using the terms in the list below, write the appropriate type of receptor in each blank. You may use a term more than once.*

Chemoreceptors   Mechanoreceptors   Nociceptors

Photoreceptors   Thermoreceptors

1. Pain receptors   _____

2. Smell and taste receptors   _____

3. Hearing receptors   _____

4. Detect temperature changes   _____

5. Detect oxygen and carbon dioxide levels in the blood   _____

6. Deep pressure receptors   _____

7. Present only in the eye to detect light   _____

8. Detect touch and pressure   _____

9. Detect chemicals dissolved in fluid   _____

10. Detect damage to nearby cells   _____

Motor Functions

Motor impulses travel from the CNS to effectors. We now look at the origins of motor control and motor pathways.

Motor Origins

Sensory signals arrive in the CNS where integration occurs before a motor response is initiated. Those integration centers are:

- **Spinal cord:** Integration centers located in the _____ matter generate somatic reflexes to stimulate skeletal muscle contraction and visceral reflexes to stimulate cardiac muscle, smooth muscle, and glands.

- **Brain stem:** Integration centers are in the three parts of the brain stem. These three parts are _____, _____, and _____. Visceral motor impulses generated here, such as coughing, sneezing, vomiting, changes in heart rate, and breathing, are considered reflexes since they require little integration.

- **Cerebellum:** Integration centers are housed in _____ matter and connected to centers in the cerebral cortex, basal ganglia, and brain stem. Sensory information (equilibrium) from the inner ear is coordinated with the cerebral cortex to generate motor impulses that control _____, balance, and coordination.

- **Basal ganglia:** Integration centers are clusters of _____ matter embedded within the cerebrum. These centers control _____ _____

- **Hypothalamus:** The integration center in the hypothalamus is for involuntary integration and control; it is an origin of motor impulses that control the autonomic nervous system over pathways to _____ muscle, _____ muscle, and glands.

- **Cerebral cortex:** The highest level of integration is housed in an area in front of the central sulcus known as the _____. Motor impulses originating here require thought, memory, body coordination, and muscle movements.

Motor Pathways

Motor impulse pathways can travel along:

1. Simple reflex arcs (Chapter 8)
2. Autonomic pathways (Chapter 8)
3. Somatic pathways

   - Somatic pathways conduct voluntary motor impulses from the motor areas, usually the primary motor cortex of the cerebrum, to skeletal muscles along a single neuron known as the _____ *motor neuron*. The impulse travels through the cerebrum and crosses to the opposite side as the impulse travels through the brain stem. The impulse exits the spinal cord, through either a cranial nerve or nuclei.
   - The _____ *motor neuron* transmits the impulse to the second neuron in the pathway, the _____ *motor neuron*.

Review Time!

I. Using the terms in the list below, write the appropriate origin for motor control in each blank. You may use a term more than once.

Basal ganglia   Brain stem   Cerebellum

Hypothalamus   Spinal cord   Cerebral cortex

1. The highest level of integration _____

2. Somatic reflex control of skeletal muscle contraction _____

3. Integration centers are housed in the midbrain, pons, and medulla oblongata _____

4. Controls semi-voluntary events like laughing, walking, and jumping _____

5. Origin for motor impulses requiring thought or memory _____

6. Initiates visceral motor reflexes such as coughing, sneezing, and breathing _____

7. Origin for motor impulses that serve the autonomic nervous system _____

8. Motor impulses control body posture, balance, and coordination _____

9. Primary motor cortex _____

10. Visceral reflex control that changes heart rate or breathing _____

CONCEPT 2

General Senses

Concept: The general senses are sensations detected by simple receptors. They include touch and pressure, temperature, pain, and body position.

LEARNING OBJECTIVE 3. Describe the structure and function of each of the general sensory receptors.

General senses, such as touch, pressure, temperature, pain, and body position, are detected by simple sensory receptors. Interpretation and processing occurs in the _____. Sensory receptors may be:

- **Encapsulated nerve endings:** _____ surrounded by layers of connective tissue to form a capsule.
- **Free nerve endings:** Dendrites are bare dendrites that lack the capsule.

Touch and Pressure

Cutaneous sensations are so called because of the numerous mechanoreceptors present in the _____ to detect touch and pressure.

Touch Receptors

- **Tactile** (Meissner) **corpuscles** are encapsulated nerve endings that detect slight movement. Where are they abundant? _____.
  Tactile corpuscles adapt to stimuli after a few minutes.
- **Tactile disc** (Merkel receptor) is a less common touch receptor that has free nerve endings in the _____.
- **Ruffini corpuscles** are found in the _____ of the skin and detect stretch.

Pressure Receptors

- **Lamellar** (Pacinian) **corpuscles** are encapsulated nerve endings that respond only to _____. They are located deep in the skin, around joints and tendons, and in certain visceral organs. These receptors also adapt to stimuli within minutes.

Temperature

Thermoreceptors are free nerve endings in the skin that detect heat and cold. Both pain receptors and thermoreceptors respond to extreme temperatures by triggering a sensation of _____.

Pain

Pain is detected by **nociceptors,** which are free nerve endings in the skin, muscles, and most visceral organs. _____ may sense chemicals released when cells are damaged or destroyed. Pain can also result when any receptors is excessively stimulated.
The different types of pain are:

- **Superficial somatic pain** comes from nociceptors in the _____.
  An example of this is _____.
- **Deep somatic pain** arises from nociceptors in skeletal muscles, joints, tendons, or fascia.

- **Visceral pain** comes from nociceptors in the walls of visceral organs that respond to widespread disturbances (stomach cramps, heartburn).

  An example of this is _____

  Visceral pain is difficult to pinpoint because the major nerve pathways are not easily distinguished by the brain. Therefore, _____ **pain** is the reason people feel heart attack pain in the arm or jaw.

The pathway of pain to the cerebral cortex along sensory neurons can be interrupted or reduced using analgesics, anesthesia, drugs, or surgery, among other treatments.

Body Position

Proprioceptors provide information on the degree of muscle contraction, tension in tendons, position of joints, and the position of the head relative to the ground. Proprioceptors enable you to control your body _____ without the use of any other sense. The primary receptors of body position are:

- **Muscle spindles** are present in _____ muscle and stimulated by stretch of the muscle.
- **Tendon organs** are situated between a tendon and a skeletal muscle and house two (or more) sensory neurons. They are stimulated by _____ in a tendon.

CONCEPT 3

Special Senses

Concept: Each special sense is detected by receptors located within supportive tissue. These receptors are highly specialized to respond to one type of stimulus, and include smell, taste, sight, and hearing and equilibrium.

The following **special sensory organs** include which receptors surrounded by support tissues?
- **Smell:** Detected by _____
- **Taste:** Detected by _____
- **Sight:** Detected by _____
- **Hearing:** Detected by _____
- **Equilibrium:** Detected by _____

Smell

LEARNING OBJECTIVE   4. Describe the special sensory structures of smell and the olfactory pathway.

The sense of smell (also known as olfaction) is detected by _____ receptors in the nasal cavity.

Olfactory Structures

Olfactory organs are situated high in the nasal cavity; they include cells and receptors.
- Why does sniffing help you detect a smell? _____

_____

Parts of the Olfactory Organ

- **Olfactory receptors** are neurons in the nasal epithelium. The axon of the neuron extends through the cribriform plate to the ———————————————— bone and terminates in the olfactory bulb of the brain.
- **Supporting cells** surround and support the olfactory receptors.
- **Basal cells** undergo mitosis to produce new receptors.
- **Olfactory hairs** are the ———————————————— on the olfactory receptors that extend into the mucus layer beyond the nasal epithelium.
- **Olfactory glands** produce ———————————————— . They are located in connective tissue deep to the olfactory organs.

Olfactory Pathway

Olfactory receptors generate an action potential as gas molecules entering the mucus layer atop the nasal epithelium and become dissolved in the mucus and then reach the olfactory hairs. The pathway follows:

- Olfactory hairs of olfactory receptor travel through the ———————————————— (ethmoid bone)
- Impulse travels to the ———————————————— , which are the origin of cranial nerve I (olfactory nerves)
- From the olfactory nerve, the impulse travels to the ———————————————— lobe for interpretation

The olfactory pathways are closely linked to the ———————————————— system of the brain.

- Do you recall what happens at the limbic system?————————————————
——

Review Time!

I.   *Provide a brief answer for each of the following questions about olfaction.*

1. Through which cranial bone do the olfactory receptors travel to transmit the sense of smell into the brain?————————————————————————————————

2. Why do familiar fragrances trigger memories?————————————————————
——

3. What is the function of the basal cells?————————————————————————
——

4. With what other sense is smell commonly linked?————————————————————

5. Where are the olfactory bulbs located?————————————————————————

6. What would happen if your olfactory receptors were not continually replaced?
——
——

7. Why does sniffing help you maximize your sensitivity to smells?————————————
——

8. What type of receptor detects the sense of smell?————————————————————

9. Why do you think a person with a dry nasal cavity may have difficulty smelling?
——
——

10. Which cranial nerve is responsible for transmitting smell sensations to the brain? Provide both the name and Roman numeral. ————————————————————————

Taste

LEARNING OBJECTIVE **5.** Describe the special sensory structures of taste and the gustatory pathway.

Taste, like smell, is detected by chemoreceptors. Taste and smell operate simultaneously when we eat.

Gustatory Structures

Taste buds, the organs of taste, are scattered through the oral cavity, on the surface of the _____ in raised hills known as **papillae,** on the roof of the mouth, and in the pharynx. The parts of the taste bud are:

- **Gustatory cells** are taste receptors surrounded by a capsule of epithelial cells. At the base of the gustatory cell are sensory nerve fiber endings.
- The free ends of the gustatory cells form **gustatory microvilli**.
- The gustatory microvilli project through an opening in the taste bud known as the **taste pore**.

Five primary taste sensations, associated with a particular type of taste bud, are:

- Sweet
- Salty
- Bitter
- Sour
- Umami (meaty)

Sensory adaptation by the _____ receptors is rapid and the burst of flavor you first taste declines within seconds.

Gustatory Pathway

Chemicals dissolved in saliva are detected by chemoreceptors in gustatory cells. If the change is great, nerve impulses are generated by sensory nerve fibers at the base of the gustatory cells. Impulses travel along cranial nerves VII, IX, and X. Do you recall the names of these cranial nerves?

- VII is _____
- IX is _____
- X is _____.

From these cranial nerves, the impulse is taken to the _____. Impulses then pass to the thalamus, which directs the impulses to the primary gustatory center in the cerebral cortex.

Review Time!

I. Provide a brief answer for each of the following questions about gustation.

1. List the five taste senses. _____
    _____

2. Since there are five taste senses, how do we experience such a wide variety of tastes?
    _____
    _____

3. What is the relationship between gustatory cells, gustatory microvilli, and taste pores?
    _____
    _____

4. What type of receptor detects the sense of taste?_____

5. What other sense is linked to the sense of taste?_____

6. Name the three cranial nerves that carry taste sensations to the brain. Provide both the name and Roman numerals. _____
    _____

7. Why do subsequent tastes of a piece of warm chocolate cake not quite match the first taste?

_____

8. Why are taste buds considered organs?_____

_____

9. What role does the thalamus play in the gustatory pathway?_____

_____

10. Mrs. Gee has damage to the primary gustatory center in her right cerebral cortex. Why do you think she has difficulty tasting food?_____

_____

Sight

The majority of the sensory receptors in the body are photoreceptors in the eye.

Accessory Structures

LEARNING OBJECTIVE 6. Describe the accessory structures and the parts of the eye.

Eyelids protect anterior surface of the eye and contain hairs known as **eyelashes.** Each eyelid has four layers: (1) thin outer skin, (2) skeletal muscle, (3) connective tissue, (4) inner mucous membrane known as the **conjunctiva.**

• What is the function of the conjunctiva?_____
• What is inflammation of the conjunctiva called?_____

Lacrimal apparatus consists of the lacrimal gland, lacrimal sac, and nasolacrimal duct.

• **Lacrimal gland** secretes _____, a dilute salt solution with an antibacterial enzyme to fight infection.
• **Lacrimal sac** is in the _____ bone. Tears are carried to the sac by **lacrimal canals.**
• **Nasolacrimal duct** carries tears from the lacrimal sac to the nose.
• **External muscles** (6) originate in the walls of the orbit and insert on the tough outer eyeball surface.

Structure of the Eye

The eye is the organ of vision and has _____ (_how many?_) layers as well as compartments filled with fluid.

Fibrous Tunic

The **fibrous tunic** is the outer, thick layer of the eye. It has two regions.

1. _____ is the "white" of the eye formed of fibrous, connective tissue. The sclera protects the eye, forms its shape, and has many blood vessels. The optic nerve emerges from the posterior surface.

2. _____ is the anterior, transparent portion through which light passes. There are _no_ blood vessels in this slightly bulged structure.

Vascular Tunic

The **vascular tunic** contains many blood vessels that nourish the eye's structures. There are three main components, and the associated lens.

1. **Choroid** is a thick, dark brown membrane that lines the internal surface of the _____. A pigmented layer underlies the choroid. Together, the dark brown layer and the pigmented layer absorb light and prevent it from reflecting back out of the eye.

2. **Ciliary body** is modified from the choroid and is composed of _____ muscle. The ciliary body is connected by string-like structures to the lens by **suspensory ligaments**.

> **TIP!** Think of the lens as a trampoline and the suspensory ligaments as the cords that attach the trampoline to the frame (ciliary body).

3. The **iris** is attached to the inner margin of the ciliary body and suspended between the _____ and the _____. Contraction of smooth muscles in the iris changes the diameter of the **pupil**, the opening in the center, to control the amount of light entering the eye.

The transparent **lens** is behind the pupil and iris. With age, the lens loses its transparency, as is evident with *cataracts*. The lens creates a division between two main compartments of the eye.

1. The anterior compartment is in front of the lens. It is divided into two *chambers* by the _____. The **anterior chamber** is between the cornea and the iris; the **posterior chamber** is between the iris and the lens. The **aqueous humor**, a clear, watery fluid, circulates within these two chambers. *Glaucoma* results when the aqueous humor is blocked from circulation.

2. The posterior compartment behind the lens is the **posterior cavity**. The thick, gel-like **vitreous humor** helps support the structure of the eye and is housed in the posterior cavity. Does the vitreous humor circulate through the eye like the aqueous humor? _____

Nervous Tunic

The **nervous tunic** consists of the **retina**. The retina is a thin layer of _____ that form the innermost lining of the eye's posterior wall. Although the retina has its own blood supply, it receives most of its nourishment from the _____ layer beneath it.

• What is the function of the retina? _____

_____

The retina has three distinct layers of neurons.

1. **Photoreceptor cells** form the layer closest to the choroid. Photoreceptor cells respond to light and include the aptly named _____ **cells** and _____ **cells**.
   • **Rod cells** are sensitive to low levels of light. Rod cells outnumber cone cells from 100 million to 6 million.
   • **Cone cells** are _____ sensitive and require more light to form a sharper image.

2. **Bipolar cells** are neurons that form a middle layer of the retina.

3. **Ganglion cells** are multipolar neurons that form the innermost layer of the retina. The long axons of the ganglion cells form the _____ nerve (cranial nerve II), which emerges from the posterior eye and extends to the brain. There are *no* _____ cells in the **optic disc** ("blind spot") at the point where the axons form the optic nerve.

Lateral to the optic disc near the center of the retina, a yellow spot known as the **macula lutea** is found. In the center, the focal point known as **fovea centralis** (central fovea) is situated with _____ only. The images formed on this depression in the middle of the macula lutea produces the sharpest images, known as **visual acuity**.

Review Time!

I. *Using the terms in the list below, label the eye illustration.*

1. _____
2. _____
3. _____
4. _____
5. _____
6. _____
7. _____
8. _____
9. _____
10. _____
11. _____
12. _____

Anterior chamber	Fovea centralis	Optic disc (blind spot)	Pupil
Choroid	Iris	Optic nerve	Retina
Cornea	Lens	Posterior chamber	Sclera

II. *Using the terms in the list below, write the appropriate part of the eye in each blank. You may use a term more than once.*

Anterior chamber	Aqueous humor	Choroid	Fibrous tunic
Iris	Lens	Macula lutea	Posterior cavity
Pupil	Retina	Vascular tunic	Vitreous humor

1. The thick, gel-like fluid found in the posterior cavity of the eye   _____
2. The thin, dark-brown membrane that is part of the vascular tunic   _____
3. Rod cells and cone cells populate this layer   _____
4. The opening in the iris   _____
5. Separates the anterior compartment of the eye from the posterior compartment   _____
6. The layer composed of the sclera and cornea   _____
7. Colored part of the eye that can be seen from the exterior   _____
8. The watery fluid found in the anterior compartment of the eye   _____
9. Transparent structure located immediately behind the pupil and iris   _____
10. Part of the anterior compartment in front of the iris   _____
11. The tunic rich in blood vessels that includes the choroid, ciliary body, and iris   _____

12. The fovea centralis sits in a depression in the middle of this yellow spot _____

13. Compartment found behind the lens _____

14. Separates the anterior and posterior chambers _____

15. Detect light and transportation of light to the optic nerve _____

III. Provide a brief answer for each of the following questions about the structures and functions of the parts of the eye.

1. Which structure of the fibrous tunic lacks blood vessels?_____

2. What divides the anterior and posterior compartments? The anterior and posterior chambers?
_____
_____

3. List the cells through which light passes on its way to the optic nerve. _____
_____

4. How does the iris regulate light entry into the eye?_____
_____

5. What purpose does the pigmented layer beneath the choroid serve? _____
_____

6. Which type of photoreceptor cell is sensitive to low levels of light?_____

7. The axon of what type of cell forms the optic nerve (cranial nerve II)?_____

8. What type of photoreceptor cell is the only type present in the fovea centralis?
_____

9. Why does the blind spot, or optic disc, exist?_____
_____

10. What part of the eye is affected when a person has cataracts?_____

11. How can glaucoma lead to blindness?_____
_____

12. Where is the greatest visual acuity in the eye?_____

13. Which type of humor circulates?_____

14. Name two parts of the vascular tunic composed of smooth muscle.
   1. _____
   2. _____

15. Name two parts of the eye that are transparent.
   1. _____
   2. _____

Refraction and Accommodation

LEARNING OBJECTIVE 7. Explain how the eye accommodates and how light is converted to a nerve impulse.

Refraction is the bending of light.

• What structures of the eye refract light? _____
_____

The refraction of light through these structures forms an inverted (upside-down), reduced in size, and reversed from left to right, image on the _____. The brain learns to rearrange image.

Accommodation is the alteration of the lens shape for near and far vision. The shape of the lens is altered by _____ ligaments, which pull and flatten the lens so we can see distance. To see nearby objects, the lens becomes more _____. The lens is the only structure of all those that refract light that accommodates. A normal eye shape, known as an *emmetropic* eye, refracts light rays onto the _____ to form a clear image of that object. Visual problems occur when a lens is too strong or too weak, or structural problems of the eyeball are present.

- **Myopia** is commonly called _____. The eyeball is too long or the refraction is too great so that an image is formed in front of the retina.
- **Hyperopia** is commonly called _____. The eyeball is too short or the lens is weak or "lazy" so that the image focuses behind the retina.
- _____ occurs when the cornea, lens, or both have unequal curvatures. Blurred vision results.

Activation of Rods and Cones

Nerve impulses are converted from patterns of light by photoreceptor cells (rods and cones) in the retina. Recall the following information about rods and cones:

- **Rods** are useful in low, dim, or night situations when little light is available. They are not sensitive to _____. Vision is limited to outlines for figures.
- **Cones** are color sensitive. Sharp images and visual _____ depend on vision from cones. Cones do not share the fiber route to the brain used by rods, which results in the brain's ability to interpret the image sharply.

Both photoreceptor cells (rods and cones) use light-sensitive pigments.

Rhodopsin (visual purple) is a light-sensitive pigment in **rod cells.** Rhodopsin is composed of retinene, which is synthesized from vitamin _____. A deficiency in this vitamin can result in _____ blindness.

- In low levels of light, rhodopsin breaks apart and triggers reactions that lead to hyperpolarization of the rods.
- Hyperpolarization of the rod triggers depolarization of the adjacent bipolar neuron, which stimulates the nearby _____ cell to produce action potentials. Rhodopsin, currently degraded, is resynthesized in preparation for the next light ray. During this time when rhodopsin is regenerated is a period of light insensitivity and we cannot see.

EXAMPLE

Have you ever walked into a dark room from well-lit room and cannot see? Explain why.

_____

Photopsin is a light-sensitive pigment in **cone cells** that react to red, green, and blue light. The decomposition of photopsin in bright light activates an enzyme that triggers reactions and lead to hyperpolarization and the generation of an action potential by ganglion cells.

EXAMPLE

Have you ever been temporarily blinded from a camera's flash? Explain why.

_____

Visual Pathway

LEARNING OBJECTIVE 8. Describe the visual pathway.

• Rods and cones (retina)
• Bipolar neurons (retina)
• _____ cells (retina) generate an action potential if the stimulation is great. enough. Axons of ganglion exit the eye by way of the optic nerve (cranial nerve II).
• Optic nerve (cranial nerve II)
• **Optic chiasma** is the point at which the optic nerves cross as they travel into the brain. Some fibers cross at the chiasma: The fibers from the medial side of the retina cross while those from the lateral side do not. What is the benefit of the mixing of fibers of the two optic nerves? _____ _____

• Optic tracts extend from the optic chiasma to the thalamus. Some fibers terminate in nuclei that control eye reflexes.
• Thalamus sends impulses to the _____ lobe of the cerebral cortex to the **visual cortex** where interpretation of visual signals occurs.

Review Time!

I.   *Provide a brief answer for each of the following questions about the process of vision.*

1. Complete this pathway of vision from the retina to the appropriate lobe of the brain where visual processing occurs: Rods and cones → _____ cells → ganglion cells → optic nerve (cranial nerve _____) → optic _____ → optic tracts → _____ → occipital lobe

2. How is an image formed on the retina different from what we actually see?
    _____
    _____
    _____

3. What structure(s) of the eye can refract light?_____
    _____

4. Which structure is the only one to accommodate for near and far vision?
    _____

5. Explain the role of the lens in the refraction of light. _____

6. What pigments are present in rods? In cones? _____
    _____

7. What accounts for the temporary insensitivity to light when you step out of your house at night to gaze at the night sky, yet you can see very little? _____
    _____
    _____

8. Explain what part of the visual pathway accounts for three-dimensional vision and depth perception? _____
    _____

9. What vitamin deficiency leads to night blindness?_____

10. What accounts for an astigmatism? _____
_____

11. What types of light are the rods and cones most sensitive to?_____
_____
_____

Hearing

The sense of hearing is combined with equilibrium, both of which are detected by mechanoreceptors.

Structures of the Ear

LEARNING OBJECTIVE 9. Identify the parts of the ear.

The organ of hearing is the ear. Sound waves produce action potentials in receptor cells that ultimately reach the brain. The three parts of the ear are the external ear, the middle ear, and the inner ear.

External Ear

1. **Auricle** is the external appendage that collects _____ and channels them into a tube that travels into the temporal bone.

2. **External auditory canal** is a tube that extends into the _____ bone created by the external auditory meatus. Glands in the canal secrete a waxy lubricant known as **cerumen** (ear wax). The canal channels sound waves to the eardrum.

Middle Ear

Middle ear (_____ cavity) is the air-filled space within the temporal bone bordered by the eardrum and one of the tiny ossicles.

1. **Auditory (eustachian) tube** is a narrow tube that allows air to pass from the throat to the tympanic cavity and enables air pressure on both sides of the tympanic membrane to equalize. Infections that travel along the mucous membrane lining from the mouth and throat to the middle ear are called _____ . If infection spreads to the air cells of the mastoid process of the temporal bone, the condition is called *mastoiditis*. Both conditions can lead to permanent hearing loss.

2. **Tympanic membrane** (eardrum) is a thin barrier separating the outer and _____ ears. It receives sound waves from the external auditory canal and transmits them to the tiny ear bones (ossicles). Sound waves cause the membrane to vibrate; the vibrations are transmitted to the auditory ossicles.

3. **Ossicles** are the **malleus** (hammer), _____ (anvil), and **stapes** (stirrup). Sound waves traveling through the ossicles are amplified (made louder). Vibrations continue to the **oval window**, which sits beneath _____ and opens into the cochlea of the inner ear. The vibrations continue in the inner ear by causing fluids to move.

Inner Ear

Inner ear is a fluid-filled **labyrinth.** There are two portions of the labyrinth: the outer **bony labyrinth** and the inner **membranous labyrinth**. The **bony labyrinth** is a series of canals that includes the semicircular canals, vestibule, and cochlea. The membranous labyrinth is a series of sacs and tubes that lies within the walls of the bony labyrinth. **Perilymph** is the fluid situated between the walls of the bony labyrinth and the walls of the membranous labyrinth. **Endolymph** is the fluid inside the _____.

1. **Semicircular canals** consist of three loops at right angles to each other.
2. **Vestibule** is a chamber between the _____ canals and the cochlea. It functions in equilibrium.
3. **Cochlea** is a snail shell–shaped structure formed by spiral and coiled canals. The bony labyrinth divides it into upper and lower compartments.
   - Upper compartment is the **vestibular duct** (scala vestibuli). The vestibular duct extends from the _____ window to the end of the cochlea.
   - Lower compartment is the **tympanic duct** (scala tympani). The tympanic duct extends in the opposite direction to the vestibular duct and travels from the end of the cochlea to the _____ window.

A third channel is seen in cross section; it is part of the membranous labyrinth.

   - The _____ **duct** is separated from the vestibular duct by the **vestibular membrane** while it is separated from the tympanic duct by the **basilar membrane.** The **organ of Corti** (spiral organ) sits atop the basilar membrane. The organ of Corti is a series of _____ cells that support hair cells. The hair cells are the mechanoreceptors of hearing. The free ends of the hair cells have cilia that extend into the endolymph of the cochlear duct. The **tectorial membrane** is a gelatinous membrane that lies over the cilia of the hair cells while the basal ends of the hair cells contact the nerve fibers of the cochlear nerve (branch of cranial nerve VIII, _____ nerve).

Review Time!

I. *Using the terms in the list below, label the parts of the ear.*

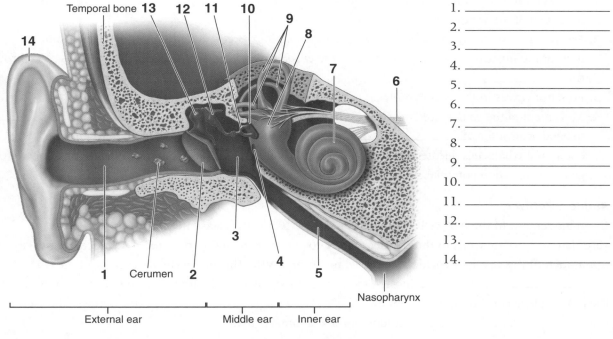

1. _____
2. _____
3. _____
4. _____
5. _____
6. _____
7. _____
8. _____
9. _____
10. _____
11. _____
12. _____
13. _____
14. _____

Auditory tube	Incus	Semicircular canals	Vestibular cochlear nerve
Auricle	Malleus	Stapes	Vestibule
Cochlea	Oval window	Tympanic cavity	
External auditory canal	Round window	Tympanic membrane	

II. *Using the terms in the list below, write the appropriate part of the ear in each blank. You may use a term more than once.*

Auditory ossicles	*Auditory (eustachian) tube*	*Auricle*	*Vestibule*
Cochlea	*External auditory canal*	*Tympanic membrane*	

1. Cerumen is a waxy lubricant present in this canal _____

2. Function is to equalize pressure on both sides of the tympanic membrane _____

3. External appendage that collects sound waves in the air _____

4. Vibrates with sound waves against the malleus _____

5. Resembles a snail shell _____

6. Malleus, incus, and stapes _____

7. Outer boundary for the middle ear _____

8. Houses the vestibular, tympanic, and cochlear ducts _____

9. Separates the outer and middle ears _____

10. Chamber situated between the semicircular canals and the cochlea _____

Physiology of Hearing

LEARNING OBJECTIVE 10. **Trace the path of sound waves through the ear to the generation of nerve impulses that reach the brain.**

Vibrations transmitted through the *tympanic membrane* land with the _____ *(malleus, incus, stapes).*

1. *Stapes* vibrates back and forth and pushes the *oval window* in and out. Waves are produced in the *perilymph* of the inner ear.

2. *Perilymph* pressure waves pass through the *vestibular duct* (*scala vestibuli*) and push the vestibular membrane inward, increasing pressure of the *endolymph* within the cochlear duct. Waves pass through the _____ *window* and into the *tympanic cavity.*

3. Pressure waves in the endolymph cause the basilar membrane to move slightly.

4. Movement of the *basilar membrane* causes the hair cells of the organ of _____ to bend against the _____ *membrane*. If the movement of the hair cells is great enough, the hair cells release neurotransmitters that stimulate sensory neurons in the cochlear nerve to generate an action potential.

Auditory Pathway

If the movement of the hair cells is great enough, the hair cells release neurotransmitters that stimulate sensory neurons in the cochlear nerve to generate an action potential. The cochlear nerve is a branch of the vestibulocochlear nerve, cranial nerve VIII. This nerve carries the impulse to the _____ in the brain stem at which point the impulses cross to the opposite side of the brain before continuing to the midbrain, _____, and to the auditory area of the _____ lobe of the cerebral cortex.

Equilibrium

LEARNING OBJECTIVE 11. Distinguish between the two mechanisms of equilibrium.

Where are the receptors for equilibrium located? _____

Equilibrium includes two types: static equilibrium and dynamic equilibrium.

Static Equilibrium

Static equilibrium is the sensation of body position, mainly the _____. Receptors are housed in the _____ of the inner ear. Static equilibrium provides information about:

• Exact position of the head needed to maintain _____

• _____ acceleration, such as riding in a car that speeds up quickly

How is static equilibrium detected? Two sacs in the membranous labyrinth of the vestibule are the _____ and _____. These sacs are connected by a duct. The **macula** is inside the walls of these two sacs and formed by two types of receptor cells: supporting _____ cells and _____ cells. These cells have microvilli and a single cilium that extend into a thick, jelly-like mass embedded with carbonate crystals known as _____. The movement of the otoliths in the macula causes the hair cells to bend and stimulate the release of neurotransmitters by the hair cells. If you tilt your head upward or downward, an action potential is transmitted in the _____ nerve (branch of the vestibulocochlear nerve, cranial nerve VIII). The impulse terminates in the cerebellum for interpretation.

Dynamic Equilibrium

Dynamic equilibrium is the sensation of rapid movements (of the head) in response to rotational acceleration (turning your head left or right). Receptors are housed in the _____ canals of the inner ear and assist in balancing the head and body when moved suddenly.

How is dynamic equilibrium detected? Dynamic equilibrium is sensed in an expanded region of the membranous labyrinth of the _____ known as the **ampulla.** The ampulla contains the **cristae,** the sensory organs that contain supporting cells and hair cells. The hair cells are the _____ and their hair-like processes extend into a jelly-like mass known as the **cupula.** When the head shifts rapidly, the shifting of the cupula causes the processes of the hair cells to bend.

• What happens to generate a nerve impulse? _____
_____

• Where within the brain is dynamic equilibrium processed? _____

Review Time!

I. Provide a brief answer for each of the following questions about the processes of hearing and equilibrium.

1. Once sound is transmitted by the tympanic membrane to the malleus, name the parts of the ear it travels through to the cochlear nerve. _____
_____
_____

2. Discuss the role of the hair cells of the organ of Corti in conducting sound waves.

_____

_____

_____

3. Discuss the functions of the oval window and round window. _____

_____

4. How do you think hearing would be affected if the auditory ossicles could not vibrate and amplify sound waves? _____

5. How do you think hearing would be affected if the hair cells of the organ of Corti were damaged from working in a loud environment? _____

_____

6. Which part of the ear is fluid filled? _____

7. Distinguish between the type of sensory information transmitted over the vestibular branch and the cochlear branch of the vestibulocochlear nerve. _____

_____

8. Where are static equilibrium receptors housed in the inner ear? _____

9. Where are dynamic equilibrium receptors housed in the inner ear? _____

10. Describe the role of otoliths in the detection of static equilibrium. _____

_____

_____

11. Explain the role of the cupula in the detection of dynamic equilibrium.

_____

_____

_____

12. What lobe of the brain interprets sound? _____

13. What role does the cerebellum play in the pathway of sensations traveling from the inner ear?

_____

_____

_____

14. Why do you think riding feverishly fast on a merry-go-round leaves you with the lingering sensation of motion once you dismount from the ride? _____

_____

_____

15. Even with your eyes shut, you can still sense the car in which you are a passenger has sped up very quickly. Is this sensation an example of dynamic equilibrium or static equilibrium? Explain your choice. _____

_____

_____

The Endocrine System

Tips for Success as You Begin

Read Chapter 10 from your textbook before attending class. Listen when you attend lecture and fill in the blanks in this notebook. You may choose to complete the blanks before attending class as a way to prepare for the day's topics. The same day you attend lecture, read the material again and complete the exercises after each section in this notebook. Spend time every day with this chapter as it will help you make sense of the material. Hormones can be difficult to remember without sufficient, frequent review. You may want to spend time creating flash cards for your studies.

Introduction to the Endocrine System

What is the primary role of the endocrine system? _____

_____

The endocrine system uses **hormones** to affect body structures. Hormones circulate through the blood until they reach a target cell. Hormone action is slower but longer-lasting than the actions of the _____ system.

- What are some of the ways in which hormones affect cells? _____

_____

_____

CONCEPT 1

Composition of the Endocrine System

Concept: The endocrine system is composed of numerous glands that secrete their products into the extracellular space, eventually diffusing into the bloodstream. These products are the hormones.

LEARNING OBJECTIVE 1. Distinguish between exocrine glands and endocrine glands.

LEARNING OBJECTIVE 2. Identify the primary endocrine glands of the body and their locations.

Glands of the endocrine system produce and secrete hormones. Recall the two types of glands, introduced in Chapter 4:

- _____ **glands** secrete products into ducts that travel into body cavities, spaces within organs, or onto body surfaces. Recall that these include oil, sweat, mucous, and salivary glands.

215

• _____ **glands** are *ductless* and secrete their products (hormones) into the surrounding space outside the cells. The hormones then diffuse into the blood stream.

As we discuss the glands of the endocrine system, add labels to the illustration below. When you are done, you should be able to identify the glands of the endocrine system listed below.

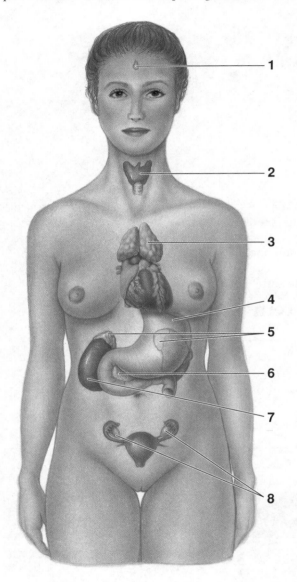

1. _____
2. _____
3. _____
4. _____
5. _____
6. _____
7. _____
8. _____

Adrenal glands	Pancreas	Thymus gland
Gonads (ovaries)	Pituitary gland	Thyroid and parathyroid gland
Kidneys	Stomach	

CONCEPT 2

Hormones

Concept: Hormones act only upon cells to which they selectively bind. The two major types of hormones are water soluble, which cannot pass through the cell membrane barrier without assistance, and lipid soluble, which can easily pass across the cell membrane.

LEARNING OBJECTIVE 3. Explain why a hormone affects only target cells.

Hormones only cause action in cells to which they can bind. Hormones can generally be classified as water soluble or lipid soluble. Water-soluble hormones cannot pass through the cell membrane without assistance while lipid-soluble hormones can easily pass.

Hormonal Action

Hormones only influence _____ **cells**. These cells have protein molecules in their cell membranes known as receptors. Receptors bind to or reject specific hormones. Does a hormone have the ability to affect cells of the target organ if there are no receptors for that particular hormone?

_____

_____

Once binding has occurred, the hormone can change the cell's activities, such as the metabolic processes or protein synthesis.

LEARNING OBJECTIVE 4. Distinguish between water-soluble and lipid-soluble hormones by their entry into the cell to cause cellular change.

Water-soluble Hormones

Let's consider the water-soluble hormones:
- What types of hormones are water soluble? _____
- Can water-soluble hormones travel across the cell membrane? _____

Water-soluble hormones use the **second-messenger system**, described next:
- The *first messenger* is the hormone. The hormone binds to a receptor on the target cell's cell _____.
- _____ is activated, which in turn activates **adenylate cyclase**.
- Adenylate cyclase converts _____ to cyclic AMP, the *second messenger*.
- Cyclic AMP diffuses throughout the cell, promoting chemical reactions that activate _____ known as **protein kinases**.
- Protein kinases react with other molecules to cause changes in the target cell.

  Examples of hormones that are water soluble and utilize the second-messenger system

_____

_____

_____

TIP! The cascading set of changes seen here with a water-soluble hormone is similar to what happens when you ring the doorbell. As the first messenger, you play the role of the hormone by binding with the receptor on the cell membrane (and ring the doorbell). As the hormone, however, you do not enter the house. The signaling chain of events begins inside the house when the person answering the door receives your message. The person who answers the door plays the role of cyclic AMP (the second messenger). Once the communication has been made by you to the person answering the door, a set of changes eventually result in the activation of protein kinases.

Lipid-soluble Hormones

Hormones that dissolve in lipids mainly include _____ hormones that can pass directly through the cell membrane. What happens next?

- Once inside the cell, the hormone binds to a protein receptor located within the _____.
- The hormone–receptor complex enters the _____.
- The complex binds a specific region of DNA and activates protein synthesis.

The result? Lipid-soluble proteins activate genes to make new proteins and enzymes.

Examples of hormones that stimulate protein synthesis are _____
_____
_____

TIP! How can lipid-soluble hormones travel directly through the cell membrane without using the second-messenger system? You may want to review Chapter 3 for information about the cell membrane structure. The phospholipids that create the bilayer of the cell membrane have nonpolar, hydrophilic heads and polar, hydrophobic tails. These phospholipids allow lipid-soluble hormones to travel through the bilayer, but not water-soluble hormones.

Prostaglandins

LEARNING OBJECTIVE 5. Describe how prostaglandins differ from hormones and how they affect the body.

Prostaglandins, or local hormones, are hormone-like lipids that regulate nearly all cells.

- What organs produce prostaglandins? _____
_____

Function: Prostaglandins travel across cell membranes by diffusion and inhibit or stimulate the formation of _____. In turn, prostaglandins affect hormones that use cyclic AMP.

- Do you recall if water-soluble *or* lipid-soluble hormones activate cyclic AMP?
_____

- Why are prostaglandins *not* considered true hormones? _____
_____

Hormonal Control

LEARNING OBJECTIVE 6. Distinguish between negative feedback, positive feedback, and nervous control of hormone secretion.

Feedback Control

Chemical signals sent to _____ glands through the blood stream tell these glands to adjust their rate of secretion. Two systems that operate in this way are negative feedback systems and positive feedback systems.

Negative feedback systems control hormone secretion by responding in the *opposite* direction of the stimulus. Hormone release or secretion is *inhibited* by this system. This is the *most common* method of feedback control.

- Explain how parathyroid hormone is an example of the positive feedback system.
_____
_____
_____

Positive feedback systems are unstable and uncommon. The response is provided by the system in the *same* direction as the stimulus in an effort to cause the endocrine gland to *increase* its rate or hormone release.

- Explain how oxytocin (OT) is an example of the positive feedback system.

_____

_____

_____

Nervous Control

Nervous control regulates only some endocrine glands, such as the adrenal _____ and the _____ .

CONCEPT 3

Pituitary Gland

Concept: The pituitary gland receives its control from the hypothalamus to produce many hormones, some of which control the activities of other glands. It includes an anterior and a posterior lobe.

LEARNING OBJECTIVE 7. Describe the anatomical features of the pituitary gland.

LEARNING OBJECTIVE 8. Identify the hormones secreted by the pituitary gland, the action of each hormone, and how the secretion of each hormone is regulated.

The pituitary gland:
- Sits in the sella turcica of the _____ bone.
- Is attached to the hypothalamus by a stalk known as the _____ .
- Produces a wide variety of hormones.
- Receives regulating hormones from the _____ .
- Has two portions: the larger glandular anterior lobe and the smaller nervous posterior lobe.

Anterior Lobe

The anterior lobe of the pituitary gland:
- Is composed of glandular epithelium.
- Has 5 types of secretory cells that produce _____ (*how many*) types of hormones. We discuss those hormones next.

Growth Hormone (GH)
Primary effects:
- Stimulates body cells to grow and divide
- Promotes _____ in cell size
- Increases rate of catabolism of carbohydrates and fats (*Recall that catabolism is* _____
_____)
- Maintains blood glucose (short term)

Regulation of release is via negative feedback:
- _____ (low blood glucose "sugar") triggers an increase in the release of GH. GH promotes the conversion of glycogen to glucose. Glucose enters the blood and raises blood glucose levels.
- _____ (high blood glucose "sugar") inhibits GH release.

Thyroid-stimulating Hormone (TSH)

Primary effects:
- Regulates cellular metabolism
- Targets the _____ gland to produce and secrete two hormones. Since TSH targets another endocrine gland, it is considered a **tropic hormone**.

Regulation of release is via negative feedback:
- Low levels of thyroid hormones stimulate the hypothalamus to produce releasing hormones that stimulate TSH production. Increases in TSH will cause an increased rate of thyroid hormone secretion.
- High levels of thyroid hormones inhibit TSH production. In turn, how is the hypothalamus affected? _____

Adrenocorticotropic Hormone (ACTH)

Primary effects:
- Targets the adrenal cortex (outer region) to produce certain hormones.

Regulation of release is via negative feedback:
- Low levels of adrenal cortex hormones stimulate the release of releasing hormones produced by the _____ to increase ACTH production.
- Various forms of stress influence release of ACTH.

Follicle-stimulating Hormone (FSH)

Primary effects:
- In females, FSH (1) stimulates egg development within the ovaries, and (2) stimulates ovaries to release _____ (female sex hormones).
- In males, FSH stimulates _____ production by testes.
- FSH is a **gonadotropic hormone** because it targets the gonads.

Regulation of release:
- Releasing hormones produced by the hypothalamus control FSH production in response to _____ (female) and _____ (male).

Luteinizing Hormone (LH)

Primary effects:
- In females, LH works with estrogen to (1) stimulate the release of an ovum (egg) from the ovary (known as ovulation) and (2) prepare the _____ for implantation of the fertilized ovum.
- In males, LH stimulates cells of the testes to produce and secrete testosterone.
- LH is a **gonadotropic hormone** because it targets the _____.

Regulation of release:
- Regulating factors released by the hypothalamus control LH secretion

Prolactin (PRL)

Primary effects:

- Stimulate and maintain milk production (part of the process known as _____. This process also involves the ejection of breast milk from mammary glands, which is controlled by a different hormone).

Regulation of release:

- Releasing hormones from the hypothalamus can inhibit or stimulate PRL production.
- PRL levels are influenced by hormonal changes occurring during menstruation, _____, and delivery of an infant.

Posterior Lobe

The posterior lobe of the pituitary gland:

- Is an extension of the hypothalamus and is thus constructed mostly of neuroglial cells that support the terminal ends of axons. The cell bodies are housed in the _____ and are called **neurosecretory cells**. These cell bodies make oxytocin (OT) and antidiuretic hormone (ADH).
- Produces no hormones. It only stores hormones made by the hypothalamus until it is time for their release.

Oxytocin (OT)

Primary effects:

- Stimulate contractions of smooth muscle in the wall of the _____.
- Stimulates cells around _____ ducts to contract, causing milk ejection.
- Readies the uterus for birth toward the end of pregnancy.

Regulation of release is via _____ feedback:

- OT increases throughout pregnancy and signals the beginning of uterine contractions for birth.
- Although levels of OT decline after birth, they rise again when an infant suckles the _____ and the hypothalamus is stimulated.

Antidiuretic Hormone (ADH)

Primary effects:

- Regulate _____ balance in the body.
- Reduce urine flow by moving water from the kidney into the bloodstream, reducing sweat production, and constricting the smooth muscle in blood vessels (vasoconstriction) to elevate _____.
- Increase body fluid volume.

Regulation of release:

- Hypothalamus detects osmotic pressure in the blood using osmoreceptors. Recall that osmotic pressure increases when you become _____ and the blood is less dilute. In other words, the more solutes in your blood, the higher the osmotic pressure.
- How does ADH promote water balance when body fluids are low? _____
  _____
  _____
- What is the effect on ADH when the blood is dilute after having drunk a large volume of water? _____
  _____
  _____

Review Time!

I. *Using the terms in the list below, write the appropriate hormone in each blank. You may use a term more than once.*

ACTH	*ADH*	*FSH*	*GH*
LH	*OT*	*PRL*	

1. Stimulates the production of some hormones by the adrenal cortex   _____

2. Regulates fluid balance in response to increased osmotic pressure   _____

3. Promotes growth and cell division   _____

4. Stored in the posterior pituitary until released to start uterine contractions   _____

5. Released in response to hypoglycemia   _____

6. Promotes milk ejection   _____

7. Stimulates and maintains milk production for breastfeeding   _____

8. Promotes ovulation   _____

9. Promotes water reabsorption from the kidney and reduces perspiration   _____

10. Type of gonadotropic hormone that stimulates sperm production by the testes   _____

11. Stimulates contraction of the smooth muscle of the uterus   _____

12. Reduces urine output   _____

13. Promotes secretion of testosterone   _____

14. Stored in the posterior pituitary; also known as vasopressin   _____

15. Operates under positive feedback control   _____

II. *Provide a brief answer for each of the following questions about the hypothalamus and pituitary gland.*

1. Name two hormones released by the posterior pituitary that are made by the hypothalamus.

   1. _____

   2. _____

2. What triggers the release of ADH? Explain. _____

   _____

   _____

3. Explain how ADH promotes fluid retention. _____

   _____

   _____

4. Why must OT and PRL work together? What is produced through the concerted efforts of these two hormones? _____

   _____

   _____

5. What differences exist between the anterior and posterior pituitary lobes in terms of types of tissue constructing each? _____

   _____

   _____

6. What is the function of a tropic hormone? Provide an example and explain how it operates as a tropic hormone. _____

_____

_____

7. What are gonadotropic hormones? Provide two examples and explain how one of your examples operates as a gonadotropic hormone. _____

_____

_____

_____

_____

8. What effect does hyperglycemia have on growth hormone production?

_____

_____

9. If the pituitary gland was removed, list the hormones and glands that would be affected as a result. _____

_____

_____

_____

10. Sarah has problems with her thyroid gland and is often tired. Her thyroid gland does not produce enough thyroid hormones. Which anterior pituitary hormone should be checked? Why?

_____

_____

_____

CONCEPT 4

Thyroid Gland and Parathyroid Glands

Concept: The thyroid and parathyroid glands are located in the neck. Thyroid gland hormones help regulate metabolism and growth, and reduce calcium and phosphate levels in the bloodstream. Parathyroid hormone increases calcium and phosphate levels.

LEARNING OBJECTIVE 9. Describe the anatomical features of the thyroid and parathyroid glands.

LEARNING OBJECTIVE 10. Identify the hormones secreted by the thyroid and parathyroid glands, the action of each hormone, and how the secretion of each hormone is regulated.

Where are the thyroid and parathyroid glands located? _____

_____

While the thyroid gland regulates metabolism, both the thyroid and parathyroid glands manage calcium and phosphorus levels in body fluids such as the blood.

Thyroid Gland

Location: The thyroid gland sits in the neck, below the larynx in front of the trachea. It has a _____ shape connected by a bridge known as the *isthmus*.

Structure: Constructed of glandular epithelium, the thyroid gland has hollow compartments called **thyroid follicles**.

- Follicular cells are simple _____ epithelium; they line the follicle walls. Colloid, a thick and clear fluid, is housed within the follicle. What hormones are made by the follicle cells? _____

- Parafollicular cells are situated between the follicular cells. What hormone is produced by the parafollicular cells? _____

Thyroxine (T_4) and Triiodothyronine (T_3)

Functions:

T_4 and T_3 target nearly every cell of the human body.

- Stimulate metabolism rate
- Promote _____ synthesis
- Increase _____ uptake
- Increase lipid metabolism
- Increase nervous system actions

Regulation of release is via negative feedback involving the hypothalamus, anterior pituitary, and thyroid gland.

- If thyroid hormone levels *decrease,* the hypothalamus secretes a releasing hormone (thyroid-releasing hormone, or TRH) to trigger the release of _____ from the anterior pituitary. As a result, TSH stimulates the follicle cells to release _____ and _____ into the bloodstream.

- What happens once levels of T_3 and T_4 are restored to normal? _____ _____ _____

> **TIP!** TRH is made by the hypothalamus; TRH targets the anterior pituitary gland and stimulates the release of TSH. TSH now travels to the thyroid gland to stimulate the release of thyroid hormones, T_3 and T_4.

Calcitonin

Do you recall what cells of the thyroid gland make and secrete calcitonin? _____

Functions:

- Lowers _____ and _____ levels in the blood.
- Works in conjunction with parathyroid hormone (PTH) to maintain normal concentrations of these ions.

Regulation of release is via negative feedback:

- If calcium levels *increase,* calcitonin secretion _____.
- Calcitonin inhibits osteoclasts from dissolving bone matrix, which in turn favors the activity of bone-producing cells known as _____.
- Calcitonin stimulates excretion and loss of calcium and phosphate ions by the _____. These ions are lost from the urine as they are removed from the blood.

Parathyroid Glands

Location: Four to five pea-sized glands sit embedded in the posterior side of the _____ gland.

> **TIP!** Remember that the parathyroid glands sit around the thyroid gland.

Structure: Constructed of _____ epithelium, the parathyroid glands secrete only one hormone, parathyroid hormone (PTH).

Parathyroid Hormone (PTH)
Functions:

- Maintain _____ and _____ levels in the blood along with calcitonin.
- PTH increases blood calcium levels by increasing osteoclasts in bone tissue. Osteoclasts break down bone matrix to release calcium ions (bone resorption). *What does calcitonin do?* _____
  _____
- PTH stimulates conversion of precursor molecules to form vitamin _____.
- PTH decreases blood phosphate levels; phosphate is excreted by the kidneys.

Regulation of release is via negative feedback with *no* influence by the hypothalamus or pituitary gland.

- Low blood _____ levels stimulate the release of PTH.

Review Time!

I. *Place a number from 1 to 3 in the blank before each statement to indicate the correct order of the release of the following hormones.*

   _____ T_3 and T_4

   _____ TSH

   _____ TRH

II. *Provide a brief answer for each of the following questions about the thyroid and parathyroid glands.*

1. Name two hormones that regulate blood levels of calcium and phosphate.

    1. _____

    2. _____

2. What is the target of thyroid-releasing hormone (TRH)? _____

3. What effect does an increase in blood calcium have on the secretion of PTH?

    _____

    _____

4. Name two hormones produced and secreted by the thyroid gland that regulate cell metabolism.

    1. _____

    2. _____

5. What hormone is made by the follicular cells of the thyroid gland? _____

6. What hormone is made by the parafollicular cells of the thyroid gland? _____

7. What effect does an increase in thyroxine (T_4) have on TRH release? _____

8. What effect does PTH have on osteoclast activity? _____
    _____

9. Explain how the effects of PTH and calcitonin are opposite to each other.

_____

_____

_____

_____

10. Under what conditions will PTH promote the reabsorption of calcium ions from the kidney?

_____

CONCEPT 5

Adrenal Glands

Concept: Each adrenal gland contains two portions, an inner medulla and an outer cortex. Hormones released by the medulla perform functions similar to the sympathetic division of the ANS, and those of the cortex have varied roles in regulating fluid balance, carbohydrate metabolism, and sexual development.

LEARNING OBJECTIVE   11. Describe the anatomical features of the adrenal glands.

LEARNING OBJECTIVE   12. Identify the hormones secreted by the adrenal glands, the action of each hormone, and how the secretion of each hormone is regulated.

The adrenal glands sit atop each _____, behind the peritoneum. The two portions of the adrenal gland are the adrenal medulla and the adrenal cortex. We discuss both parts next.

Adrenal Medulla

Structure: Modified nervous tissue that forms the adrenal medulla arose from the sympathetic division of the autonomic nervous system.

Function: The adrenal medulla secretes two hormones:

1. _____

2. _____

Epinephrine and norepinephrine (NE) are functionally similar and have the same effect on the body as the neurotransmitters. As neurotransmitters, these chemicals promote the _____ response. As hormones that travel in the blood, epinephrine (adrenaline) and norepinephrine (noradrenaline) have a long-lasting effect than neurotransmitters because hormones are removed more slowly from blood than neurotransmitters are from synapses. Since epinephrine and norepinephrine cause changes that mimic the sympathetic nervous system, they are called _____. The effects they promote include:

- ↑ metabolic rate (↑ *means* "increased")
- ↑ heart rate
- ↑ alertness
- ↑ enlargement of the airways
- routing of blood to vital organs (such as _____, _____, _____ muscles)

Regulation of release: Nervous system control increases release of epinephrine and norepinephrine during times of _____ (such as injury, disease, or pain). The hypothalamus detects anxiety, then conducts a message along sympathetic preganglionic neurons to the adrenal medulla to increase secretion.

Adrenal Cortex

Structure: The adrenal cortex is composed of glandular epithelium. Cells are arranged in three distinct layers (outer, middle, and inner).

Function: Steroid hormones, derived from _____ are made by each layer.

> **TIP!** As you learn the adrenal cortex hormones, remember that "corticoid" reminds us of a "steroid hormone from the cortex" while the prefix tells us what is being regulated. Mineralocorticoids regulate "minerals" such as sodium and potassium while glucocorticoids regulate "*sugar*" (gluco).

Mineralocorticoids

Aldosterone is the primary mineralocorticoid.

Functions: Aldosterone maintains the balance of body fluids by regulating the concentration of

_____ and _____ ions. Aldosterone promotes target

organs to retain _____ and to remove _____.

- If sodium is retained, then water will also be retained since water follows sodium by osmosis. Water retention increases blood volume and in turn, blood pressure.
- If sodium is lost in the urine, _____ will also be lost. Since loss of fluids reduces blood volume, blood pressure will also decrease.

Target organ: Aldosterone targets the kidneys, sweat glands, salivary glands, and digestive tract.

Regulation of release: Aldosterone is released in response to:

- Decrease in blood pressure due to a decrease in blood pressure. *Renin–angiotensin mechanism* is the regulatory mechanism that helps to restore blood pressure.
- Decrease in _____ ion concentration in the blood. Renin–angiotensin mechanism is the regulatory mechanism that helps to restore sodium ion concentration.
- Increase in _____ levels of the extracellular fluids.

Glucocorticoids

Glucocorticoids include **cortisol, corticosterone**, and **cortisone**. _____ is the most abundant.

Functions:

- Promote an increase in glucose in blood through the breakdown of proteins into amino acids by

  the _____ (*what organ?*), a process known as *gluconeogenesis*.

> **TIP!** Break down the term: *gluco* = sugar, *neo* = new, *genesis* = beginning

- Inhibit allergic reactions (by suppressing the _____ system).
- Decrease inflammation (by suppressing the _____ system).

Regulation of release: ACTH (from the pituitary gland) stimulates the release of glucocorticoids from the adrenal cortex, under negative feedback control.

Androgens

Androgens are produced by both males and females throughout life in small quantities. Here are some androgens and disorders related to them:

- **DHEA** produces masculinizing effects in a young male before puberty. It is replaced

  by _____ during and after puberty. Females secrete a different androgen.

• **Masculinization** in females is called *virilism* and is due to a disease called *congenital adrenal hyperplasia (CAH)*. What physical effects would a female experience? _____

_____

_____

CONCEPT 6

Pancreas

Concept: The pancreatic islets produce two primary hormones that have opposing effects. Together they help maintain glucose levels in the blood to stay within the range of homeostasis.

LEARNING OBJECTIVE   13. Describe the anatomical features of the pancreatic islets.

LEARNING OBJECTIVE   14. Identify the hormones secreted by the pancreatic islets, the action of each hormone, and how the secretion of each hormone is regulated.

Location: The pancreas is situated in the _____ cavity behind the stomach.

Function: The pancreas has a dual function. As an endocrine gland, it secretes two hormones (insulin and glucagon) that regulate blood _____ levels. As an exocrine gland, it secretes digestive enzymes into the small intestine.

Structure: Pancreatic islets produce two hormones:

• *Alpha* cells secrete glucagon.
• *Beta* cells secrete insulin.

Glucagon

Function: Glucagon raises blood glucose levels in response to a decline in blood glucose.

Target organ: Glucagon targets the _____ to break down glycogen into glucose. Do you recall what type of organic compound glycogen is? _____

Regulation of release: Negative feedback. How does the pancreas respond to blood glucose levels that are too low? The alpha cells release glucagon. Glucagon is inhibited by _____ (*low* or *high?*) blood glucose levels.

Insulin

Functions: Insulin also regulates blood glucose levels by:

• Lowering blood glucose levels in response to an increase in blood glucose (opposing glucagon).
• Inhibiting _____.
• Facilitating uptake of glucose by binding to receptors on the cell membranes of skeletal muscle, cardiac muscle, and adipose cells. If the glucose is no longer in the blood stream, then the glucose levels are effectively lowered.

Regulation of release is by negative feedback.

• How does the pancreas respond to blood glucose levels that are too high? The beta cells release _____. Insulin is inhibited by low blood glucose levels.

• **Diabetes mellitus** is a disease that occurs when the _____ cannot produce normal insulin levels or there is a failure of the cell membrane receptors to recognize and bind insulin.

Review Time!

I.   *Using the terms in the list below, write the appropriate hormone in each blank. You may use a term more than once.*

Aldosterone   Cortisol   Epinephrine and norepinephrine

Glucagon   Insulin

1. Released by the beta cells of the pancreatic islets   _____
2. Regulated by the renin–angiotensin pathway   _____
3. Increases blood volume and blood pressure through reabsorption of sodium ions and water   _____
4. Increases alertness, metabolic rate, and blood flow to vital organs   _____
5. Released in response to high blood glucose levels   _____
6. Release by the alpha cells of the pancreatic islets   _____
7. Mimics the effects of the "fight or flight" response   _____
8. Anti-inflammatory effect   _____
9. Inhibits allergic reactions   _____
10. Produced by the adrenal medulla   _____

II.   *Provide a brief answer for each of the following questions about the adrenal glands and the pancreas.*

1. Compare the effects of growth hormone, glucocorticoids, epinephrine, norepinephrine, and glucagon on glucose levels. _____
   _____
   _____
   _____
   _____

2. Name the hormone responsible for gluconeogenesis. _____
3. What hormone inhibits gluconeogenesis? _____
4. What are the three primary effects of aldosterone? _____
   _____
   _____
   _____

5. What effect does an increase in potassium levels have on aldosterone secretion? Where does the excess potassium go? _____
   _____
   _____

6. Which hormonal insufficiency is the cause of diabetes mellitus? _____
7. Name the hormone responsible for lowering blood glucose levels. _____
8. April was alarmed to learn she has testosterone in her blood. Which gland secretes it?
   _____
   _____

9. Explain how prolonged stress can lead to increased blood pressure and heart rate.

_____

_____

_____

10. Although both aldosterone and ADH influence fluid balance, they operate differently. Discuss how these hormones operate and what triggers each to be released. _____

_____

_____

_____

11. An 18-wheeler truck just nearly missed hitting Sam head-on while he was driving. Exasperated, he pulls over to the side of the road with his heart pounding. What other symptoms do you think he is experiencing as a result of the effects of adrenaline and noradrenaline? _____

_____

_____

CONCEPT 7

Gonads, Pineal Gland, and Thymus Gland

Concept: The gonads—the testes and ovaries—are the sex glands that produce the sex hormones. The pineal gland is located within the cranial cavity and secretes a hormone that regulates day and night cycles, and the thymus gland in the thoracic cavity secretes a hormone that plays a role in the immune response.

LEARNING OBJECTIVE 15. Describe the anatomical features of the gonads, pineal gland, and thymus gland.

LEARNING OBJECTIVE 16. Identify the hormones secreted by the male and female gonads, the pineal gland, and the thymus gland, and the action of each hormone.

Gonads

The gonads are paired reproductive organs: _____ in females and _____ in males.

- **Females:** The ovaries are located in the pelvic cavity and secrete estrogen and progesterone starting at puberty under the direction of FSH. What are some of the effects of estrogen on a female?

_____

- **Males:** The testes are located in a sac, the scrotum, outside the pelvic cavity and start secreting testosterone. What are some of the effects of testosterone on a male? _____

_____

Pineal Gland

Location: The pineal gland is located in the cranial cavity, in the brain, as part of the _____.

Structure: The pineal gland is composed of modified neurons and neuroglial cells and innervated by neurons of the sympathetic nervous pathway.

Function: One hormone, **melatonin**, is secreted by the pineal gland. What are the three functions of melatonin?

1. _____

2. _____

3. _____

Thymus Gland

Location: The thymus gland lies in the mediastinum superior to the heart. It is prominent early in life, but diminishes in early adulthood.

Function: The thymus gland secretes a group of hormones called _____ which stimulate and promote the development and maturation of certain white blood cells known as T lymphocytes.

Review Time!

I.   *Provide a short answer to the following questions about the gonads, pineal gland, and thymus gland.*

1. What other gland of the body, besides the gonads, produces androgens?

_____

2. At what point in life is the thymus gland most active? _____

3. At what point in life do the gonads start producing sex hormones? _____

4. What role does the hypothalamus play in controlling the production of hormones by the gonads?

_____

_____

5. People who travel west to east can experience jet lag and exhaustion. One solution is to have the traveler sit in front of a light box once he or she has arrived in the new location. Why might this work? What hormone is being stimulated to be released? _____

_____

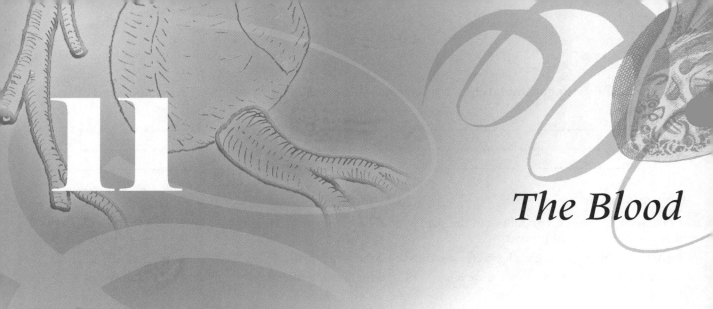

11

The Blood

Tips for Success as You Begin

Read Chapter 11 from your textbook before attending class. Listen when you attend lecture and fill in the blanks in this notebook. You may choose to complete the blanks before attending class as a way to prepare for the day's topics. The same day you attend lecture, read the material again and complete the exercises after each section in this notebook. Spend time every day with this chapter as it will help you make sense of the material. You'll likely want to spend a significant amount of time practicing the blood typing information at the end of this chapter.

Introduction to the Blood

What type of tissue is blood? _____

Blood contains:

1. **Formed elements**, which are the _____ elements of blood.
2. **Plasma**, which is the watery matrix of blood.

CONCEPT 1

Characteristics of Blood

Concept: Blood performs three main functions that are each important in maintaining homeostasis. They are transportation, protection, and regulation. The properties of blood are universal in all people, and are often used as indicators of the state of health.

LEARNING OBJECTIVE 1. Identify the three primary functions of blood.

Functions of Blood

Functions: Transportation, protection, and regulation.

1. **Transportation:** What are some examples of substances that travel in the blood?

   _____

   _____

2. **Protection:** What does blood protect our bodies from? _____

   _____

3. **Regulation:** What does blood help regulate? _____

   _____

Properties of Blood

LEARNING OBJECTIVE **2. Describe the physical properties of blood.**

- **Color** of blood is due to a pigment that is an iron-rich protein known as **hemoglobin**. The crimson-red color results from oxygen bound to the iron on hemoglobin, typical of _____ blood. The dark-red color (not truly blue) results when the iron is not as saturated with oxygen, as is typical of _____ blood.
- **Volume** of blood accounts for 8% of our body's weight. Males have _____ to _____ liters on average, while females have 4 to 5 liters on average.
- **Viscosity** is the resistance a substance has to flow. Blood is more viscous than water, meaning it is slower to flow than water. Blood is also stickier than water.
- **pH** of blood ranges between 7.35 and 7.45, slightly alkaline on the pH scale. Buffers help to maintain pH.
  - If pH falls below 7.35, a condition known as _____ arises.
  - If pH rises above 7.45, a condition known as _____ arises.

CONCEPT 2

Plasma

Concept: Plasma consists of water and a small amount of dissolved substances. It provides a watery transport medium for solutes and formed elements.

LEARNING OBJECTIVE **3. Distinguish between plasma and the formed elements.**

LEARNING OBJECTIVE **4. Identify the dissolved substances in plasma.**

Plasma forms the majority of blood (about 55%). Plasma is the liquid portion of the blood. Plasma includes:
- Water (_____%)
- Dissolved substances (solutes) such as proteins, breakdown products of metabolism, gasses, nutrients, and hormones.

Plasma Proteins

Most **plasma proteins** are made in the _____. Three main groups include the albumins, globulins, and fibrinogen:

1. **Albumins** are the majority of plasma proteins. They are made by the _____ and help to increase the viscosity of the blood by increasing osmotic pressure. (_Do you need to review osmotic pressure from Chapter 3?_)

- Osmotic pressure pulls water into the blood stream, so an increase in _____ causes an increase in osmotic pressure of the blood and pulls more fluids into the blood stream.
- Liver problems that decrease production of albumins can cause fluids to be lost from blood vessels, resulting in excess fluids in the _____ space. *Ascites* is a condition resulting from low osmotic pressure. Severe malnutrition and liver disease can cause the appearance of a swollen belly, commonly seen with ascites.

2. **Globulins** are the second most common type of plasma protein. _____ globulins serve as antibodies in the immune response.

3. **Fibrinogen** constitutes a small percentage of the plasma proteins. It is a precursor to _____, used in the blood clotting mechanism. When fibrinogen and other clotting factors are removed, the remainder is called **blood serum**. Blood serum is useful if blood needs to be stored and reused. *Why?* _____

Other Plasma Solutes

- **Nonprotein nitrogen (NPN) substances** are byproducts of metabolism such as amino acids, urea, and uric acid.
- **Gasses** such as the respiratory gasses _____ and _____, and other gasses inhaled by the lungs, such as nitrogen.
- **Nutrients** absorbed by the digestive system, including glucose, lipids, and amino acids.
- _____ absorbed by the digestive system or released by metabolism, including sodium, chloride, bicarbonate, potassium, calcium, phosphate, sulfate, and magnesium ions. Their functions include maintaining the osmotic pressure of the blood, acid–base balance, muscle contraction, and bone maintenance.

CONCEPT 3

Formed Elements

Concept: The formed elements include red blood cells, white blood cells, and platelets. They perform most of the functions of blood.

LEARNING OBJECTIVE 5. Describe two ways that blood can be analyzed.

LEARNING OBJECTIVE 6. Distinguish between the formed elements on the basis of their concentrations in blood, their structure, and their primary function.

Formed elements are cells and cell fragments that account for about _____% of the total blood volume. A centrifuge can separate the three types of formed elements.

Two ways blood can be analyzed:

1. **Hematocrit** is the percentage of _____ blood cells in a sample.

2. A _____ involves taking a sample of blood and smearing it across a microscope slide and staining it with dye.

What are the three formed elements?

1. _____

2. _____

3. _____

Hematopoiesis is the process of making formed elements.

• Before birth, where does hematopoiesis occur? _____

• After birth, where does hematopoiesis occur? _____

All blood cells come from one group of bone marrow stem cells called *pluripotent hematopoietic stem cells*. These stem cells can go on to produce all other types of formed elements through one of two lines:

1. *Myeloid stem cell*s give rise to red blood cells, most white blood cells, and megakaryocytes.

2. *Lymphoid stem cells* give rise to _____ (one specific type of white blood cell).

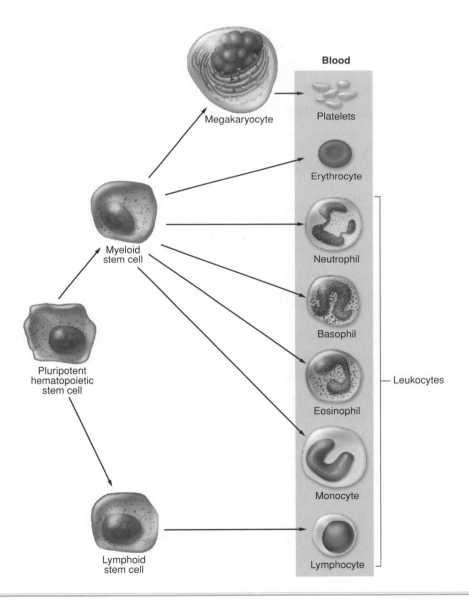

TIP! Use the prefix to help you remember each type of blood cell. Eryth- means red while leuk- means white. Erythrocytes are red blood cells while leukocytes are white blood cells.

Red Blood Cells (RBCs or Erythrocytes)

LEARNING OBJECTIVE   7. Describe the structure and function of hemoglobin.

LEARNING OBJECTIVE   8. Identify the function of red blood cells.

Red blood cells are the most abundant of all formed elements. Normal RBC concentration in blood is 4.6 million to 6.2 million per cubic millimeter of blood (males) or 4.2 million to 5.4 million per cubic millimeter of blood (females).

Structure

Red blood cells:

- Are small, flexible cells shaped like biconcave discs. The shape increases the surface area for increased
  _____.

- Are thin in the center and thicker at the edges, allowing RBCs to stack like plates as they flow through
  _____.

- Have no _____, which allows the cell to hold more pigment molecules (hemoglobin).

Function

Red blood cell functions include:

- Transport _____ *from* the lungs (primary function). Iron in hemoglobin binds to oxygen molecules. When oxygen levels are *low* in tissues, iron releases oxygen which diffuses into the tissues.
- Transport of small amounts of _____ *to* the lungs. Carbon dioxide diffuses into RBCs and binds to a different section on the hemoglobin from oxygen. Carbon dioxide is transported *to* and unloaded at the lungs.
- _____ is any reduction in the number of RBCs or their ability to transport gasses.

Life Cycle

Erythropoietin is a hormone released by the _____ and liver in response to a decrease in oxygen levels in the blood. The process starts as a *myeloid stem cell* in the red marrow divides and forms a large cell with a nucleus. This nucleated cell has organelles and begins to produce hemoglobin. The cell ejects its nucleus and most organelles and enters the bloodstream, but continues to produce hemoglobin using ribosomes. A day or two after entering the bloodstream, the cell stops producing hemoglobin and its ribosomes are degraded. The transformation to a mature RBC is complete.

- **Target organ:** Erythropoietin travels to the red marrow and stimulates RBC production.
- **Control of release:** This hormone is controlled by _____ feedback. Once RBC volume is normal, an increase in oxygen inhibits erythropoietin release.
- **Life span of RBC:** _____ (*how many?*) days. Why is the life span so short?

_____

_____

Recycling of RBC

RBCs are removed from circulation and parts of the cell and hemoglobin are recycled.

- **Macrophages** (white blood cells) remove damaged RBCs by phagocytosis. *What is phagocytosis?*

_____

- Hemoglobin is broken down by enzymes into heme and globin groups.
  1. Heme loses its _____ and is converted into **biliverdin**. Biliverdin (greenish pigment) may be further converted into **bilirubin** (orange pigment). Both pigments are released into the liver which excretes them as bile pigments into bile. These pigments are also the main source of color of the stool.
  2. Iron, part of the heme group, is taken to the _____ to make new hemoglobin.
  3. Globin is broken down into _____ which are taken to the red marrow for the manufacturing of new hemoglobin.

White Blood Cells (WBCs or Leukocytes)

LEARNING OBJECTIVE 9. Distinguish between the types of white blood cells on the basis of their structural and functional differences.

Features of white blood cells:
- Fewer in number than _____.
- The least common of the formed elements. Normal WBC concentration in blood is 5,000 to 10,000 per cubic millimeter of blood.
- **Function** in fighting disease.

Types of WBCs

All white blood cells:
- Possess a _____
- Can wander outside the circulatory system
- Can be distinguished by _____ in the cytoplasm. The cells are known as granulocytes and agranulocytes.

Granulocytes

Granulocytes are white blood cells. They have visible granules (pebble-like objects) in the cytoplasm and lobed nuclei. They are about two times larger than an RBC.

Granulocytes are produced in red marrow with the RBCs. They are distinguished on the basis of the color their granules stain. The three types are _____, _____, and _____. The suffix ending -*phil* ("loving") is for the type of stain they "love."

Neutrophils

- Most abundant of the WBCs
- Granules stain _____
- Nucleus has 2 to 5 lobes with a narrow bridge
- First at the site of injury or infection
- Destroy invaders by _____
- Help activate acute inflammation, a response to injury or infection accompanied by swelling, pain, heat, and redness

Eosinophils

- Granules stain _____ in acid stain
- Nucleus has _____ lobes only
- Not as mobile as neutrophils
- Response to parasitic infections
- Remove particles that cause allergic reactions, such as pollen and mold, by _____

Basophils

- Least common of the WBCs
- Large granules stain _____ in basic stain
- Nucleus is S-shaped with 2 lobes
- Produce histamine during _____ reactions. Histamine causes itching and inflammation.

Agranulocytes

Agranulocytes are white blood cells. They feature few or small cytoplasmic granules and are produced by the bone marrow and organs of the lymphatic system (spleen, lymph nodes, and thymus). The two types are _____ and _____.

Monocytes

- Largest cell in the blood
- Nucleus is round, oval, or U-shaped, and occupies most of the cell volume
- Mature into _____, which help clean up dead and dying RBCs
- Destroy foreign material through _____.

Lymphocytes

- Smallest WBC
- Nucleus is large and round and occupies nearly all of the cell volume
- Defend against microorganisms and cancer cells by promoting an _____ response
- Some produce antibodies, the basis for immunity

> **TIP!** To remember the types of white blood cells from most common to least common, keep in mind "**N**ever **L**et **M**onkeys **E**at **B**ananas." The first letter of each word represents the neutrophils, lymphocytes, monocytes, eosinophils, and basophils.

Function

Although WBCs have specialized functions, their common function is to protect the body from disease. This function is dependent on the ability of most WBCs to travel where they are needed.

- WBCs travel across capillary walls by **diapedesis** so they can reach the site of infection. Once outside the bloodstream, WBCs extend _____ (pseudopodia) in the direction of travel. WBCs are attracted to infections by chemicals and often destroy by phagocytosis.
- What three WBCs serve as phagocytes? _____, _____, _____
- Phagocytes release chemical signals to direct other WBCs to the site of infection. A collection of living, dead, and broken cells is referred to as _____.

Platelets (Thrombocytes)

Platelets (**thrombocytes**) are:

• Fragments formed from a _____ that breaks apart in the bone marrow. Each fragment has cytoplasm surrounded by a cell membrane.

• Less numerous than red blood cells, ranging from 150,000 to 360,000 per cubic millimeter of blood.

• Important for prevention of fluid loss by initiating the formation of _____.

Review Time!

I.   *Using the terms in the list below, write the appropriate type of white blood cell in each blank. You may use a term more than once.*

   Basophil   Eosinophil   Lymphocyte   Monocyte   Neutrophil

   1. Least abundant of the white blood cells   _____

   2. Phagocytes dead and dying red blood cells   _____

   3. Produces histamine   _____

   4. Produces antibodies   _____

   5. Most abundant of the white blood cells   _____

   6. Smallest of the white blood cells   _____

   7. Responds to parasitic infections   _____

   8. Matures into macrophages   _____

   9. Largest of the white blood cells   _____

   10. Granules stain blue with a basic stain   _____

II. *Using the terms in the list below, write the appropriate type of formed element in each blank. You may use a term more than once.*

   Erythrocyte or red blood cell   Leukocyte or white blood cell   Platelet or thrombocyte

   1. Cell fragment   _____

   2. Anucleate cell at maturity   _____

   3. May contain granules   _____

   4. Protects the body from disease   _____

   5. Formed from a megakaryocyte   _____

   6. Transports oxygen and carbon dioxide   _____

   7. Initiates blood clots   _____

   8. Travels by diapedesis to the site of infection   _____

   9. Contains a pigment called hemoglobin   _____

   10. Most numerous of the formed elements   _____

   11. Life span is approximately 120 days   _____

   12. Many serve as phagocytes   _____

   13. A lack of these cells is called anemia   _____

   14. Used to determine hematocrit   _____

   15. Can be categorized as granulocytes or agranulocytes   _____

III. Provide a brief answer for each of the following questions about plasma and formed elements.

1. A blood test shows 3.4 million RBC per cubic millimeter of blood for a male. Is this within the normal range? Explain your answer. _____

_____

2. How do granulocytes and agranulocytes differ? _____

_____

3. How can anemia be a stimulus for erythropoietin production? _____

_____

_____

4. Rank the formed elements from most common to least common per cubic millimeter of blood.

_____

_____

5. Describe the primary functions of the erythrocytes, leukocytes, and platelets.

_____

_____

_____

_____

6. What are the target organs of erythropoietin? _____

7. What happens to the heme and globin groups when red blood cells are recycled?

_____

_____

_____

8. Describe the structure of a red blood cell. _____

_____

_____

9. Through a microscope, you see a cell with granules that stain red and a nucleus with two lobes. What type of cell (*be specific!*), have you seen? What is the function of this cell?

_____

_____

_____

10. Explain how you could differentiate between a neutrophil and a monocyte if you saw these cells through a microscope. _____

_____

_____

CONCEPT 4

Hemostasis

Concept: The stoppage of bleeding following a blood vessel accident is called hemostasis. It involves three steps: blood vessel spasm, platelet plug formation, and coagulation.

---

10. Identify the role of platelets in blood clot formation.

11. Describe blood vessel spasm, platelet plug formation, and coagulation, and relate each to the prevention of excessive blood loss.

Hemostasis is the process that occurs when a blood vessel ruptures and large amounts of plasma and formed elements may escape. What is the main threat to homeostasis? _____

_____

The three steps of hemostasis (*not to be confused with* homeostasis) follow.

Blood Vessel Spasms

When cut or torn, smooth muscle in the wall of a blood vessel contracts.

- What is the function of contraction when the vessel is cut or torn? _____

_____

- What chemical helps to prolong the spasm? _____

_____

Platelet Plug Formation

When a blood vessel wall is damaged, platelets increase in size and surface area and become sticky.

- What do platelets stick to? _____

_____

A **platelet plug** forms as platelets accumulate with collagen.

- What is the purpose of the platelet plug? _____

Platelet plug formation is usually accompanied by coagulation.

Coagulation

Coagulation is the most effective and complex of the blood clotting mechanisms. It is a series of events resulting in the formation of a blood clot (also known as *blood clot formation*). The main event ultimately involves the formation of _____.

1. Injured blood vessel and platelets release **thromboplastin**.
2. Thromboplastin interacts with calcium ions and other substances to convert _____ into **thrombin**.
3. Thrombin combines soluble fibrinogen elements to form an insoluble protein molecule called **fibrin**.
4. Fibrin sticks to surfaces of the blood vessels. Fibrin forms a meshwork that traps blood cells. A blood clot = _____ + _____.

TIP! To help you keep the steps here in order, remember that *pro* = before, *thromb* = clot, *and gen* = form.

Coagulation takes 2 to 8 minutes. A lack of any factors can lead to a decreased ability of blood to clot. Clotting factors may be lacking due to vitamin _____ deficiency, liver disease, or genetic conditions such as hemophilia. Permanent repair begins after the clot has formed.

- Fibroblasts strengthen the clot and seal the tear.
- *Fibrinolysis* is the removal of the blood clot by enzymes that digest fibrin threads, returning fibrinogen to the plasma for later reuse.

Some blood clot formations are undesirable.

- _____ is a clot that may form in a blood vessel when it is not needed and block circulation to a vital organ. It may be a result of atherosclerosis, an accumulation of fatty deposits.
- _____ is a free-floating clot (thrombus) that has detached; it may lodge in a blood vessel supplying a vital organ and cut off its blood supply.

Review Time!

I. *Provide a brief answer for each of the following questions about hemostasis.*

1. For how long do vascular spasms typically occur? What can cause them to last longer?

_____

_____

_____

2. Immediately upon cutting yourself shaving, you place a tissue onto the cut. Ten minutes later, you remove the tissue. Why does bleeding restart? Explain. _____

_____

_____

3. What constitutes a blood clot? _____

4. What type of muscle forms the wall of a blood vessel? _____

5. What step is mimicked by applying pressure to a cut? _____

6. Why do you think fibrinolysis is necessary? _____

_____

7. Why would liver disease impair clotting ability? _____

_____

8. What does serotonin promote during the process of hemostasis? _____

_____

9. What is the difference between a thrombus and an embolus? _____

_____

10. Is a platelet plug the same as a blood clot? Explain. _____

_____

_____

CONCEPT 5

Blood Groups

Concept: Blood grouping is based upon the reaction between surface proteins on the cell membranes of red blood cells and special plasma proteins. The two major systems are ABO and Rh.

LEARNING OBJECTIVE 12. Describe the interaction between antigens and antibodies during the mixing of incompatible blood types.

LEARNING OBJECTIVE 13. Distinguish between the ABO system and the Rh system, including the optional blood types and their interactions.

Blood groups are based upon the reaction between surface proteins present on cell membranes of RBC and special plasma proteins. Before we discuss the ABO blood group and Rh blood group, you'll need to clearly understand the following terms:

- **Antigens** (agglutinogens) are _____ present on the surface of an RBC. They can trigger an immune response.
- **Antibodies** (agglutinins) disable unwanted molecules in an immune reaction.
- **Agglutination** occurs when incompatible blood types clump together. Agglutination means that two types of blood are not compatible with one another for transfusion. If there is no agglutination, the samples of blood are compatible.
- **Blood typing** involves the identification of _____ to determine compatibility for transfusions.

> **TIP!** Agglutination should not be confused with coagulation (blood clot formation). Agglutination occurs when antibodies bind to and clump antigens. Coagulation occurs as part of the process of hemostasis.

ABO System

The ABO system is based on two **antigens**, A and B, which are inherited.

- If both antigens are inherited, the blood type is AB.
- If antigen A is inherited, the blood type is _____.
- If antigen B is inherited, the blood type is _____.
- If no antigens are inherited, the blood type is O.

> **TIP!** There are only two antigens, A and B, in the ABO blood groups. If you have one or both of these antigens, then you have the blood type that corresponds. If you have antigen A, you have blood type A. Keep in mind that blood type O has no antigens—neither antigen A nor B.

Antibodies (formed early in life) react only with antigens that a person does not have.

- Anti-A antibodies are formed to react with the _____ antigen. Type O and B have these anti-A antibodies.
- Anti-B antibodies are formed to react with the _____ antigen. Type O and A have these anti-B antibodies.
- A person with AB blood has neither antibody. Do you know why? _____

	Red blood cell	Plasma
Type A	Antigen A	Antibody B (anti-B)
Type B	Antigen B	Antibody A (anti-A)
Type AB	Antigens A and B	No antibodies
Type O	No antigens	Antibodies A and B (anti-A and anti-B)

Blood Transfusions

Transfusion reactions occur when blood types are not compatible and agglutination occurs. Matching must be done to prevent reactions.

- Blood type A cannot receive B or AB. Why? _____
- Blood type B cannot receive A or AB. Why? _____
- Blood type O cannot receive A, B, or AB. Why? _____
- Can a person with AB blood receive types A, B, or O? Why?

_____

_____

> **TIP!** There is a pattern to determining who can receive what blood type in a transfusion. When typing blood, we cannot receive blood **against** which we have built antibodies. For instance, blood type A cannot receive type B since it carries antibodies against type B. We do not form antibodies against type O. Why? Blood type O carries **no** antigens.

Safe Practice

It is safest practice to give the person requiring blood the same type of donor blood as he or she has. In emergencies, type _____ (formerly called the *universal donor*) can be used. Type O has no AB surface antigens, but it does have anti-A and anti-B antibodies. Type AB blood can receive any blood in small amounts.

- Why could type O potentially cause problems if transfused to a person with type B blood?

_____

_____

Rh System

The Rh system is based on one inherited antigen, known as the Rh antigen.

- If the Rh antigen is inherited (the majority of us) = Rh-positive
- If the Rh antigen is *not* inherited = Rh-negative

Rh antibodies are only formed upon exposure to the antigen and a person becomes sensitized during transfusion. These antibodies are not automatically present as with the anti-A and anti-B antibodies in the ABO system.

- *First transfusion:* An Rh-negative person receives blood from an Rh-positive person and becomes sensitized to the Rh antigen. Why does an agglutination reaction not usually occur with the first incompatible combination of blood types? _____

_____

- *Subsequent transfusions:* The donor's blood will agglutinate when it contacts the anti-Rh antibodies found in the recipient's blood. Why will agglutination occur for the second incompatible combination, but not the first? _____

_____

Rh and Pregnancy: An Example of Rh Sensitization

Rh sensitization occurs when a mother is Rh-negative and is carrying an Rh-positive fetus for the first time.

- Why is this first pregnancy usually not problematic? _____

_____

- Why is RhoGAM administered? _____

_____

- How does the mother become sensitized to the Rh antigen from the fetus? _____

_____

- What happens the next time a mother becomes pregnant with another Rh-positive infant? The anti-Rh antibodies cross the placenta and cause an _____ reaction with the fetal red blood cells.
- What condition results? _____

_____

Review Time!

I. Using the terms in the list below, write the appropriate blood type in each blank. You may use a type more than once.

   Blood type A   Blood type B   Blood type AB   Blood type O

   1. Carries the A antigen only   _____
   2. Carries no antigens   _____
   3. Carries anti-A and anti-B antibodies   _____
   4. Cannot receive type A, B, or AB due to antigens present   _____
   5. Carries antigens A and B   _____
   6. Can receive any blood type in small amounts   _____
   7. Can give to any blood type in small amounts   _____
   8. Carries the B antigen only   _____
   9. Has no antibodies   _____
   10. Formerly called the universal donor   _____

II. *Provide a brief answer for each of the following questions about blood groups and compatibility.*

1. What distinguishes the processes of agglutination and coagulation? _____
_____
_____

2. What is the difference between an antigen and an antibody? _____
_____
_____

3. Why don't we form anti-O antibodies? _____
_____

4. List the antigens associated with the ABO system. List the antigen associated with the Rh system.
_____
_____
_____

5. Why doesn't agglutination occur when a person with type AB blood receives type A blood during a transfusion? _____
_____

6. Why does agglutination occur when a person with type A blood receives type AB blood during a transfusion? _____
_____

7. If a mother is Rh-positive and her fetus is Rh-negative, is RhoGAM necessary?
_____
_____

8. Alex's friend is going into surgery and he wants to donate blood in case she needs it. He has type A; she has type B. Are these blood types compatible? Explain. _____
_____

9. Why and when is the RhoGAM shot administered? _____
_____

10. Why does the first transfusion of Rh-positive blood to a person with Rh-negative blood usually not cause agglutination? _____
_____

III. *For each of the following questions, fill in the correct blood types in the space provided.*

1. What blood type(s) can type B blood receive?   _____
2. What blood type has the B antigen only?   _____
3. What blood type(s) can type O receive?   _____
4. What blood type(s) can type AB receive?   _____
5. What blood type has no antigens?   _____
6. What blood type(s) can receive type A blood?   _____
7. What blood type(s) agglutinate with type B blood?   _____
8. What blood type(s) carry anti-B antibodies?   _____
9. What blood type(s) can give blood to type AB blood?   _____
10. What blood type(s) agglutinate with type O blood?   _____

The Cardiovascular System

12

Tips for Success as You Begin

Read Chapter 12 from your textbook before attending class. Listen when you attend lecture and fill in the blanks in this notebook. You may choose to complete the blanks before attending class as a way to prepare for the day's topics. The same day you attend lecture, read the material again and complete the exercises after each section in this notebook. To learn the path of blood flow through the heart, use a visual aid such as a picture or heart model as you trace the pathway. You'll also find learning the systemic blood vessels will be easier if you have pictures or a model to view. Since many vessels are named by location, use their names as clues to help you learn their locations.

Introduction to the Cardiovascular System

LEARNING OBJECTIVE 1. Identify the general function of the cardiovascular system.

The **function** of the cardiovascular system is to move blood continuously through the body to deliver oxygen and nutrients to cells while removing wastes.

The **organs** of the cardiovascular system include the (1) heart and (2) blood vessels. The cardiovascular system is a closed system of vessels in which blood is confined to travel. Blood leaves the heart and travels through the:

- Aorta branches into _____ that carry blood to the body (except the lungs)
- Pulmonary trunk branches into arteries that carry blood to the lungs
- _____ for the exchange of gasses and other substances
- Veins to carry blood back to the heart

The color scheme for vessels is that veins are typically colored *blue* (blood is low in oxygen, deoxygenated blood) while arteries are colored *red* (blood is oxygenated).

TIP! Remember this rhyme: The body's arteries are red, and its veins are blue. In the heart and lungs, there's an exception of two: Pulmonary arteries are blue while pulmonary veins are red. (You'll find out why the pulmonary vessels are colored different shortly.)

CONCEPT 1

Heart Structure

Concept: The heart is located in the center of the thoracic cavity and is surrounded by two serous membranes. The heart wall is composed of three layers, dominated by the middle myocardium. The myocardium surrounds the four inner chambers and pushes blood through one-way valves during their contraction.

LEARNING OBJECTIVE 2. Identify the location and general features of the heart.

The heart is:

- A fist-sized muscular pump that propels blood through the thoracic cavity
- Oriented with its pointed **apex** positioned inferiorly. The apex rests on the _____. The **base** is the heart's flattened superior margin
- Situated with two-thirds on the _____ side of the midline of the chest and one-third on the _____ side

Coverings of the Heart

LEARNING OBJECTIVE 3. Describe the layers of the pericardium.

The **pericardium** is a double-layered serous membrane surrounding the heart and the blood vessels that attach to the heart.

- **Parietal pericardium (pericardial sac)** is divided into two layers.
  1. The outer fibrous layer is constructed of _____ tissue and anchors the heart to the diaphragm, sternum, and blood vessels attached to the heart.
  2. The inner, thin serous layer is composed of _____ epithelium with connective tissue underneath.
- **Visceral pericardium (epicardium)** is anchored to the heart. This innermost layer also plays a double role as the outermost heart wall.
- The space between the parietal pericardium and the visceral pericardium creates the _____ **cavity**. The pericardial cavity contains a small amount of fluid that is secreted by the serous cells of the pericardium. The function of this fluid is _____.
  _____
  _____

Pericarditis is a situation in which the pericardium becomes swollen and the fluid production by the serous cells is inhibited. The serous membranes stick together, causing severe chest pain, and can impede heart activity.

List the layers surrounding the heart from outermost to innermost. _____
_____
_____
_____

TIP! Think of the two layers of the parietal pericardium as the front and back of two pieces of paper glued together. The outer, fibrous pericardium is the outer side that, when peeled back from the heart's surface, exposes the parietal pericardium. The visceral pericardium can be imagined as shrinkwrap that covers the heart. If you tried to remove the visceral pericardium (epicardium), you'd also be plucking away the heart muscle underneath.

The Heart Wall

LEARNING OBJECTIVE   **4. Identify the layers of the heart wall.**

There are three layers in the heart wall (not to be confused with the *membranes* surrounding the heart).

1. **Epicardium** (*What is the other name for this wall?* _____). The epicardium is the outermost layer of the heart wall. It often contains fat deposits.

2. **Myocardium** is constructed of _____ muscle tissue that is responsible for pumping blood. A **fibrous skeleton** of connective tissue fibers link parts of the heart together.
   - What is the function of this fibrous skeleton? _____

3. **Endocardium** is the inner lining of the heart wall that covers the chambers and valves. _____ epithelium with a thin layer of connective tissue underneath creates the **endothelium** that also lines major blood vessels leaving the heart.

> **TIP!** How do you remember the location of these three walls? The prefix *epi-* means "upon" or "over," while the "*m*" in myocardium serves as a reminder of the "middle" layer. Of course, *myo* means "muscle." Last, the prefix *endo-* means "within."

Heart Chambers

LEARNING OBJECTIVE   **5. Describe the structure of the atria and ventricles.**

Four chambers are found in the heart: two superior atria (*atrium* is singular) receive blood while two inferior ventricles contract and propel blood out of the heart.

> **TIP!** Remember that "a" comes alphabetically before "v." So, atria are superior chambers of the heart while ventricles are inferior chambers of the heart.

Atria

The atria are the superior, receiving chambers of the heart. That means these chambers receive blood from blood vessels returning blood to the heart.

> **TIP!** Anatomy is like learning a different set of vocabulary terms. An *atrium* is a single chamber while the term *atria* refer to both the right and left chambers.

Some features of the atria:

- An **auricle** is a flap-like appendage found on both the atria. The function of the auricle is to

_____

- Myocardium in the atria is thin.
- _____ **muscles** are ridges of the myocardium.
- **Interatrial septum** separates the two _____.
- **Foramen ovale** is a hole in the heart of a fetus that allows blood to pass from the right atrium to the left atrium while the lungs develop. After birth, the hole closes and a small oval depression remains, known as the _____. Incomplete closure after birth is a problem called *interatrial septal defect.* Cyanosis occurs in babies with this defect. What are "blue babies?" _____

_____

> **TIP!** There are built-in clues to these names: *Auricle* means ear (and it really does look like an ear!) while *pectinate* means chest. *Interatrial septum* means wall between the atria. *Foramen ovale* means oval-shaped hole while *fossa ovalis* means oval-shaped depression.

Ventricles

The ventricles push blood out of the heart with their forceful contractions. Some features of the ventricles:

- The ventricles are muscular chambers with thick myocardium. The left ventricle is the thickest of the two chambers. Why? _____

_____

- Where does the right ventricle send blood? _____

- **Interventricular sulcus** is a groove on the external surface of the heart. This groove separates the right and left _____.

- **Coronary sulcus** is a groove on the posterior external surface. This groove separates the _____ from the _____.

- **Trabeculae carneae** are prominent ridges on the internal _____ walls.

- _____ **muscles** are projections associated with the trabeculae carneae. Some heart valves are attached to these muscles by way of white cords ("heart strings") known as **chordae tendineae**.

- **Interventricular septum** is a muscular wall that internally separates the right and left ventricles. The septum parallels the externally visible interventricular _____.

- *Ventricular septal defect* is an unwanted opening that allows blood to move back and forth between the ventricles during their contractions. Why is this opening problematic? _____

_____

_____

> **TIP!** More built-in clues are seen in these names: *Interventricular sulcus* is a groove (sulcus) between the ventricles, like the *coronary sulcus* is a groove on the heart's surface. *Trabeculae carneae* means fleshy beams and *papillary muscles* are nipple-like extensions of muscle projecting from the ventricles' interior surface. *Chordae tendineae* are literally "heart strings." *Interventricular septum* is a wall (septum) dividing the two ventricles.

Heart Valves

LEARNING OBJECTIVE   6. Describe the structure and function of the heart valves.

Heart valves ensure that blood flows in *one* direction through the heart: from the atria to the ventricles and from the ventricles out through _____. These valves prevent the backflow of blood.

Atrioventricular (AV) Valves

The **AV valves** are located between each atrium and ventricle. There is one on each side of the heart.

- **Tricuspid valve** is the right AV valve. It has _____ (*how many*) leaflets or cusps that anchor in the right ventricle by chordae tendineae to _____ muscles.

- **Bicuspid valve (mitral valve)** is the left AV valve. It has _____ (*how many*) leaflets or cusps that anchor in the left ventricle by chordae tendineae to papillary muscles.

> **TIP!** Having trouble keeping the tricuspid valve and the bicuspid valve locations straight? Remember to "try (tri) before you buy (bi)." The tricuspid valve is on the right side while the bicuspid valve is on the left side. Also, the tricuspid name has an "r" to remind you of the right side of the heart.

How the AV Valves Work

- When the atrium has filled with blood, its walls contract and blood is pushed through the AV valve into the _____.

- The AV valve is open and allows blood to flow through since the papillary muscle is relaxed. *Where are the papillary muscles?* _____
- Once the ventricle begins to contract, blood is forced up against the cusps of the AV valve.
- Chordae tendineae are kept tight. The cusps invert, preventing blood from back flowing into the atria.
- Blood pushes into the next available space: the large arteries (_____ and _____).

AV Valve Problems
- Chordae tendineae rupture and allow backflow of blood into the atria from the ventricles.
- *Heart* _____ results from minor failure of the AV valve to close completely.

Semilunar (SL) Valves

The **SL valves** are situated within the base of the large arteries emerging from the heart near the union with the ventricles.
- **Pulmonary valve** is the right SL valve. It lies within the base of an artery called the pulmonary trunk near the right ventricle.
- **Aortic valve** is the left SL valve. It lies within the aorta near its origin at the left ventricle.

How the SL Valves Work
- The valves are dense connective tissue covered with endocardium. Both have three half-moon cusps with the bottom of the bowl facing the ventricles.
- When the SL valve is *closed,* the cusps contact one another and close off the vessel.
- The SL valves *open* in response to blood flow and pressure changes as the ventricles contract. As blood is pushed against the SL valves, they open and blood flows through the vessels (aorta and pulmonary trunk) out of the heart.
- When the ventricles relax, the SL valves *close,* preventing the backflow of blood into the _____ (*which chambers?*).
- Heart murmurs can occur if SL valve closure is incomplete. AV valve heart murmurs are more common.

> **TIP!** Think of the SL valves as trap doors. Trap doors stay closed unless you walk over them, then they suddenly open. The SL valves stay closed unless the force and pressure of blood pushes them open. Then, they slam shut after the ventricles relax.

Blood Flow Through the Heart

LEARNING OBJECTIVE 7. Trace the flow of blood through the chambers of the heart.

Practice the flow of blood through the heart with a picture or heart model nearby. You'll find the flow easiest to learn when you can *see* the chambers, valves, or vessels through which the blood flows.
- Superior vena cava (SVC), inferior vena cava (IVC), and coronary sinus return blood to the right atrium
- Right atrium (*blood is low in oxygen and high in carbon dioxide*)
- Tricuspid valve
- Right ventricle
- _____ valve
- Pulmonary trunk (an artery)
- Lungs (*gas exchange restores oxygen to blood in exchange for the removal of carbon dioxide*)
- Pulmonary veins (4)
- _____ atrium
- Mitral (bicuspid) valve

- Left ventricle
- Aortic valve
- Aorta
- Blood vessels carry blood to the body
- Returned to right atrium

As we discuss the parts of the heart, add labels to the illustration below and practice saying aloud the flow of blood through the heart. When you are done, you should be able to identify the parts of the heart listed below.

1. _____
2. _____
3. _____
4. _____
5. _____
6. _____
7. _____
8. _____
9. _____
10. _____
11. _____
12. _____
13. _____
14. _____
15. _____
16. _____
17. _____
18. _____

Aorta	Left pulmonary artery	Pulmonary valve
Chordae tendineae	Left ventricle	Right atrium
Fossa ovalis	Mitral (bicuspid) valve	Right ventricle
IVC	Papillary muscle	SVC
Interventricular septum	Pectinate muscle	Trabeculae carneae
Left atrium	Pulmonary trunk	Tricuspid valve

Supply of Blood to the Heart

Coronary circulation is the flow of blood through the heart's own blood vessels that service the heart muscle (myocardium).

- Oxygenated blood from the _____ travels through the right and left **coronary arteries**. These arteries branch off the base of the aorta and carry oxygenated blood to the myocardium of the heart. Blockage of a coronary artery is the most common cause of a heart attack.
- Capillaries pick up _____ and wastes and transport blood to **coronary veins**.
- Most blood drained from the heart is collected by the **coronary sinus** which returns blood to the _____ atrium of the heart.

Review Time!

I. *Using the terms in the list below, label the parts of the heart.*

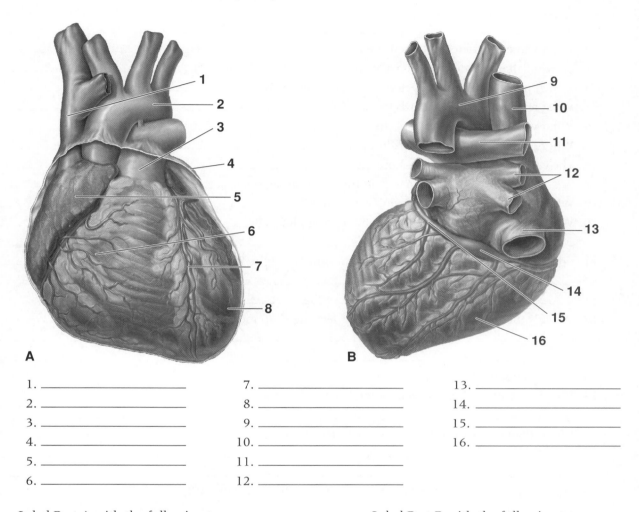

A   B

1. _____   7. _____   13. _____
2. _____   8. _____   14. _____
3. _____   9. _____   15. _____
4. _____   10. _____   16. _____
5. _____   11. _____
6. _____   12. _____

Label Part A with the following terms: Label Part B with the following terms:
  Aorta   Aorta
  Auricle of the right atrium   Coronary sinus
  Interventricular sulcus   Coronary sulcus
  Left ventricle   IVC
  Parietal pericardium (cut)   Pulmonary artery
  Pulmonary trunk   Pulmonary vein
  Right ventricle   Right ventricle
  SVC   SVC

II. *Provide a brief answer for each of the following questions about heart anatomy and circulation.*

   1. Name three veins that return blood to the right atrium.

      1. _____

      2. _____

      3. _____

   2. What valve is situated between the right atrium and the right ventricle? _____

   3. To what chamber do pulmonary veins carry oxygenated blood? _____

   4. Which heart wall is constructed of cardiac muscle tissue? _____

   5. What are the thin white cords that anchor the AV valves? _____

   6. What valve guards the base of the pulmonary trunk? _____

   7. Where is the apex of the heart located? _____

   8. The coronary sulcus separates the _____ and _____ on the external heart surface.

   9. Where does the pulmonary trunk carry blood? _____

  10. Where are the papillary and pectinate muscles located? _____

      _____

  11. From superior to deep, list the layers that surround the heart. _____

      _____

      _____

  12. What is the name of the opening in the fetal heart found between the right and left atria?

      _____

      _____

  13. What is the function of the AV valves? _____

  14. Which side of the heart (*right* or *left*) deals with blood that is low in oxygen?

      _____

  15. When the ventricles contract, what happens to the AV valves? Why? _____

      _____

      _____

  16. When the ventricles contract, what happens to the SL valves? Why? _____

      _____

      _____

  17. When the left ventricle contracts, through what valve will the blood pass?

      _____

  18. Where is the coronary sulcus located? _____

  19. What role do the auricles play in heart function? _____

  20. Trace blood flow through the heart by starting with the three veins that empty blood into the right atrium. _____

      _____

      _____

      _____

CONCEPT 2

Heart Function

Concept: The heart moves blood through the blood vessels. It does so by a carefully regulated sequence of contractions known as the cardiac cycle. Each cardiac cycle is triggered by an electrical event that originates from modified heart tissue called the sinoatrial (SA) node, and is regulated by the autonomic nervous system.

The heart's **function** is to propel blood through the body through rhythmic contractions of the myocardium.

Cardiac Cycle

LEARNING OBJECTIVE 8. Define cardiac cycle.

The **cardiac cycle** is the time to complete a single heartbeat. The cycle includes (1) the contraction of the atria, followed by (2) the contraction of the ventricles.

- **Systole** is the state of contraction.
- **Diastole** is the state of relaxation.

Let's take the *contraction of the atria* first and examine what's happening in the heart. This time period is known as ventricular diastole.

- Atria are contracting, pressure rises, and blood is forced into the _____.
- Ventricles are relaxed (diastole) and volume is expanded, pressure is falling, and blood is drawn in from the major vessels.

Once the atria have contracted, they relax and it's time for the ventricles to contract. This time period is known as ventricular systole.

- Atria have relaxed, pressure is falling, and blood is drawn in from the major vessels.
- Ventricles contract (systole), pressure rises, and blood is pushed out through the large _____ (aorta and pulmonary trunk).

We have now completed one cardiac cycle.

Heart Sounds

LEARNING OBJECTIVE 9. Identify the sounds of the heart, and relate them to the cardiac cycle.

The heart sounds "lubb–dupp" come from the _____ in blood flow caused by the closure of the heart valves.

- **"Lubb"** is a sound that comes from the closure of the AV valves. The ventricles are contracting, known as ventricular systole. What does *systole* mean? _____
- **"Dupp"** is a sound that comes from the closure of the SL valves. The sound is heard during ventricular diastole. What does *diastole* mean? _____

Auscultation is the procedure of listening to the internal sounds of the body, including heart sounds, with a _____.

Heart Conduction System

LEARNING OBJECTIVE 10. Describe the components and function of the heart conduction system.

The heart does not require external stimulation to contract. It has the ability to beat on its own due to a built-in system called the *heart conduction system.* Specialized cardiac cells send _____ impulses to each cardiac muscle cell; the cell with the fastest rhythm sets the pace for the HR.

- **SA node** is located in the _____ atrium and is known as the "pacemaker." The SA node initiates each cardiac cycle by generating an electrical impulse that spreads over both atria along the **internodal pathway**. As a result of the stimulation, the atria contract (*atrial systole*).
- **AV node** is located in the inferior part of the interatrial septum on the right side. It receives impulses from the SA node via the internodal pathway. It sends the message to the _____ to contract after a short delay. The delay allows the atria to contract and the ventricles to fill with blood. If there are problems with the delay, the ventricles may pump an insufficient supply of blood to vital organs. This condition is known as _____.
- **AV bundle (bundle of His)** receives the message from the AV node and then sends it on to branches known as _____.
- **Purkinje fibers** pass into the myocardium to reach cardiac cells of the ventricles. These fibers stimulate the ventricles to _____ (*ventricular systole*). By the time the ventricles have contracted, the atria have completed their contraction and returned to a relaxed state.

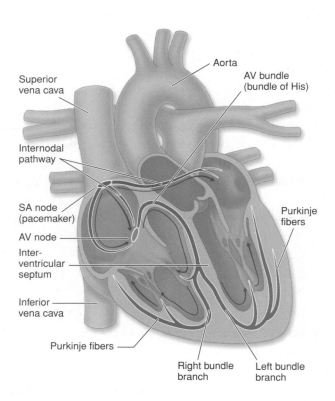

Electrocardiogram (ECG or EKG)

LEARNING OBJECTIVE   11. Identify the electrical events measured in a normal electrocardiogram.

An **electrocardiogram** (**ECG** or **EKG**) is a recording of the measurement of the _____ activity of the heart. Each wave indicates a cycle of depolarization (upward tracing) and repolarization (downward tracing). Let's take a moment to review depolarization and repolarization.

- *Depolarization:* Sodium channels open on the cell membrane. Sodium ions rush in the cardiac muscle cell to begin an _____.
- *Repolarization:* Sodium channels close and _____ channels open while muscle contraction occurs.

The waves of the ECG are:

• **P wave:** SA node depolarizes the _____ (*which chambers?*) and the atria contract.

• **QRS complex** includes the Q, R, and S waves. This complex mainly represents depolarization of the ventricles, which leads to ventricular contraction. Why is the QRS complex greater than the P wave?

_____

• **T wave** is the repolarization of the ventricles. Why can't we see a wave for atrial repolarization?

_____

ECG helps to analyze problems such as:

• *Cardiac arrhythmia* is any abnormal pattern of cardiac electrical activity.

• Large P wave indicates an enlarged _____.

• Flat T wave suggests insufficient _____ is reaching the heart muscle.

• Long Q–T interval may occur if there has been myocardial damage.

Review Time!

I. *Place a number from 1 to 5 in the blank before each step of the pathway to indicate the correct order of the conduction of nerve impulses of the heart's conduction system.*

_____ AV bundle (bundle of His)

_____ AV node

_____ Internodal pathway

_____ Purkinje fibers

_____ SA node

II. *Provide a brief answer for each of the following questions about heart function.*

1. What valves close during "lubb" and "dupp?" _____

_____

2. What does one cardiac cycle represent? _____

3. What wave on an ECG corresponds to an impulse sent from the SA node? _____

4. Why is there a delay when the AV node fires an impulse? _____

_____

5. Why is the QRS complex larger than the P wave? _____

_____

6. What is an ECG? _____

_____

7. Where is the SA node located? _____

8. What is the function of the SA node? _____

9. What does an impulse from the AV node cause to happen? _____

_____

10. What does the T wave on an ECG represent? _____

11. What are the atria doing during atrial systole? _____

12. Which node sends an impulse to promote atrial systole? _____

13. What happens during ventricular systole? _____

14. When the atria are in systole, what is happening with the ventricles? _____

_____

15. Which valves close during ventricular systole? _____

_____

16. Which valves open during ventricular systole so blood can leave the heart? _____

_____

III. *Using the terms in the list below, label the parts of the ECG tracing.*

1. _____
2. _____
3. _____
4. _____
5. _____

P wave   T wave

Q, R, and S waves

Cardiac Output (CO)

LEARNING OBJECTIVE   12. Define cardiac output, and describe how it is regulated.

The heart must be able to adjust to demands by changing:

- **Heart rate (HR):** Usually _____ beats per minute.
- **Stroke volume (SV):** Usually _____ milliliters of blood per heartbeat. SV is the amount of blood ejected by one ventricle during a single contraction.

CO is calculated by multiplying HR and SV:

HR (75 beats per minute) × SV (70 mL/beat) = CO (5,250 mL/min)

At rest, approximately 5,250 milliliters or 5.250 liters of blood are pumped by the heart. During exercise, SV and HR can increase greatly.

- Why does a person who is a conditioned athlete have a competitive edge over someone who is not?

_____

- **Cardiac reserve** is the difference between a resting heart and a heart that is at its maximum CO. For a person who does *not* exercise regularly, the cardiac reserve is _____ to

_____ liters. For a person who is a conditioned athlete, the cardiac reserve is

_____ to _____ liters.

- **Starling's law of the heart:** The greater the stretch of the cardiac muscle, the greater its strength in contraction (think of a rubber band). How does this law relate to an athlete and the effect of exercise on CO?

_____

Regulation of Heart Activity

The **cardiac center** in the medulla oblongata of the brain can alter heart activity by way of nerve fibers of the autonomic nervous system.

- Parasympathetic fibers travel by way of the vagus nerve (cranial nerve X) to the SA and AV nodes. Parasympathetic fibers _____ (*slow* or *speed?*) the HR by the release of acetylcholine (ACh).

- Sympathetic fibers also travel from the medulla oblongata to the SA and AV nodes; some fibers terminate in the myocardium of the ventricles. Sympathetic fibers _____ (*slow* or *speed?*) both HR and SV by the release of norepinephrine (NE).

How does the medulla oblongata manage a balance between these two autonomic branches?

- At rest, which type of autonomic impulse is favored? _____
- During exercise, which type of autonomic impulse is favored? _____

How does the medulla oblongata know which type of impulse to favor?

- **Baroreceptors** are sensitive to the stretch, or changes in pressure, that comes with changes in blood pressure. These baroreceptors are mainly located _____
_____

- When there is an *increase* in blood pressure, the baroreceptors signal the cardiac center in the medulla oblongata to send parasympathetic impulses to the SA node of the heart. Why?
_____
_____

- **Cerebrum** or **hypothalamus** may also send signals to the medulla oblongata so that HR can be altered in response to emotions, sensory stimuli, or conscious thought.

Review Time!

I. Provide a brief answer for each of the following questions about heart function.

1. What is HR at rest? _____
2. What is SV at rest? _____
3. What is the average CO at rest? _____
4. Where is the cardiac center housed? _____
5. What do baroreceptors monitor? _____
6. What is Starling's law of the heart? _____
_____

7. Relate Starling's law of the heart to how exercise benefits the heart. _____
_____
_____

8. What can the cardiac center modify? _____
9. What neurotransmitter and which autonomic impulse decreases HR? _____
_____

10. What neurotransmitter and which autonomic impulse increase both HR and SV?
_____
_____

11. What cranial nerve travels to the SA and AV nodes to slow HR? What Roman numeral represents this cranial nerve? _____
_____

CONCEPT 3

Blood Vessels

Concept: Arteries and arterioles are three-layered tubes that carry blood away from the heart, with properties of contractility and elasticity. Capillaries are microscopic tubes that serve as the site of material exchange between blood and interstitial fluid, due to their very thin wall. Veins and venules are not contractile or elastic, and carry blood toward the heart.

LEARNING OBJECTIVE 13. **Distinguish between the types of blood vessels on the basis of their structure.**

Blood vessels form a closed system to transport blood to and from the heart.

Arteries and Arterioles

Arteries and arterioles are strong, elastic tubes that begin as the major arteries of the heart (the aorta and pulmonary trunk). They extend away from the heart and branch into _____, which are thinner and have a smaller diameter. The three-layered wall of arteries and arterioles (from deep to superficial) include:

1. **Tunica interna:** Endothelium of the tunica interna is enveloped by connective tissue with elastic fibers. This tunica is the site of vascular disease, such as *atherosclerosis*. This layer surrounds a hollow interior known as a _____.

2. **Tunica media:** Thick smooth muscle and elastic fibers compose this middle layer. This layer is critical to the function of arteries as it provides contractility and elasticity to the artery. *Contractility* is the ability to contract while *elasticity* is the ability to _____.
   Sympathetic nerve fibers of the autonomic nervous system (called **vasomotor fibers**) travel to this layer of smooth muscle and can change the diameter of the vessel lumen.
   - **Vasoconstriction** occurs when the vessel contracts due to stimulation by sympathetic fibers. The diameter of the vessel _____ (*decreases* or *increases?*)
   - **Vasodilation** occurs when the vessel relaxes due to inhibition of stimulation. The recoil effect of elastic fibers returns the size of the lumen. The diameter of the vessel _____ (*decreases* or *increases?*)

3. **Tunica externa:** Thin connective tissue layer anchors this layer to other structures.

> **TIP!** Use the obviously named layers of the vessels as hints to their locations. Tunica interna is the **internal** layer; tunica **m**edia is the **m**iddle layer; and tunica externa is the **external** layer.

Capillaries

Capillaries are the smallest vessels in the body. The diameter of capillaries is so small that red blood cells (RBCs) can pass through one at a time.

- **Structure:** Only made of endothelium (tunica _____). Endothelium forming the walls is semipermeable so that some movement occurs by diffusion, osmosis, facilitated diffusion, and active _____.

- **Function:** Gas and nutrient exchange occurs between blood of capillaries and interstitial fluid by *diffusion*. _____ and nutrients move into the interstitial fluids while _____ and wastes move into the plasma of the blood.

How Do Substances Travel Across the Wall of the Endothelium?

- *Pores of intermediate size* permit fluid to be leaked from blood into the surrounding space. Such fluid, once leaked, is referred to as _____ **fluid**.
- *Large pores* permit bulk transport of molecules (small intestine and kidney)
- *Tight junctions* prevent bulk transport of molecules since there are small or no pores (_____ barrier)

How Do Capillaries Carry Blood to Cells?

Capillary beds are networking branches of capillaries that are present in most tissues. Capillary beds feature:

- **Thoroughfare channels:** Present in capillary beds, thoroughfare channels are direct connections between an arteriole and a venule, with _____ in between.
- **Precapillary sphincter:** This valve regulates the flow of blood into the true capillaries. It is innervated by _____ fibers. Blood may fill the capillary bed, or the bed may be empty.

Venules and Veins

Venules are vessels that are smaller than veins, but have a larger lumen than capillaries. Venules lead to veins and both vessels carry blood that is low in oxygen and high in carbon dioxide and waste materials *toward* the heart.

- **Systemic veins** carry blood *low* in oxygen (known as deoxygenated blood) back to the heart. Do you remember which heart chamber this blood is returned to? _____
- Recall that systemic veins are colored blue on models.
- **Pulmonary veins** carry blood *high* in oxygen from the lungs back to the heart. Do you remember which heart chamber this blood is returned to? _____
- Recall that pulmonary veins are colored red on models.

Structural and Functional Features of Venules and Veins

- Consist of three walls: (1) thin tunica interna, (2) sparse tunica media, and (3) thicker tunica externa.
- Compared to arteries, veins have thinner walls and a larger lumen. Specifically, tunica media is thinner since it contains less _____ muscle and fewer _____ fibers. Therefore, veins mostly lack the properties of contractility and elasticity that the arteries have.
- Veins house _____% of the blood supply. Veins are not fully expanded unless there is strenuous activity. *Distensibility* means the walls can expand or distend when the vessel fills with blood. Distensibility allows for variations in blood _____ and blood _____.
- Blood pressure drops by the time the flow of blood reaches the veins.

Adaptations to veins assist with the return of blood to the heart:

- **Valves** are formed from the tunica _____. The one-way valves resemble the SL valves of the heart and prevent the _____ and _____ of blood in the extremities. Overstretched valves are called *varicose veins.*
- **Pumps** are either respiratory or skeletal muscle in nature.
  1. The *respiratory pump* occurs when you inhale. Upon inhalation, the pressure increases in the _____, which squeezes local veins.
  2. The _____ *pump* occurs whenever you move your limbs. Skeletal muscles contract and relax, pushing blood back toward the heart.

Review Time!

I. *Using the terms in the list below, write the appropriate type of vessel in each blank. You may use a term more than once.*

    Arteriole or artery   *Capillary*   *Venule or vein*

    1. May possess valves   _____

    2. Constructed of tunica interna only   _____

    3. Site of gas, nutrient, and waste exchange   _____

    4. Possesses a thinner tunica media   _____

    5. Often carries blood low in oxygen toward the heart, except
       for the pulmonary vessels   _____

    6. Often carries oxygenated blood away from the heart, except
       for the pulmonary vessels   _____

    7. Vessel with the smallest diameter   _____

    8. Distensible, but not elastic, vessels   _____

    9. Operate under low blood pressure   _____

   10. Contractility and elasticity are features of these vessels   _____

CONCEPT 4

Blood Pressure

Concept: Blood pressure is the primary force that pushes blood through vessels. It is influenced by CO, peripheral resistance, and blood volume, which are regulated by nervous, hormonal, and kidney factors.

Blood pressure is the force exerted by blood against the inner walls of the vessels.

• Why is blood pressure important? _____

• In which vessels is it most important? _____

• How is blood pressure measured? _____

Blood pressure is the **highest** in arteries and arterioles, lower in capillaries and venules (where blood flow is slower, too). Blood pressure plays a minor role in the veins. Thus, valves, respiratory activity, and skeletal muscle activity provide what's needed to move blood back to the heart.

Measuring Blood Pressure

Blood flows from *high* pressure to *low* pressure. The highest pressure is in the _____. Why? _____

• **Systolic pressure** is normally _____ mm Hg or less when the ventricles are contracting (ventricular systole) and the aorta stretches.

• **Diastolic pressure** is normally _____ mm Hg or less when the aorta walls recoil to their original shape and pressure falls. Elasticity of the aortic wall prevents pressure from falling further, so blood is moved along. This pressure occurs during ventricular diastole.

Blood pressure is measured using a **sphygmomanometer**. Here's how this device works:

- The cuff is wrapped around the brachial artery (arm).

- _____ is pumped into the cuff and the flow of blood into the brachial artery is cut off.

- A release valve is slightly opened so that pressure in the cuff drops.

- Through a stethoscope, a tapping sound (_____ sounds) may be heard as soon as blood begins to squeeze through the artery. The pressure at this moment is *systolic pressure.*

- As pressure begins to drop, more blood spurts through the artery and the sound becomes louder before becoming inaudible. At the moment the sounds become inaudible, the pressure is the _____ *pressure.*

Measuring Pulse

Which vessels expand and stretch, then recoil to the original shape with the passage of blood through their lumen? This rhythmic contraction and relaxation can be felt in arteries as a **pulse**. The pulse is generated by ventricular systole each time the heart contracts (one heartbeat).

- In which arteries is the pulse commonly felt? _____

- What is the average resting pulse rate in *adults*? _____

- What is the average resting pulse rate in *children*? _____

- If the HR exceeds **100** beats per minute, the condition is _____

- If the HR drops below **60** beats per minute, the condition is _____

Factors Affecting Blood Pressure

LEARNING OBJECTIVE 14. Describe the factors influencing blood pressure.

Three main factors influence arterial blood pressure:

1. Cardiac output (CO)

2. _____ resistance

3. Blood volume

Role of Cardiac Output

Recall that:

$$CO = HR \times SV$$

If HR or SV changes, CO changes and the amount of blood that can be pushed is affected.

- If CO ↑, blood pressure ↑ (*where* ↑ *means increase*).

- If CO ↓, blood pressure ↓ (*where* ↓ *means decrease*).

Role of Peripheral Resistance

Peripheral resistance is the friction or drag encountered as blood flows through a vessel. Peripheral resistance slows blood flow and is determined by:

1. **Vessel diameter:** The _____ the vessel diameter, the greater the peripheral resistance and the slower the flow of blood.

   - Vasoconstriction of a vessel causes ↓ diameter, ↑ peripheral resistance, and ↑ blood pressure.

   - Vasodilation of a vessel causes ↑ diameter, ↓ peripheral resistance, and ↓ blood pressure (*where* ↓ *means decrease and* ↑ *means increase*).

2. **Viscosity of the blood:** Thicker, more viscous blood _____ peripheral resistance which leads to an increase in blood pressure. Thinner, less viscous blood _____ peripheral resistance and leads to a decrease in blood pressure.

The bottom line: Increases in peripheral resistance lead to increases in blood pressure while decreases in peripheral resistance lead to decreases in blood pressure.

TIP! Let's think of an analogy for the two types of peripheral resistance we've covered.

1. Vessel diameter: You have the option of drinking your milkshake through one of two straws—a very small, thin straw (like a coffee stirrer) or a large straw with a wide diameter. Which straw provides the least peripheral resistance to flow? The large straw with a wide diameter makes for easier drinking due to decreased peripheral resistance.

2. Viscosity: Which milkshake is easier to drink—a thin milkshake (less viscous) or a thicker milkshake (more viscous)? The thinner milkshake provides less peripheral resistance to flow. What's the bottom-line message? Wider vessels and less viscous blood provide less peripheral resistance to the flow of blood.

Role of Blood Volume

Blood volume is a measure of the amount of plasma and formed elements present in the cardiovascular system. The average blood volume is _____ liters. Changes in blood volume directly influence blood pressure. For instance:
- If blood volume ↓, blood pressure ↓ (*where ↓ means decrease*).
- If blood volume ↑, blood pressure ↑ (*where ↑ means increase*).

Review Time!

I.   *Provide a brief answer for each of the following questions about blood pressure.*

1. Why is systolic pressure heard first when listening through a stethoscope during use of a sphygmomanometer? _____
   _____

2. What is a normal value for systolic pressure? _____

3. In what type of vessel does blood pressure play its primary role?_____

4. Since blood pressure plays a minor role in veins, discuss two adaptations that assist with the return of blood to the heart. _____
   _____
   _____

5. What effect on blood pressure does vasoconstriction have? _____

6. What effect does a great loss of blood volume, say through hemorrhage, have on blood pressure?
   _____

7. Which tunic of the artery has the ability to constrict? _____

8. If HR increases, how are SV and CO affected? _____

9. Aaron, a non-athletic 43-year-old adult, has a resting pulse rate of 45 beats per minute. Is this rate normal? Explain. _____
   _____

10. Nicotine in cigarettes causes vasoconstriction. How does vasoconstriction affect peripheral resistance and blood flow? _____

II. Using the figure below, answer the following questions about blood pressure.

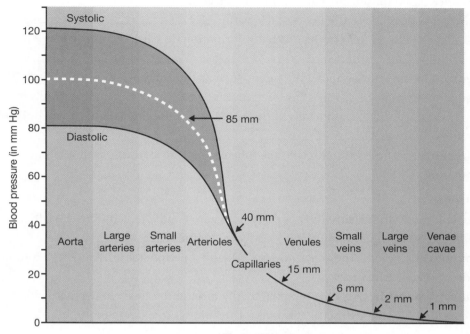

1. In which blood vessel is the blood pressure the highest? _____
2. In which blood vessels does blood pressure make the
   steepest drop? _____
3. What is the blood pressure as blood flows into capillaries? _____
4. What is the blood pressure as blood flows into large veins? _____
5. By the time blood flows from the vena cavae into the right
   atrium of the heart, what is the pressure of the blood? _____

Regulation of Blood Pressure

LEARNING OBJECTIVE 15. Describe how blood pressure is regulated.

Nervous system, hormonal, and kidney factors control blood pressure. We'll explore each factor next.

Nervous System Controls

Blood pressure can be controlled when the nervous system adjusts CO and peripheral resistance. How does the nervous system accomplish this task?

- **CO** may be increased or decreased by autonomic nervous system activity that travels between reflex centers in the medulla oblongata and the SA node of the heart. If the fibers are parasympathetic, how is the HR affected? _____ If the fibers are sympathetic, how is the HR affected?

  _____

- **Peripheral resistance** is controlled by a reflex center in the medulla oblongata known as the *vasomotor center*. Nerve fibers travel from the vasomotor center to the smooth muscle in tunica _____ of arterioles. An increase in the rate of nerve impulse transmission stimulates *vasoconstriction* of the arterioles; a decrease in the rate of nerve impulse transmission causes *vasodilation*.

The vasomotor center in the medulla oblongata determines when to stimulate and when to inhibit CO or peripheral resistance based on sensory information received from:

- **Baroreceptors** in vessels above the heart (such as the _____ and the _____ arteries). What information do baroreceptors convey to the medulla? _____

- **Chemoreceptors** in the arteries above the heart, such as the aorta and carotid arteries. They are sensitive to sudden drops in _____ levels or increases in _____ ion levels in the blood and send impulses to the medulla oblongata to stimulate blood pressure. _____

- **Higher brain centers:** These influence the medulla oblongata, so your emotional state can influence blood pressure, too!

Hormonal Controls

- **Epinephrine** and **norepinephrine (NE)** are stress triggered and released from the adrenal medulla. These hormones enhance the fight or flight response activated by the _____ division of the autonomic nervous system. These hormones ↑ HR and ↑ peripheral resistance by promoting arteriole vasoconstriction (*where ↑ means increase*).

- **Atrial natriuretic peptide (ANP)** is secreted by the atria of the heart to decrease blood volume, which leads to a decrease in blood pressure. It stimulates the kidneys to excrete more _____ ions and water to promote a decrease in blood volume. *Remember, water follows salt!*

- **Antidiuretic hormone (ADH)** is produced by the hypothalamus (and secreted by the _____ pituitary lobe) and stimulates the kidneys to conserve water. What effect does water retention have on blood volume and thus, blood pressure? _____

Kidney Controls

The kidneys provide two long-term mechanisms of blood pressure control.

Blood Volume Mechanism

- If there is an **increase** in blood volume or in blood pressure, the kidneys allow more water to leave the body as urine. **ANP**, a hormone we previously discussed, can promote the loss of _____ ions and water in the urine.

- If there is a **decrease** in blood volume or in blood pressure, the kidneys may reduce the amount of water leaving the body as urine. **ADH**, a hormone we previously discussed, can restore blood volume and pressure to a more favorable level.

Renin–Angiotensin Mechanism

- If blood pressure decreases, special kidney cells release **renin** (an enzyme) into the blood.
- Renin triggers the formation of another chemical called **angiotensin II**, a strong

  _____.

- Angiotensin II stimulates the release of another hormone called **aldosterone**, which is produced by the adrenal gland.

  1. What does aldosterone stimulate the kidneys to do? _____

  2. How does an increase in sodium and water reabsorption by the kidneys restore blood pressure? _____

TIP! Do you have the renin–angiotensin mechanism straight in your head? Low blood pressure triggers the release of renin. Renin leads to the formation of angiotensin II. Angiotensin II leads to the formation of aldosterone. Aldosterone reabsorbs sodium and water to increase blood volume and blood pressure.

Review Time!

I. *Provide a brief answer for each of the following questions about the regulation of blood pressure.*

1. What information do baroreceptors transmit to the medulla oblongata?
   _____

2. What information do chemoreceptors transmit to the medulla oblongata?
   _____

3. Where are baroreceptors and chemoreceptors located? _____

4. Where is the vasomotor center housed? _____

5. Name three hormones that can increase blood pressure and one hormone that decreases blood pressure. _____
   _____
   _____
   _____
   _____

6. What triggers the release of renin? _____

7. What does aldosterone stimulate the kidneys to do? _____
   _____

8. Describe two ways the nervous system controls blood pressure. _____
   _____
   _____

9. Describe how aldosterone and ADH can both accomplish an increase in blood pressure but through different mechanisms. _____
   _____
   _____

10. How does the vasomotor center respond to increased blood pressure to restore homeostasis?
    _____
    _____

11. Maggie is so excited that she has a winning lottery ticket. She is experiencing the effects of the sympathetic nervous system enhanced by two hormones, _____ and _____. Explain the effects of these hormones on blood pressure.
    _____
    _____

CONCEPT 5

Circulatory Pathways

Concept: Circulatory pathways channel blood in a closed loop throughout the body. They include the pulmonary circulation that transports blood to the lungs and back to the heart, and the much larger systemic circulation that carries blood to all other body structures and returns to the right atrium.

LEARNING OBJECTIVE 16. Distinguish between the pulmonary and systemic pathways in terms of function.

LEARNING OBJECTIVE 17. Identify the major arteries and veins in the pulmonary and systemic pathways.

There are two distinct pathways of the circulatory system:

1. **Pulmonary circulation** is the route blood travels from the heart to the lungs and back.
2. **Systemic circulation** is the route blood travels from the heart to the remaining areas of the body and back again.

Pulmonary Circulation

Pulmonary circulation is the route of blood flow from the heart to the _____ and back to the heart. What is the purpose of the pulmonary circuit? _____

_____

• What blood gas diffuses into the blood during pulmonary circulation? _____
• What blood gas diffuses out of the blood during pulmonary circulation? _____
Can you complete the pathway of pulmonary circulation?
• **Pulmonary trunk** carries blood from the right ventricle of the heart.
• **Right pulmonary artery** and **left pulmonary artery** travel to their respective lungs.
• Right and left pulmonary arteries divide into smaller arteries and then _____.
• Pulmonary capillaries form networks around the air sacs of the lungs. The pulmonary capillaries are *the site of gas exchange*. What gas is loaded into the RBCs? _____
• Pulmonary _____ drain the capillary beds and eventually form the pulmonary veins.
• **Pulmonary veins** (2) exit each lung and carry blood to the _____ atrium of the heart.

As we discuss the blood vessels and structures of the heart and lungs, add labels to the illustration below. When you are done, you should be able to identify the vessels and structures listed below.

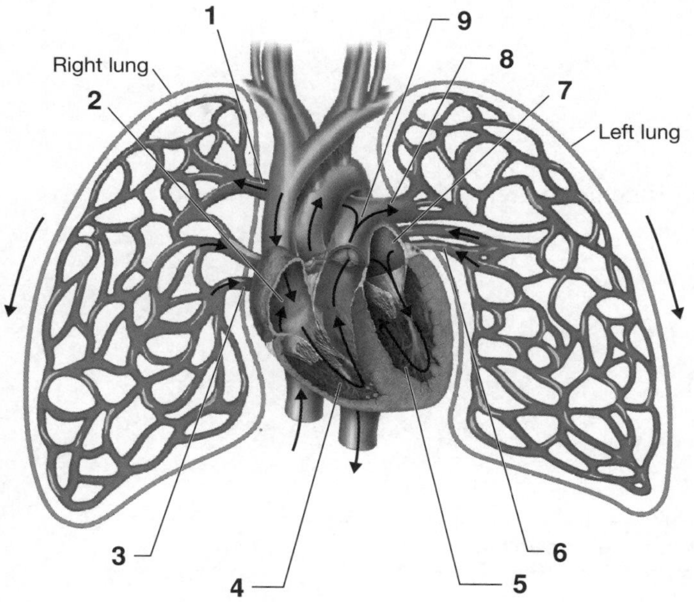

1. _____

2. _____

3. _____

4. _____

5. _____

6. _____

7. _____

8. _____

9. _____

Left atrium

Left ventricle

Left pulmonary artery

Left pulmonary vein

Pulmonary trunk

Right atrium

Right pulmonary artery

Right pulmonary vein

Right ventricle

Systemic Circulation

Systemic circulation is the route of blood flow to all body organs and tissues (except for the lungs—we just completed their circulation).

• What is the purpose of the systemic circuit? _____

_____

_____

• What blood gas begins this route? _____

• What color is blood that is highly oxygenated (on models)? _____

• What blood gas returns to the heart? _____

• What color is blood that is low in oxygen (on models)? _____

Can you complete the pathway of systemic circulation?

• Major and smaller arteries

• _____

• Capillaries

• Venules

• Smaller, then major _____

The arteries and veins of the body are often named according to the body region they supply; they usually travel parallel to one another as they feed and drain various body parts.

Systemic Arteries

The aorta originates from the left ventricle of the heart. Systemic arteries arise from the aorta.

Branches of the Aorta

The parts of the aorta are:

- Ascending aorta
- Aortic arch
- Thoracic aorta
- Abdominal aorta
- Descending aorta

The arteries that arise from each part of the aorta (listed next) are:

Ascending Aorta

- Right _____ artery
- Left _____ artery

Aortic arch supplies three branches.

- **Brachiocephalic artery** (B)
- Left **common** _____ **artery** (C)
- Left _____ **artery** (S)

TIP! Remember the three arterial branches of the aortic arch as "BCS."

Thoracic Aorta
Abdominal Aorta

- **Celiac artery** is the first branch of the abdominal aorta. It serves the liver, stomach, spleen, and

  _____.

- **Superior** _____ artery supplies the small intestine and part of the large intestine.
- **Suprarenal arteries** (2) serve each _____ gland atop each kidney.
- **Renal arteries** (2) serve each _____.
- **Gonadal arteries** (testicular arteries in males, ovarian arteries in females) supply the _____.
- **Inferior** _____ **artery** is the last major branch; it serves most of the large intestine.

Descending aorta splits at the point of L_2 vertebra into:

- Right **common iliac artery** serves the _____.
- Left **common iliac artery** serves the _____.

Arteries of the Head and Neck

The common carotid (major supplier) and subclavian arteries supply the head and neck regions with blood. The right **common carotid artery** arises from the brachiocephalic artery while the left **common carotid artery** originates from the aortic arch. At the point where the common carotid artery branches, a dilation known as the **carotid sinus** houses baroreceptors that detect changes in blood pressure.

Each common carotid artery branches into:

- **External carotid artery:** Supplies parts of the neck, face, jaw, and scalp by way of smaller branches.
- **Internal carotid artery:** Enters the cranial cavity to supply the _____.

The right **subclavian artery** originates from the brachiocephalic artery while the left **subclavian artery** arises from the _____. Each subclavian artery branches into:

- **Vertebral arteries** pass through the transverse foramina of the cervical vertebrae and enter the cranial cavity to the brain through the foramen magnum of the _____ bone.
- **Thyrocervical arteries** travel to the neck and supply the _____ and _____ glands, larynx, trachea, esophagus, pharynx, and muscles of the region.

Arteries of the Shoulder and Upper Limbs

The **subclavian arteries** entirely supply the shoulder and upper limbs. The subclavian artery approaches the armpit, or axilla, and continues downward as the **axillary artery** which branches and supplies muscles and other structures in the _____ and thoracic wall.

- The axillary artery continues into the upper arm (brachium) as the **brachial artery**.
- The **brachial artery** follows along the _____ to the elbow where it divides into ulnar and radial arteries:
    1. **Ulnar artery** travels along the ulnar side of the forearm to the wrist.
    2. **Radial artery** travels along the radial side of the forearm to the wrist.

Arteries of the Pelvis and Lower Limbs

The branches of the **common iliac arteries** supply the pelvis and lower limbs with blood. Each common iliac artery branches into:

- **Internal iliac artery** travels into the _____ wall. Its branches supply parts of the pelvic cavity and external genitals.
- **External iliac artery** carries the main supply of blood to the _____. As this vessel passes under the inguinal ligament and enters the thigh, it becomes the **femoral artery** which travels down the _____ side of the thigh.

The femoral artery branches into the **deep femoral artery** which supplies the flexor muscles of the thigh (most important femoral artery branch). The femoral artery continues behind the knee as the **popliteal artery** which branches into the:

- **Anterior tibial artery** travels between the _____ and _____.
- **Posterior tibial artery** extends behind the calf muscles.

Review Time!

I. *Provide a brief answer for each of the following questions about blood flow and systemic arteries.*

1. Where does the right subclavian artery originate? The left? _____
    _____
    _____

2. What artery is the major supplier of the head? _____

3. What three arteries arise from the aortic arch?
    1. _____
    2. _____
    3. _____

4. What does the celiac artery supply with blood? _____
    _____

5. At the point of vertebra L_2, what does the descending aorta split into? _____
    _____

6. What organs do the renal arteries serve? _____

7. What are the two branches of the brachial artery?
    1. _____
    2. _____

8. What does the external iliac artery become upon entering the leg? _____

9. What is the most important branch of the femoral artery? _____

10. What artery gives rise to the anterior and posterior tibial arteries? _____

II. *Using the terms in the list below, label the systemic arteries. The branches of the aorta (ascending aorta, aortic arch, thoracic aorta, and abdominal aorta) are labeled for you.*

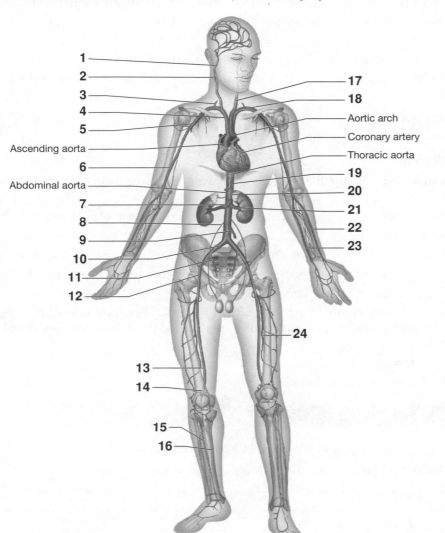

1. _____
2. _____
3. _____
4. _____
5. _____
6. _____
7. _____
8. _____
9. _____
10. _____
11. _____
12. _____
13. _____
14. _____
15. _____
16. _____
17. _____
18. _____
19. _____
20. _____
21. _____
22. _____
23. _____
24. _____

Branches of the Aortic Arch

Brachiocephalic artery

Common carotid artery

Subclavian artery

Branches of the Abdominal Aorta

Celiac artery

Superior mesenteric artery

Suprarenal artery

Renal artery

Gonadal artery

Inferior mesenteric artery

Branches of the Common Carotid Artery

External carotid artery

Internal carotid artery

Branch of the Subclavian Artery

Vertebral artery

Arteries of the Shoulder and Upper Limbs

Axillary artery

Brachial artery

Radial artery

Ulnar artery

Arteries of the Pelvis and Lower Limbs

Common iliac artery

External iliac artery

Internal iliac artery

Deep femoral artery

Femoral artery

Anterior tibial artery

Posterior tibial artery

Popliteal artery

Systemic Veins

Systemic veins form when smaller veins and venules drain blood from capillary networks (except the lungs). The blood in systemic veins is carried toward the heart, eventually draining into the SVC and IVC. The veins will be covered from those distal to as they drain into the major veins.

Veins Draining into the Superior Vena Cava

The SVC receives blood from veins in all areas superior to the diaphragm (except the lungs).

* Into which chamber of the heart will the SVC return blood?

_____

Head and Neck

* Right and left **external jugular veins** drain blood from the face, scalp, and superficial regions of the

_____.

* The external jugular veins merge with the **subclavian veins** along with the right and left **internal jugular veins**, which carry blood from the brain and deep areas of the head and neck.
* The internal jugular veins unite with the subclavian veins and form the _____ **veins** (right and left).
* The brachiocephalic veins drain blood into the **SVC**. The SVC also receives the single **azygos vein** which drains the thoracic and abdominal walls. Into which chamber of the heart does the SVC deliver blood?

_____

Upper Limbs

* Deep veins of the upper limbs parallel the pathway of the arteries and are named similarly: the **ulnar vein**, the **radial vein**, the **brachial vein**, and the **axillary vein**.
* Superficial veins of the upper limbs provide alternate routes for blood to travel. The _____ **vein** travels from the forearm to the middle of the upper arm, the _____ **vein** extends upward from wrist to shoulder, and the _____ **vein** (used during a procedure known as *phlebotomy* for blood withdrawal) interconnects the basilic and cephalic veins. At the shoulder, the cephalic vein joins the axillary vein. The axillary vein continues to join the **subclavian vein**. The subclavian vein joins the _____ jugular vein to form the brachiocephalic vein.

Veins Draining into the Inferior Vena Cava

The IVC receives blood from veins in all areas of the body below the heart.

* Into which chamber of the heart will the SVC return blood? _____

In the lower limbs, veins travel either a deep pathway or a superficial pathway:

Deep veins parallel the arteries serving the leg and share the same name, such as:

* **Anterior tibial vein**
* **Posterior tibial vein**
* **Popliteal vein**
* **Femoral vein**
* **External iliac vein**

Superficial veins interconnect with one another and the deep veins to form a network extending from foot to upper thigh. The main vessels are:

* **Great saphenous vein** is the longest vein in the body that runs from the ankle to the thigh along the _____ side of the leg.
* **Small saphenous vein** travels the lateral side from the foot, calf muscles, and into the _____ vein at the knee.

In the abdomen, several veins parallel arteries of the same name:

- **Right** _____ **vein** (right testicular vein or right ovarian vein) drains the gonads.
- **Renal vein** drains the _____.
- **Suprarenal vein** drains the _____ glands.
- **Left gonadal vein** joins the left renal vein rather than the IVC.
- **Hepatic veins** drain the liver into the IVC.

As we discuss the systemic veins, add labels to the illustration below. When you are done, you should be able to identify the systemic veins listed below.

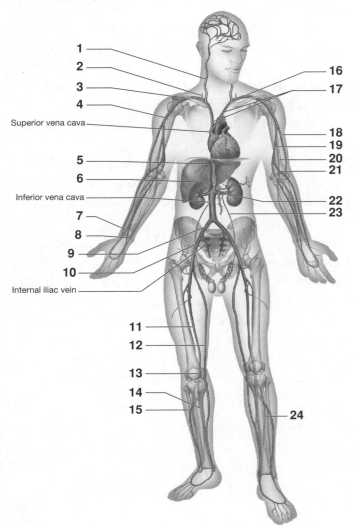

1. _____
2. _____
3. _____
4. _____
5. _____
6. _____
7. _____
8. _____
9. _____
10. _____
11. _____
12. _____
13. _____
14. _____
15. _____
16. _____
17. _____
18. _____
19. _____
20. _____
21. _____
22. _____
23. _____
24. _____

Head and Neck Veins Draining into the SVC

External jugular vein

Internal jugular vein

Left subclavian vein

Left and right brachiocephalic veins

Upper Limb Veins Draining into the SVC

Ulnar vein

Radial vein

Brachial vein

Axillary vein

Basilic vein

Cephalic vein

Median cubital vein

Lower Limb Veins Draining into the IVC

Anterior tibial vein

Posterior tibial vein

Popliteal vein

Femoral vein

External iliac vein

Great saphenous vein

Small saphenous vein

Abdominal Veins Draining into the IVC

Gonadal vein

Renal vein

Hepatic vein

Hepatic portal vein

Hepatic Portal System

The **hepatic portal system** shunts blood from the capillaries of the digestive tract to the capillaries of the
_____ before returning the blood to the IVC via the _____
vein. As blood flows through the capillaries of the liver, materials needed for metabolic functions can be
removed. Phagocytic cells can remove bacteria and other foreign materials that penetrated the intestinal
lining and entering the blood.

The flow of blood *into* the liver is as follows:

• **Hepatic portal vein** transports nutrient-rich blood low in _____ into the
liver from the digestive tract (intestine).

• **Hepatic artery** carries oxygenated blood into the liver.

The flow of blood *out* of the liver is as follows:

• **Hepatic vein** carries deoxygenated blood to the IVC.

Review Time!

I.   *Provide a brief answer for each of the following questions about blood flow and systemic veins.*

1. What does the union of the subclavian vein and the internal jugular vein form?

   _____

   _____

2. What two veins are interconnected by the median cubital vein?

   1. _____

   2. _____

3. What vein drains blood from the axillary vein? _____

4. What is the longest vein in the body? _____

5. Which vein in the arm is commonly used during phlebotomy? _____

6. The hepatic portal system is a blood pathway through which organ? _____

7. What organs do the suprarenal veins drain? _____

8. What vein carries nutrient-rich blood into the liver? _____

9. Which vein drains the liver of blood? _____

10. What vein drains blood from the brain? _____

11. Into which chamber of the heart do both the superior and inferior vena cavae return blood?

    _____

13

The Lymphatic System and the Body's Defenses

Tips for Success as You Begin

Read Chapter 13 from your textbook before attending class. Listen when you attend lecture and fill in the blanks in this notebook. You may choose to complete the blanks before attending class as a way to prepare for the day's topics. The same day you attend lecture, read the material again and complete the exercises after each section in this notebook. Spend time every day with this chapter as it will help you make sense of the material. The body's defenses can be complicated to learn; frequent study will help you to differentiate among the types of cells and processes involved in immunity.

Introduction to the Lymphatic System

- What system is closely associated with the lymphatic system? _____
- Define lymph. _____
  _____

- **Immunity** is defined as the defensive response to unwanted substances in the body.
- Two key roles of the lymphatic system are:
  1. Maintain fluid balance by carrying fluid from the _____ environment and recycling it back into the bloodstream.
  2. Perform the primary role in _____.

The specialized organs of the lymphatic system include:

- Lymph nodes
- _____
- _____
- _____

CONCEPT 1

The Lymphatic Network

Concept: The lymphatic network is a series of tubes that recycle body fluids by transporting lymph and returning it to the bloodstream.

LEARNING OBJECTIVE 1. Identify the function of the lymphatic network.

Recall from Chapter 12 that **interstitial fluid** is formed as plasma is pushed from the bloodstream through capillary walls. Most (90%) of the interstitial fluid returns back to the blood in the capillaries, but 10% does not return. This remaining fluid must be returned to the blood, or _____ problems arise such as:

• Abnormal accumulation of fluid in tissues
• Reduction of _____ volume in the blood

LEARNING OBJECTIVE 2. Distinguish between plasma, interstitial fluid, and lymph.

How does this remaining fluid rejoin circulation? **Lymphatic network** of veinlike tubes, such as capillaries, vessels, trunks, and collective ducts, drain fluid. This fluid moves by way of a one-way flow toward the heart to return to the bloodstream.

Lymph is the name given to the fluid that is found within the lymphatic network.

• When is the fluid called plasma? _____
• Where is interstitial fluid located? _____

Lymphatic Capillaries

Lymphatic capillaries are:

• Microscopic dead-end tubes
• Vessels found between cells, among capillary beds of nearly all tissues and organs
• Absent from the brain, _____, bone tissue, and
_____ of the skin.

Structure of Lymphatic Capillaries

Lymphatic capillaries are made up of a single layer of _____ with loosely joined cells that overlap. Protein filament bundles connect cells of the lymphatic capillary to the extracellular space. Why? _____
_____

• How does the lymphatic capillary prevent fluid from leaking back out to the interstitial space?
_____

Lymphatic Vessels

Lymphatic vessels are formed as lymphatic capillaries merge. The lymphatic vessels:

• Have thicker walls than lymphatic capillaries.
• Have a larger _____ than lymphatic capillaries.
• Are situated closer to the heart.

Structurally, lymphatic vessels are similar to veins of the cardiovascular system.
- Both lymphatic vessels and veins have the same _____ (*how many?*) layers of tissue.
- Both lymphatic vessels and veins have valves to prevent the _____ of fluids.

Lymphatic vessels converge into small organs known as **lymph nodes**.

Lymph Trunks and Collecting Ducts

Lymphatic trunks are formed by the merging of numerous lymphatic vessels. There are two major lymphatic trunks.

1. **Thoracic duct** drains lymph from the LEFT side of the head, neck, and thorax, LEFT upper limb, and the ENTIRE body below the diaphragm. It empties into the left _____ vein; a valve prevents blood from entering the thoracic duct.

2. **Right lymphatic duct** drains lymph from the RIGHT side of the head, neck and thorax, and the RIGHT upper limb. It empties into the right _____ vein, with which it unites.

Movement of Lymph

What factors influence the pressure gradients that affect the flow of lymph through the lymphatic network?
- Proteins in the _____ fluid
- _____ muscle contraction
- Breathing movements

Lymph Formation

How do proteins get into interstitial fluid? Smaller proteins can leak through the capillary wall at the arterial end and join the interstitial fluid. They may not reenter the venous end of the capillary when most interstitial fluid is reabsorbed. Osmotic pressure rises when proteins accumulate in the interstitial fluid.
- What is osmotic pressure? _____

What is typically housed in interstitial fluid? Interstitial fluid contains water and dissolved substances in addition to small _____ escaped from the blood.

How does interstitial fluid enter the lymphatic capillaries? Osmotic pressure in the interstitial fluid rises when solutes or proteins accumulate in the interstitial environment. When osmotic pressure rises, reabsorption into the venous end of the capillary slows due to a decrease in the pressure difference. The increased osmotic pressure forces open the lymphatic capillary pores and interstitial fluid moves into the lymphatic capillary.
- At what point is the interstitial fluid called lymph? _____

Flow of Lymph

LEARNING OBJECTIVE 3. Describe the pathway of lymph by identifying the structures through which it passes.

As pressure increases in the interstitial space, fluid flows into lymphatic capillaries along a _____. Once inside the lymphatic capillaries, the pressure provides the force needed to move the lymph along. Beyond this point, other forces assist the movement of lymph.
- _____ **pump:** Skeletal muscles contract and act as a pump to squeeze both blood vessels and lymph vessels.
- _____ **pump:** Breathing rhythmically squeezes and opens vessels as the diaphragm pushes visceral organs.
- **Valves** in lymphatic vessels allow the flow of lymph toward the heart.

Review Time!

I. *Provide a brief answer for each of the following questions about lymph and the lymphatic network.*

1. Describe the two major functions of the lymphatic system. _____

    _____

    _____

2. How are plasma and lymph similar? What makes these two fluids different?

    _____

    _____

    _____

3. How does the presence of proteins in the interstitial fluid affect osmotic pressure of the interstitial fluid? _____

    _____

4. Into what veins is lymph returned? _____

5. Describe two pumps that assist in the return of both blood and lymph to the heart.

    _____

    _____

    _____

    _____

6. In what organs or tissues are lymphatic capillaries *not* found? _____

    _____

7. Describe how lymphatic capillaries prevent trapped fluids from leaking back into the interstitial space. _____

    _____

8. Describe how circulatory veins and lymphatic vessels are similar in both structure and function.

    _____

    _____

    _____

9. From what parts of the body do the thoracic duct and right lymphatic duct collect lymph?

    _____

    _____

    _____

10. During a mastectomy of Tameka's left breast, her surgeon also removed nearby lymph nodes and lymphatic vessels. Why do you think she now experiences swelling in her left arm?

    _____

    _____

    _____

CONCEPT 2

Other Lymphatic Organs

Concept: Lymphatic organs other than the vessels consist mostly of packed lymphocytes that perform defensive functions, and include lymph nodes, spleen, thymus, and mucosa-associated lymphoid tissue.

LEARNING OBJECTIVE 4. Describe the structure and function of lymph nodes.

LEARNING OBJECTIVE 5. Identify the organs of the lymphatic system by their structures and functions.

Lymphatic organs contain lymphoid tissue, a special connective tissue with numerous lymphocytes. Recall that lymphocytes are _____

The lymphocytes initiate an immune response against disease-causing microorganisms. Other organs include the lymph nodes, spleen, thymus, and mucosa-associated lymphoid tissue (MALT).

Lymph Nodes

Lymph nodes are kidney-bean–shaped organs of lymphatic tissue.

Location: Lymph nodes are scattered along lymphatic vessels. Clusters are commonly found in a few main areas:

- Neck (_____ region)
- Armpit (_____ region)
- Groin (_____ region)
- Deep within the _____ cavity

Structure: Lymph nodes are sending and receiving stations for lymph.

- **Afferent lymphatic vessels** bring lymph into the lymph node at the _____
  (concave margin of the lymph node).
- _____ **lymphatic vessels** carry lymph away from the lymph node and onward toward the heart.

The lymph node is encapsulated by a **fibrous capsule** of dense connective tissue that also divides the lymph node into compartments. Within each compartment are **lymph nodules**, clusters of _____, that form the main structure. A **germinal center** is the center of each lymph nodule; it functions as the site of lymphocyte maturation.

The two main portions of a lymph node are the:

- **Cortex:** The outer area where lymphocytes and macrophages are located. Do you recall what these white blood cells do? _____
- **Medulla:** The inner part that contains strands of lymphocytes known as _____ cords.

Function: Lymph nodes filter and remove microorganisms (such as bacteria and viruses) and foreign particles from lymph. Lymphocytes and macrophages are present to either inactivate or engulf damaged cells and debris.

Review Time!

I. Using the terms in the list below, label the parts of the lymph node.

1. _____
2. _____
3. _____
4. _____
5. _____
6. _____
7. _____
8. _____
9. _____
10. _____
11. _____

Afferent lymphatic vessels

Efferent lymphatic vessels

Fibrous capsule

Germinal center

Hilus

Lymph continuing toward
   venous system

Lymph from body tissues

Lymph node artery and vein

Lymph nodule

Medullary cords

Valve

Spleen

The **spleen** is the largest lymphoid organ.

Location: The spleen is situated on the left side of the abdominal cavity just below the _____.

Structure: The spleen is enclosed by a **fibrous capsule** whose fibers divide the spleen into compartments with lymphocytes and macrophages. The two regions of the spleen are:

• **Red pulp:** Area filled with many _____.

• **White pulp:** Region that contains lymphoid tissue with _____.

Functions: The *primary* job of the spleen is to filter foreign particles, old and defective _____ blood cells, and platelets from the bloodstream. White blood cells within the _____ pulp accomplish this job. The *secondary* job of the spleen is to act as a blood reservoir by storing large volumes of blood in case of blood loss. The _____ pulp performs this function.

TIP! The lymph nodes filter lymph while the spleen filters blood.

Thymus

The **thymus** plays a role in the endocrine system; it is reduced in size and function in adults, but large in infants.

Location: The thymus is a large, bilobed gland located in the _____ cavity behind the sternum.

Structure: The thymus is composed of lymphoid tissue divided into clusters of lymphocytes known as _____.

Function: The cells of the thymus are only active during times when the immune system is rapidly developing, between 6 months and _____ years of age. Thymus cells promote maturation of lymphocytes into T lymphocytes.

Mucosa-associated Lymphoid Tissue (MALT)

MALTs are lymphoid organs *not* surrounded by a capsule.

Location: MALTs are scattered through lymphatic tissue of mucous membranes of the following tracts:

* _____
* _____
* _____
* _____

Types of MALT Organs

Tonsils (5) are located in the mouth and throat and are partially embedded within the mucous membranes. They enlarge during an infection due to the proliferation of _____ and white blood cells.

* **Palatine tonsils** (2) are at the back end of the palate (roof of the mouth).
* **Pharyngeal tonsil** (**adenoid**) (1) is situated against the nasopharynx (upper throat wall).
* **Lingual tonsils** (2) are found at the base of the tongue.

Peyer patches are found in the wall of the _____ intestine. They prevent the migration of bacteria from the intestinal lumen.

Review Time!

I. *Using the terms in the list below, write the appropriate lymphoid organ or tissue in each blank. You may use a term more than once*

   MALT   Spleen   Thymus   Tonsils

   1. Found in clusters in the neck, armpit, groin, and deep within the abdominal cavity   _____
   2. Most active between the ages of 6 months and 5 years   _____
   3. Located on the left side of the abdominal cavity below the diaphragm   _____
   4. Filters foreign particles from blood   _____
   5. Two examples are the tonsils and Peyer's patches   _____
   6. Red pulp and white pulp perform the main functions   _____
   7. Located in mucous membranes lining the digestive, reproductive, urinary, and respiratory tracts   _____
   8. Removes old and defective red blood cells and platelets from the bloodstream   _____
   9. Located in the thoracic cavity behind the sternum   _____
   10. Filter and remove foreign particles from lymph   _____

II. *Provide a brief answer for each of the following questions about lymphoid organs and tissues.*
   1. How are MALTs structurally different from other lymphoid organs? _____
   _____
   2. During what time of life is the thymus most active? Why? _____
   _____

3. What are the two functions of the spleen? _____

_____

4. List the functions of the red pulp and the white pulp of the spleen . _____

_____

_____

5. List the locations of the five tonsils. _____

_____

_____

6. How are the functions of the lymph nodes and the spleen similar? _____

_____

_____

7. Where is the spleen located? _____

_____

8. Where are the main clusters of lymph nodes? _____

_____

9. What two white blood cells are commonly found in lymphoid organs?

_____

_____

10. What do you think would happen if the lymph nodes could not effectively do their jobs?

_____

_____

_____

CONCEPT 3

Defense Mechanisms of the Body

Concept: The defense mechanisms of the body defend against unwanted substances to prevent disease. Their activities are mainly based on a recognition system that determines what belongs in the body, called self, and what does not, called nonself.

Pathogens cause disease and can disrupt homeostasis. Some examples of pathogens are

_____

_____

• What problems can arise if pathogens destroy large numbers of our cells? _____

_____

Self versus Nonself

LEARNING OBJECTIVE   6. Distinguish between self and nonself by describing the role of MHC proteins.

The body's defensive strategies rely on an ability to differentiate proteins. White blood cells can distinguish between proteins on the basis of the distribution and type of surface membrane proteins on a cell _____.

- **Self** are proteins that belong to the body.
- **Nonself** are proteins that do *not* belong to the body.

The distribution of proteins is genetically determined by **major histocompatibility complex (MHC)** genes. MHC proteins prescribe a code for your white blood cells to either recognize proteins as self and ignore them, or destroy them if the proteins are nonself.

- What can cause an abnormal sequence of MHC proteins? _____

_____

- What happens to cells with an abnormal sequence of MHC proteins? _____

_____

Innate versus Adaptive Immunity

LEARNING OBJECTIVE 7. Distinguish between innate and adaptive immunity.

Two defense strategies employed by the body involve lymphocytes and macrophages and are called innate (nonspecific) and adaptive (specific) immunity.

- **Innate immunity:** The skin, enzymes in saliva, and other innate defenses help prevent many kinds of _____ from entering the body.
- **Adaptive immunity:** The body mounts a defense to a specific pathogen by adapting to it. The adaptation involves _____ memory of the invader, known as a *memory cell*.

> **TIP!** Innate means "from birth." You are born with innate defenses such as skin, enzymes, and other defenses that prevent entry of pathogens into the body. But, upon exposure to specific pathogens, your body will adapt to it to create a memory of it.

CONCEPT 4

Innate Immunity

Concept: Innate immunity protects the body by forming barriers and by employing nonspecific strategies including phagocytosis, the action of natural killer cells, the production of certain proteins, and inflammation.

LEARNING OBJECTIVE 8. Identify the major strategies of innate immunity.

Barriers

Innate immunity provides barriers to the entry of pathogens into the body and strategies to destroy them if they make their way into the body. Physical and chemical barriers include:

- **Skin** is the body's first line of defense. Keratin is impenetrable to bacteria, viruses, and most toxins. Recall from Chapter 5 that keratin is _____

_____

- **Mucous membranes** provide a second important physical barrier. Mucous membranes line the body cavities that open to the exterior. Mucus traps microorganisms in the respiratory and digestive tracts.

> **TIP!** Notice the difference in spelling—it's no error. *Mucus* is the sticky substance secreted by *mucous* membranes.

_____ results when a pathogen successfully penetrates through the body's physical and chemical barriers.

Phagocytosis

Phagocytosis is the ingestion and destruction of particles by specialized cells called phagocytes. Explain how a phagocyte accomplishes phagocytosis. _____

_____

_____

_____

Phagocytosis is innate because white blood cells do not distinguish between different types of foreign cells. They only ingest cells with special proteins that identify the cell or particle as nonself.

What types of white blood cells perform phagocytosis? _____

- **Macrophages** arise from _____. They transform into "large eaters" when they approach an infection. Macrophages can also stand guard at the infection (called fixed macrophages) or wander the blood stream (called wandering macrophages).

- **Neutrophils** squeeze through blood vessel walls to reach sites of infection or inflammation.

Natural Killer (NK) Cells

NK cells do _not_ phagocytize unwanted cells. These white blood cells work by a different method:

1. NK cells secrete an arrow-shaped protein that punctures a hole in the cell membrane of cancer cells or virus-infected cells. The cell dies quickly because it loses _____ (a process called _cytolysis_).

2. NK cells secrete protein-digesting enzymes that destroy targeted cells.

How do NK cells identify unwanted cells? _____

_____

Proteins

Two important proteins for innate immunity are:

1. **Complement:** Plasma proteins (20 or more) circulate in blood plasma in the inactive state. When an infection is present, complement is activated (in other words, the protein is activated). The protein labels substances as nonself. Complement also increases the movement of phagocytes into an area of infection and stimulates their destructive abilities. What kind of white blood cells will eat the cells labeled as nonself? _____

2. **Interferons** are secreted by cells that have been infected by viruses. The interferons diffuse to nearby cells and bind to their membranes, "interfering" with the virus' ability to proliferate in those cells. Interferons are being used in the treatment of a specific type of bone marrow cancer (called _hairy cell leukemia_).

Inflammation

LEARNING OBJECTIVE   9. Describe the process of inflammation, its benefits, and its drawbacks.

Inflammation is a nonspecific response to stress, a disruption of homeostasis. Inflammation's benefit is

_____

_____

_____

The inflammation response starts when a damaged cell, a basophil (type of _____ blood cell), or a fixed connective tissue cell known as a _____ cell releases substances, such as histamine and serotonin, in the bloodstream in response to stress. These chemicals produce two main responses by local tissues:

1. **Vasodilation** of blood vessels (another way to say this is an increase or widening in the _____ of a blood vessel)
2. **Increased permeability** of blood vessels (widening of pores in capillary walls)

These responses produce four symptoms that are characteristic of inflammation.

1. _Redness_ is due to vasodilation of local blood vessels, which increases blood flow to the site of injury. What is the benefit of increased blood flow? _____
   _____
2. _Swelling_ results from fluids leaking across the capillary walls into the extracellular space. The extracellular space fills with fluid and causes swelling (called _____).
3. _Heat_ is related to the increased blood flow from deeper areas of the body where body temperature is warmer.
4. _Pain_ is caused by pressure on local pain receptors due to the increased _____ in the area of injury.

With vasodilation and increased blood flow to the site of injury come white blood cells. White blood cells fight invading microorganisms and accumulate. _____ is a thick fluid that contains living and nonliving white blood cells, bacteria and their products, and interstitial fluid.

> **TIP!** Have you ever experienced the inflammation response—such as from a bee sting or a paper cut? Remember the four symptoms that accompany inflammation: red, hot, swollen, and painful skin.

Review Time!

I. _Provide a brief answer for each of the following questions about defense mechanisms and innate immunity._

1. Explain what pathogens are and provide some examples. _____
   _____
   _____

2. How does the body tell the difference between self and nonself proteins?
   _____
   _____

3. Which type of immunity is nonspecific to pathogens—innate or adaptive?
   _____

4. What are MHC proteins? What type of blood cell checks MHC proteins to determine self or nonself? _____
   _____

5. What are the two physical barriers to the entrance of foreign substances into the body?
   1. _____
   2. _____

6. Why is phagocytosis considered a type of innate immunity and not adaptive immunity?
   _____
   _____

7. How are phagocytes different from NK cells? _____
_____
_____

8. How do NK cells accomplish cytolysis? _____
_____

9. Describe two methods NK cells use to kill cells. _____
   1. _____
   2. _____

10. What does vasodilation accomplish during the inflammation process?
_____
_____

11. What type of protein responds to virus-infected cells to prevent further infection?
_____
_____

12. How does the activation of complement help control an infection? _____
_____

13. List and describe four symptoms of inflammation. _____
   1. _____
   2. _____
   3. _____
   4. _____

14. What is pus? _____
_____

15. Why do you think people use cold compresses when an area of the body is inflamed?
_____
_____
_____

CONCEPT 5

Adaptive Immunity

Concept: Adaptive immunity relies upon the ability of specialized cells to recognize specific antigens. Once they are recognized, two very effective weapons become activated: cell-mediated immunity and antibody-mediated immunity.

Adaptive immunity is specific against pathogens. Responses involve proliferation of a certain type of lymphocyte or production of a protein called an antibody. Two types of adaptive immune responses are:
1. **Cell-mediated immunity**
2. **Antibody-mediated immunity**

Components of Adaptive Immunity

LEARNING OBJECTIVE 10. Describe the components of adaptive immunity.

Both types of adaptive immune responses involve at least some of the following: antigens, antibodies, cytokines, phagocytic cells such as antigen-presenting cells, and the two primary types of lymphocytes.

Antigens

Antigens are chemical substances that provoke an immune response when they enter the body. Antigen means *anti*body *gen*erator. White blood cells recognize antigens as nonself.

What is considered an antigen?

- Large molecules such as _____, _____, or _____ , bound to proteins.
- Microorganisms or _____ molecules they release
- Chemicals from insect bites and stings
- Molds, certain foods, and airborne particles
- _____ cells and tissues

Autoimmune disease occurs when the immune system mistakenly identifies a person's own proteins as antigens. Healthy cells and tissues can be destroyed.

Antibodies

Antibodies are protein molecules produced by lymphocytes in response to a specific antigen. The antibody binds to the antigen to form an antigen–antibody complex. Antibodies are also known as *immunoglobulins* (or *Ig*). There are five classes of antibodies. Each has a distinctive structure and specific response to specific antigens.

Cytokines

Cytokines are signaling chemicals secreted by cells such as lymphocytes, monocytes, macrophages, _____ cells, and _____ cells. Cytokines bind to receptors on a cell membrane of a lymphocyte *and simultaneously* with an antigen–MHC protein complex. Cytokines promote cell _____ and cell _____ , part of the cell's adaptive response called *activation*. The most common cytokine is _____

Lymphocytes

Lymphocytes are the most important type of white blood cell in adaptive immunity. Recall from Chapter 11 that these cells originate _____ .

Once these cells are formed, they are ready for the maturation process.

- **T cells** are lymphocytes that migrate to the thymus and mature (**T** cells for **t**hymus).
- **B cells** are lymphocytes that remain in the red **b**one marrow, or migrate to the spleen or to MALT (wall of small intestine) and mature.

Programming to recognize self cells and distinguish them from nonself cells occurs in lymphoid tissue such as lymph nodes, the spleen, MALT, and red bone marrow. Once the lymphocytes have developed this ability, they are **mature** or _____ .

> **TIP!** Remember where T cells and B cells mature by the first letter of their locations: T cells mature in the thymus while B cells can remain in the bone marrow to mature.

T Cells

- You have specific T cells programmed to attack the specific antigens you have been exposed to during your lifetime.
- T cells mature after birth. They migrate from the thymus to join circulation or reside in lymphoid tissue in the _____, _____, or _____.
- Once established, T cells continue undergoing _____ to maintain the colony and send new T cells throughout the body.
- T cells can be either helper T cells or _____ (killer) T cells (play important roles in *cell-mediated immunity* and *antibody-mediated immunity*).

B Cells

- As is true of T cells, you have a specific type of B cell for every antigen you have been exposed to during your lifetime.
- Lymphocytes remain in the _____, _____, or _____ for development after maturation.
- Like T cells, B cells migrate to lymph nodes or other lymphoid tissue. However, they do not enter circulation like T cells.
- B cells are the primary cells involved in *antibody-mediated immunity*.

Antigen-presenting Cells (APCs)

APCs are usually monocytes or macrophages that remove unwanted substances by phagocytosis. The role of these cells in adaptive immunity involves *presentation of antigen* molecules to a special type of lymphocyte (called a helper T cell). These phagocytes wander the body surveying cells and molecules in search of antigens. Once an APC finds an antigen, the phagocyte _____

_____

After the phagocyte engulfs the antigen:

- APC processes the antigen within vesicles in the cytoplasm by digesting it and packaging some of its molecules along with MHC proteins produced by the APC cell.
- The _____ molecules bind to MHC proteins produced by the APC.
- The vesicle exits the cell by exocytosis. The vesicle merges with the cell membrane and attaches the antigen–MHC protein complex onto the external surface of the APC.
- Now that the antigen–MHC protein complex is on the external surface, it can be *presented* to a _____.
- The presentation of the antigen stimulates the helper T cell into action (we'll cover helper T cells *later*).

Review Time!

I. *Using the terms in the list below, write the appropriate type of lymphocyte in each blank. You may use a term more than once.*

   B cells   T cells   Both B cells and T cells

   1. Can be a helper or a killer   _____
   2. Reside in lymph nodes and other lymphoid tissue   _____
   3. Provides antibody-mediated immunity   _____
   4. Less common in circulation   _____
   5. Provides cell-mediated immunity   _____
   6. Trained to detect MHC proteins on the membranes of self cells _____

7. Important in adaptive immunity   _____

8. Originate from the bone marrow before birth   _____

9. Matured in the thymus   _____

10. Become immunocompetent after gaining the ability to
    distinguish self from nonself cells   _____

II.   *Place a number from 1 to 5 in the blank before each statement to indicate the correct order of the steps in the process of antigen presentation by APCs.*

_____ Antigen–MHC protein complex is presented to a helper T cell.

_____ APC digests the antigen within a vesicle in the cytoplasm.

_____ The antigen molecules chemically bind to MHC proteins produced by the APC.

_____ The vesicle undergoes exocytosis; the vesicle merges with the cell membrane.

_____ The antigen–MHC protein complex is attached onto the external surface of the APC.

Cell-mediated Immunity

LEARNING OBJECTIVE   11. Distinguish between cell-mediated and antibody-mediated immunity.

LEARNING OBJECTIVE   12. Describe the roles of the various forms of T cells during cell-mediated immunity.

Helper T cells and cytotoxic T cells provide cell-mediated immunity, but must be *activated* first. Once activated, the helper or cytotoxic T cells undergo _____. The cell gains special properties that allow the activated T cell to react against particular antigens. The properties are passed on to descendent cells known as **clones**.

Helper T Cells

Helper T cells (CD4 T cells) stimulate defensive activities of other cells.

What is the process of cell-mediated immunity with helper T cells?

• APC identifies an antigen in the body and phagocytizes the antigen.

• APC processes the antigen and expresses it on the _____.

• APC presents the antigen to an *inactive* helper T cell.

• Upon receipt of a second signal from a cytokine, the helper T cell is activated.

• The activated helper T cell enlarges and divides into two secondary clone lines: *active helper T cells* and *memory helper T cells.*

  1. **Active helper T cells** secrete _____ (such as interleukin-2). The cytokines provide a trigger for continued helper T cell proliferation, cytotoxic T cell activation and proliferation, and stimulation of NK cells.

  2. **Memory helper T cells** are not engaged against the infection. A *secondary infection* that occurs when an antigen appears in the body a second time may trigger _____ helper T cells to proliferate and change into new clone lines of _____ helper T cells and more memory helper T cells.

Cytotoxic T Cells

Cytotoxic T cells (CD8 T cells) attack infected body cells and destroy them (*seek and destroy*).

What is the process of cell-mediated immunity with cytotoxic T cells?

• Inactive cytotoxic T cells are activated when they recognize an antigen–MHC protein complex on the surface of an infected body cell.

- Cytotoxic T cells require cytokines to stimulate activation, as do helper T cells.
- Activated cytotoxic T cells enlarge and divide into two secondary clone lines: _____ cytotoxic T cells and _____ cytotoxic T cells.
   1. **Active cytotoxic T cells** actively seek cells infected with the antigen in all body tissues in addition to seeking out cancer cells and transplanted cells. Once found, the active cytotoxic T cell binds to the target cell and secretes _____ proteins, protein-digesting enzymes, and _____ (lymphotoxins)—all of which destroy the cell.
   2. **Memory cytotoxic T cells** remain in the blood in case of a secondary infection by the same antigen. Once activated, they rapidly proliferate active cytotoxic T cells and additional memory cytotoxic T cells, reducing the time to defeat the antigen.

Antibody-mediated Immunity

LEARNING OBJECTIVE   13. Describe the roles of the various forms of B cells during antibody-mediated immunity.

Antibody-mediated immunity (humoral immunity) is provided by _____ cells. B cells remain in lymph nodes, the spleen, or MALT. B cells are _not_ seeking and destroying antigens while in circulation throughout the body.

Antibody-mediated immunity operates as follows:

- An antigen passing through a lymphatic organ binds to a _____ on the B cell's membrane. The B cell is now activated.
- The B cell draws the antigen into its cytoplasm where it is processed within _____ (similar to APC processing).
- The B cell breaks the antigen into fragments and combines some with MHC proteins produced by the cell.
- The antigen–MHC protein complex is expressed on the outside of the cell membrane of the B cell.
- A helper T cell recognizes the antigen–MHC protein complex and binds to it, activating the B cells and stimulating the helper T cell to secrete _____ to activate more B cells.
- How is adaptive immunity affected if there are few helper T cells for B cell activation? _____ _____

- Activated B cells divide and two clone lines are produced.
   1. **Plasma cells** secrete antibodies.
   2. **Memory B cells** do not secrete antibodies.

Plasma Cells

Plasma cells secrete _____ that saturate body fluids (blood and lymph) upon exposure to an antigen. Several days after the exposure, one plasma cell can secrete hundreds of millions of antibodies each day for 4 or 5 days until it dies. Antibody levels peak about _____ (_how many?_) weeks after the initial activation. Antibodies bind to antigens forming an antibody–antigen complex. A phagocyte removes the complex.

Memory B Cells

Memory B cells do _not_ secrete antibodies. These inactive cells remain for years in lymph nodes and other lymphoid tissues. If the same antigen is encountered later, memory B cells form _____ cells and more memory B cells. The response time to the infection is reduced. **Active immunization** is he ability of the immune system to respond to _____
_____

Allergic Response

Allergic response is antibody-mediated immunity that involves the activation of _____ cells, which results in the production of IgE antibodies. IgE antibodies interact with mast cells, which cause local inflammation, instead of attacking an antigen (known as an *allergen*). Secondary responses to allergens can trigger reactions such as *asthma* or *systemic anaphylaxis.*

Review Time!

I. *Provide a brief answer for each of the following questions about adaptive immunity.*

1. What are some examples of chemical substances that serve as antigens?
    _____
    _____
    _____

2. Where are T cells and B cells matured? _____
    _____
    _____

3. What is the most common cytokine produced by lymphocytes? _____

4. How does a lymphocyte become immunocompetent? _____
    _____
    _____

5. Describe the role of APCs in innate immunity. _____
    _____
    _____

6. What is the purpose of antigen presentation? _____
    _____

7. How would cell-mediated immunity be affected if antigen presentation did not occur?
    _____
    _____
    _____

8. To which cell is the antigen–MHC protein complex presented to initiate cell-mediated immunity?
    _____

9. What is activation? _____

10. What two clone lines are created when T cells are activated?
    1. _____
    2. _____

11. Which type of T cell seeks and destroys infected cells? _____

12. How is the helper T cell involved with the activation of a B cell? _____
    _____
    _____

13. Contrast the functions of cytotoxic T cells and helper T cells. _____
    _____
    _____

14. What kind of T cell remains in the blood in case of a secondary infection by the same antigen?
    _____

15. How do B cells and T cells work together to provide the body with antibody-mediated immunity?

_____

_____

_____

16. What two clone lines are created when B cells are activated?

1. _____

2. _____

17. What specific type of B cell secretes antibodies? _____

18. What is active immunization? _____

_____

19. Describe two ways the body prepares for secondary infections of the same antigen.

_____

_____

_____

20. What kind of immunity is associated with allergic response? Which Ig class of antibodies is involved?

_____

_____

21. Briefly explain how cell-mediated immunity differs from antibody-mediated immunity.

_____

_____

_____

Acquired Immunity

LEARNING OBJECTIVE   **14. Contrast the routes of acquired immunity.**

Acquired immunity includes ways to introduce antigens and antibodies into the body to stimulate an immune response.

Naturally Acquired Active Immunity

Naturally acquired active immunity develops from pathogen exposure during daily living in which the disease and its symptoms are experienced. Immunity is acquired through the process of having the disease, such as _____, _____, and _____. Immunity may be lifelong or short-lived.

Naturally Acquired Passive Immunity

Naturally acquired passive immunity involves the transfer of antibodies from a person with immunity to a person without immunity, such as during _____ and _____. IgG antibodies cross the placenta to the fetus during pregnancy while IgA antibodies are conferred in breast milk. The effects are short-lived as the infant's body breaks down the antibodies.

Artificially Acquired Active Immunity

Artificially acquired active immunity is the deliberate, artificial introduction of an antigen to stimulate the immune system through a _____, which may be by injection or may be administered orally. Effects of the vaccine produce long-lasting protection without the symptoms of the disease. What is the benefit of a booster shot (vaccine)? _____.

Artificially Acquired Passive Immunity

Artificially acquired passive immunity is the transfer of foreign, active antibodies by injection. The effects are short-lived.

• These antibodies don't last very long because _____
_____

The foreign antibodies are called *immune serum globulins* (formerly called _____) and are used for conditions such as snake bites, rabies, hepatitis, and tetanus.

Review Time!

I. *Using the terms in the list below, write the appropriate type of acquired immunity in each blank. You may use a term more than once.*

Naturally acquired active immunity   *Naturally acquired passive immunity*

Artificially acquired active immunity   *Artificially acquired passive immunity*

1. Passes through the breast milk   _____

2. Administered to prevent the symptoms of disease
    such as polio   _____

3. Used for life-threatening conditions such as snake bites   _____

4. Long-lived, but may involve booster shots   _____

5. Being sick from influenza   _____

6. Vaccine   _____

7. Administered in response to a diagnosed disease
    such as hepatitis   _____

8. Passes through the placenta to the fetus   _____

9. Administered for rabies   _____

10. Immune serum globulins   _____

The Respiratory System

14

Tips for Success as You Begin

Read Chapter 14 from your textbook before attending class. Listen when you attend lecture and fill in the blanks in this notebook. You may choose to complete the blanks before attending class as a way to prepare for the day's topics. The same day you attend lecture, read the material again and complete the exercises after each section in this notebook. Spend time every day with this chapter as it will help you make sense of the material. As you learn about the respiratory system, think about the structure (anatomy) for each organ as you consider its function (physiology).

Introduction to the Respiratory System

LEARNING OBJECTIVE 1. Identify the main function of the respiratory system.

LEARNING OBJECTIVE 2. Distinguish between pulmonary ventilation, external respiration, and internal respiration.

Why is breathing necessary? _____
_____
_____

Discuss the function of the respiratory system. _____
_____
_____

Three events are involved in the process of respiration.

1. **Pulmonary ventilation** is breathing in and out; it is the movement of air between the external environment and the air sacs of the lungs.
2. **External respiration** is the gas exchange that occurs when gas molecules diffuse between air sacs of the lungs and the capillaries surrounding them.
3. **Internal respiration** is the gas exchange that occurs when gas molecules diffuse between the bloodstream and body cells.

> **TIP!** Use the obvious names (internal and external) to help you keep straight *where* internal respiration and external respiration occur. External respiration occurs where the gas from *outside* (external) the body first contacts the bloodstream. Internal respiration occurs *inside* the body where the bloodstream exchanges gasses with surrounding cells and tissues.

List the organs of the respiratory system.
- Nose
- Pharynx
- _____

- Trachea
- Bronchial tree
- _____

295

CONCEPT 1

Upper Respiratory Organs

Concept: The upper respiratory organs conduct air between the external environment and the entry into the lower respiratory organs.

LEARNING OBJECTIVE **3. Identify the organs of the upper respiratory tract on the basis of their location, structure, and functions.**

The respiratory system is *structurally* divided into two portions.

- **Upper respiratory tract:** Includes the head and neck, and following organs:
  _____, _____, and _____.
- **Lower respiratory tract:** Begins at the base of the neck and includes the trachea, bronchi and their branches, and alveoli (tiny _____ of the lungs). The lungs include the network of bronchial branches, alveoli, and supporting tissues.

The respiratory system is divided according to the organ *function*.

- **Conduction zone:** Includes organs that (1) conduct air from the external atmosphere to air sacs in the lungs, and (2) warm and humidify air. The organs of the conduction zone are the nose, pharynx, trachea, bronchi, and _____.
- **Respiratory zone:** The actual site of gas exchange that occurs between _____ and a vast capillary network.

Nose

The nose is the initial receiving chamber for inhaled air.

Structure: The following are parts of the nose.

- **Nasal cavity** is the space created by two _____ bones and cartilage.
- **Nasal chambers** (2) are within the nasal cavity. The chambers are divided into two by the
  _____.
- **External nares** are the _____ or openings into the nose.
- **Nasal vestibule** is the small entryway into which air passes after entering the nares.
  _____ filter particles from inhaled air.
- **Nasal conchae** are three bony projections attached to the lateral walls of both nasal chambers. These projections increase the _____ of the nasal cavity and increase the physical contact between inhaled air and the nasal cavity walls.
- **Nasal meati** are narrow passageways between the nasal _____.
- **Paranasal sinuses** are associated with the nasal cavity that communicates by way of small ducts that can become plugged during inflammation and infection (called *sinusitis*). They are lined with
  _____.

TIP! Anatomy is like learning a foreign language. For instance, *meatus* is a singular narrow passageway while *meati* are multiple narrow passageways. Likewise, a *concha* is a singular bony projection while *conchae* are multiple bony projections. A *naris* is a singular opening to the nose while *nares* are the two openings we have to the nose.

Functions: The nose serves to:

- *Warm air* due to the nearby bloodstream as air passes through the _____.
- *Moisten air* by the evaporation of water from the mucous membrane lining the entire nasal cavity.
- *Clean air* by the action of cilia in the mucous membrane. Mucus traps small particles such as _____ and _____. Cilia move the contaminated mucus to the pharynx (throat) where it is swallowed.

Pharynx

The pharynx is the throat.

Structure: The pharynx is a tube-shaped chamber that extends from the back of the nasal cavity to the larynx. Mucous membrane lines walls formed of skeletal muscle. The pharynx has three segments:

1. **Nasopharynx** is the superior part. It receives the (1) internal nares and the (2) openings to the two _____ tubes that travel to the middle ear.
2. **Oropharynx** is visible when you open your mouth wide.
3. **Laryngopharynx** is the inferior segment below the tongue. It unites with the larynx in the neck. What is the function of this segment? _____ _____ _____

> **TIP!** Use the clues found in the names of the segments for the pharynx regions: *naso-* means nose, *oro-* means oral (mouth), and *laryngo-* means larynx.

Function: The pharynx transports _____ to the larynx and _____ to the esophagus.

Larynx

The larynx is the voice box that connects the pharynx to the trachea.

Structure: Since the larynx is mostly cartilage lined with ciliated mucous membrane, our discussion of its structure starts with the major cartilages in the larynx.

- **Thyroid cartilage** is the large, _____-shaped piece of cartilage in the front (also known as the *Adam's apple*).
- **Cricoid cartilage** is the piece of cartilage inferior to the thyroid cartilage.
- **Epiglottis cartilage (epiglottis)** is a tongue-shaped piece of cartilage that is covered with mucous membrane. It is supported by muscles and ligaments over the opening into the larynx. During swallowing, the epiglottis _____ _____ _____

Other parts of the larynx include:

- **Glottis** is the opening into the larynx. What role does the epiglottis play in preventing the passage of food or liquid into the lower respiratory tract? _____ _____
- **False vocal cords** are the _____ *pair* of vocal folds. They do not function in sound production, but are the two pairs of mucous membrane that extend inward in a horizontal position.
- **True vocal cords** are the _____ *pair* of vocal folds. They house elastic fibers that vibrate when air rushes past. The vibrations are converted to speech. There are no cilia covering the true vocal cords to remove mucus that may accumulate. The pitch of the voice depends on the _____ of the true vocal cords. The larger the cartilages and vocal cords, the lower the vibrational frequency, and the lower (deeper) the pitch of the voice. _____ influences the growth of the larynx in males and is responsible for the enlarged cords.

Functions: The larynx:

- Provides a _____ for air traveling between the pharynx and the trachea.
- Prevents solid material from entering the trachea.
- Produces _____.

Review Time!

I. *Using the terms in the list below, label the parts of the upper respiratory tract.*

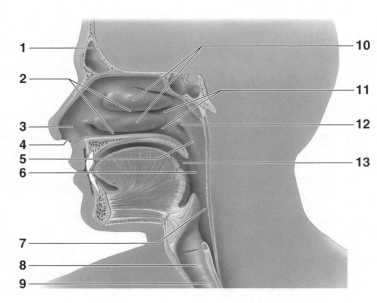

1. _____
2. _____
3. _____
4. _____
5. _____
6. _____
7. _____
8. _____
9. _____
10. _____
11. _____
12. _____
13. _____

External naris	Larynx	Nasopharynx	Palatine tonsils
Frontal (paranasal) sinus	Nasal conchae	Oropharynx	Trachea
Internal nares	Nasal meati	Opening into auditory tube	
Laryngopharynx	Nasal vestibule		

II. *Using the terms in the list below, label the parts of the larynx.*

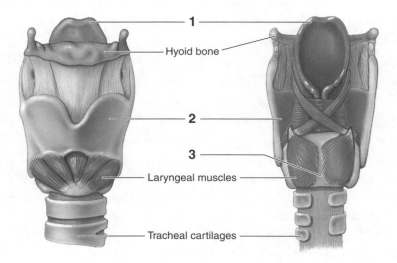

1. _____
2. _____
3. _____
4. _____

Cricoid cartilage	Glottis
Epiglottis	Thyroid cartilage

III. *Using the terms in the list below, write the appropriate upper respiratory organ in each blank. You may use a term more than once.*

Larynx   Nose   Pharynx

1. Warms, moistens, and cleans incoming air   _____

2. Divided into three segments   _____

3. Houses glottis and epiglottis   _____

4. Formed by the nasal bones and numerous cartilages   _____

5. Serves as a common passageway for both food and air   _____

6. Prevents solid material from entering the trachea   _____

7. Includes the thyroid and cricoid cartilages   _____

8. Receives mucus and other fluids from the paranasal sinuses   _____

9. Produces sound due to the vibrations of the true vocal cords   _____

10. The external openings are called the external nares   _____

IV. *Provide a brief answer for each of the following questions about the upper and lower respiratory organs.*

1. List the organs of the two structural divisions of the respiratory system.

_____

_____

2. Describe the functions of the conduction zone and the respiratory zone of the respiratory system.

_____

_____

_____

3. How does the nose help prepare air for the lower respiratory organs?

_____

_____

_____

4. What happens to contaminated mucus in the nasal cavity? _____

_____

5. What is the function of cilia in the nasal cavity? _____

_____

6. Name the three segments of the pharynx from superior to inferior. _____

_____

7. Which vocal cords, the *true* or the *false,* produce sound? _____

8. Describe the role of the epiglottis during swallowing. _____

_____

_____

9. What part of the larynx lacks cilia? Why is this significant? _____

_____

10. What is the effect of testosterone on the growth of cartilages and vocal cords of the larynx?

_____

_____

CONCEPT 2

Lower Respiratory Organs

Concept: The lower respiratory organs include the trachea, the bronchi and their branches, and the lungs. External respiration occurs within the lungs between tiny alveoli and the capillaries surrounding them.

LEARNING OBJECTIVE 4. Identify the organs of the lower respiratory tract on the basis of their location, structure, and functions.

LEARNING OBJECTIVE 5. Describe the structure and function of alveoli and the respiratory membrane.

The lower respiratory organs include the trachea, bronchi and branches, and the lungs. The function of the lower respiratory organs is external respiration. What happens during external respiration?

_____

_____

Trachea

The **trachea** (windpipe) is an air passageway (12 centimeters or 4.5 inches long; 2.5 centimeters or 1 inch wide). It is anterior to the _____ in the neck and extends from the larynx to the point at which it divides into the _____ in the thoracic cavity.

Structure: The histology (tissues) of the trachea includes **hyaline cartilage**s and **pseudostratified ciliated columnar (PSCC) epithelium**.

- **Hyaline cartilage**s formed in C-rings provide an open, rigid frame to prevent the trachea from collapsing and closing off the air passageway. Smooth muscle (trachealis muscle) and connective tissue connect the open ends of the rings so that the esophagus can expand as food travels downward.

- **PSCC epithelium** lines the trachea. It is embedded with _____ cells that produce mucus and glands that produce mucus. Cilia move this mucus toward the pharynx to be swallowed or expelled as sputum. This system of mucus transport is called the **mucociliary transporter**.

  1. What is the benefit of this transporter system? _____

     _____

  2. How does smoking affect the transporter? _____

     _____

     _____

Function: The trachea serves as a passageway for air.

Bronchial Tree

The **bronchial tree** is a branching network that resembles the branches of a tree and includes the divisions of the bronchi within the lungs:

1. **Primary bronchi** (right and left) branch off the distal end of the trachea.
   - **Right primary bronchus** is wider and shorter than the left. The right primary bronchus enters the lung more vertically. Why is the shape clinically significant? _____

     _____

2. **Secondary** (_____) **bronchi** are the first branches of the primary bronchi.
3. **Tertiary** (_____) **bronchi** are the second branches of the primary bronchi.
4. _____ **bronchioles** are the third branches of the primary bronchi.

5. **Respiratory bronchioles** are branches of the terminal bronchioles. They are only supported by a band of smooth muscle, elastic tissue, and lined with thin mucous membrane. Describe what is missing from the respiratory bronchioles. _____

6. **Alveolar ducts** are continuations of the respiratory bronchioles. These smaller tubes terminate in alveoli.
   - **Alveoli** are round, microscopic pouches that surround the alveolar ducts.

Structure: The bronchial tree is structurally similar to the trachea.

- **Hyaline cartilage** forms incomplete rings, diminishes in size and number to form partial rings or plates, and then disappears altogether.
- _____ **muscle** supports the primary bronchi.
- **PSCC** _____ **mucous membrane** lines the internal surface. It too becomes progressively thinner.

Function: The bronchial tree provides a passageway for air between the trachea and the alveoli.

- _____ involves an immune response that results in bronchial inflammation, muscle spasms of the bronchiolar walls, and the production of thickened mucus.

Lungs

The right and left **lungs** are composed of the bronchial tree, alveoli, capillary networks, and support tissue.
Function: The lungs are the site of gas exchange between the atmosphere and the bloodstream. Would you classify this gas exchange as *internal respiration* or *external respiration*? _____

General Characteristics

The lungs are pyramid-shaped organs that occupy most of the thoracic cavity from the diaphragm to the clavicles. The ribs border their surfaces to the front and back.

- Why is the right lung somewhat thicker and broader than the left lung? _____
  _____

Shape and Structure

- **Apex** is the narrow superior portion.
- **Base** is the broad inferior portion.
- **Costal surface** is the surface that lies against the _____ to the front and back.
- **Medial surface** is the surface that faces the midline (where the heart is situated). Connections to the _____ and _____ are on the medial surfaces.
- **Root** is the collection of attachments on the medial surface of each lung, including the _____ bronchus, pulmonary blood vessels, and nerves.

Serous Membranes

The **pleurae** are two layers of serous membrane surrounding each lung.

- **Parietal pleura** lines the thoracic wall and _____ and continues around the heart and between the lungs. It forms a ligament that supports the lungs by surrounding the root.
- **Visceral pleura** is an inward fold of the parietal pleura. It surrounds the lung and is firmly attached to the _____.

TIP! Think of the visceral pleura as shrinkwrap around each lung.

Pleural fluid is situated between the two layers in the **pleura cavity**, the potential space between the two pleural layers. What is the function of pleural fluid? _____ _____

Describe the condition known as pleurisy. _____ _____ _____

Divisions

Each lung is divided into smaller compartments.

1. **Lobes** are separate compartments of each lung. Each lobe is supplied by a major branch of the bronchial tree. **Fissures** are lines of division that extend completely through the lung.

   • **Right lung** has _____ lobes (upper, middle, and lower); the right lung is larger than the left lung. The right lung has two fissures. The *horizontal* fissure divides the upper and middle lobes while the *oblique* fissure divides the middle and lower lobes.

   • **Left lung** has _____ lobes (upper and lower). The oblique fissure divides the lobes from one another.

   > **TIP!** Why the difference between the right lung and the left lung? The left lung has only two lobes since it has to accommodate for the apex of the heart.

2. **Segments** are further subdivisions of each lobe. Each segment is supplied by a smaller branch of the _____ enclosed by connective tissue.

3. **Lobules** are present within each segment. Each lobule contains a single _____ and its branches, alveolar ducts, alveoli, an arteriole, a venule, capillary networks, and a lymphatic vessel.

Alveoli and Respiratory Membranes

Alveoli in the lungs of an average adult number between 300 and 500 million; that's enough surface area to cover a tennis court!

Function: Alveoli perform gas exchange between the _____ and the bloodstream. Do you recall if this gas exchange is termed *internal respiration* or *external respiration*?

_____

Structure: The wall of each alveolus is composed of a single layer of squamous epithelium. Special cells produce a layer of **surfactant** that lines the inner surface of the alveolar wall.

• Surfactant is a detergent-like lipid molecule that accompanies a thin layer of watery fluid. The watery fluid is required to keep the alveolar surface moist for _____. Recall that water molecules are attracted to one another and create surface tension that causes alveolar walls to collapse during deep exhalation. Surfactant *decreases* surface tension.

• *Infant respiratory distress syndrome (IRDS)* or *hyaline membrane disease (HMD)* occurs because premature infants have not yet developed the ability to produce surfactant. Why do these infants risk death by suffocation? _____ _____ _____

Respiratory membrane is composed of the _____ wall (simple squamous epithelial tissue + a basement membrane of connective tissue) and the _____ wall (simple squamous epithelial tissue). The close association of these walls allows for rapid diffusion of gasses during *external respiration*.

Review Time!

I. Using the terms in the list below, label the parts of the respiratory system.

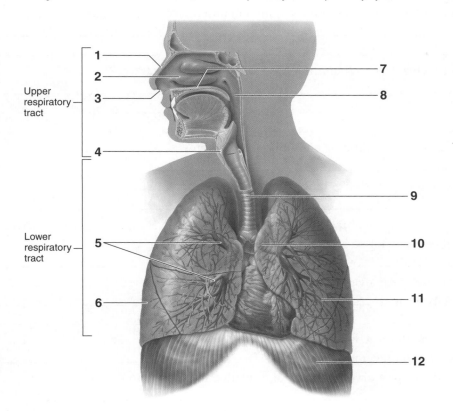

1. _____
2. _____
3. _____
4. _____
5. _____
6. _____
7. _____
8. _____
9. _____
10. _____
11. _____
12. _____

Diaphragm	Left primary bronchus	Pharynx
External nares	Nasal cavity	Right lung
Larynx	Nose	Secondary bronchi
Left lung	Palate	Trachea

II. Provide a brief answer for each of the following questions about the lower respiratory organs.

1. Why is it significant that the hyaline cartilage rings forming the trachea are C-shaped?

_____

_____

_____

2. How are goblet cells and mucous glands functionally similar? _____

_____

3. Explain the effects of smoking on the mucociliary transporter. _____

_____

_____

4. Why do aspirated items more often become trapped in the right primary bronchus?

_____

_____

5. What is the first branch of tubes that emerge from the distal end of the trachea?

_____

_____

6. Describe the role of cilia and mucus in respiratory system maintenance. _____

_____

_____

7. What is included in a bronchial tree? What is the function of the bronchial tree?

_____

_____

_____

8. How many lobes are found in the right lung and how many fissures? _____

_____

9. What is the significance of the root of each lung? _____

_____

10. What part of the lung rests on the diaphragm? _____

11. What is the relationship between lobes, segments, and lobules of the lung?

_____

12. What type of tissue composes each alveolus? _____

13. Where is the pleural cavity located? _____

_____

14. Which pleural layer lines the thoracic wall and the mediastinum? _____

15. What do the alveoli produce to prevent lung collapse? _____

16. Explain the structure of the respiratory membrane and relate the structure to the function.

_____

_____

_____

17. How does surfactant prevent lung collapse?_____

_____

18. What disease is developed by premature infants who do not yet have the ability to produce surfactant? _____

_____

19. How does asthma affect the passage of air between the trachea and the alveoli?

_____

_____

20. List the order of the structures through which air travels as it passes from the nares into the upper respiratory organs. End your pathway with the alveoli. _____

_____

_____

CONCEPT 3

Mechanics of Breathing

Concept: Inspiration requires the contraction of the respiratory muscles to expand the volumes of the thorax and lungs. Expiration requires no muscle activity, but rather the recoil of elastic tissue, while forced expiration requires muscle contraction to push air outward.

LEARNING OBJECTIVE 6. Describe the events involved in inspiration, including the roles of respiratory muscles and pressure gradients.

LEARNING OBJECTIVE 7. Describe the events involved in expiration.

Pulmonary ventilation is breathing. Breathing involves two events.

1. **Inspiration** is inhalation or breathing in.
2. **Expiration** is exhalation or breathing out.

Inspiration

Before we discuss inspiration, you'll need to understand the concepts of pressure and volume as they relate to the respiratory system.

- Air (atmospheric) pressure is _____ mm of mercury (Hg) at sea level. Pressure may be varied by changing the temperature, changing the number of molecules present in a space, or changing the *volume* of a space. If a pressure gradient forms due to changes in these factors, then air molecules rush from *high* to *low* pressure.
- *Increasing* the volume of the lungs causes a _____ in pressure (1 to 3 mm Hg below atmospheric (external) pressure). Air is drawn into the alveoli.

How does an increase in volume promote a decrease in pressure and inspiration? Let's outline the steps to inspiration.

1. The **diaphragm** and **external intercostal muscles** contract (requires energy). Contraction presses the diaphragm downward and the ribs and sternum are elevated.
2. The thoracic cavity expands (*volume* _____).
3. The pleural cavity *pressure* _____.
4. The lung surface is pulled _____, causing alveolar volume to increase.
5. Alveolar pressure decreases below atmospheric levels by 1 to 3 mm Hg.
6. Air rushes _____ the alveoli to restore equilibrium in pressure.

> **TIP!** In summary, the contraction of muscles leads to changes in volume that leads to changes in pressure. To inspire, your thoracic cavity volume must increase so that pleural cavity pressure can decrease.

Expiration

Expiration is a _____ process because it does not rely on muscle contraction. However, it does depend on the ability of the lungs and thoracic cavity to recoil, like a rubber band, after having been stretched.

How does the relaxation of muscles promote a decrease in volume, an increase in pressure, and expiration?

1. The diaphragm and external intercostal muscles relax.
2. The thoracic cavity decreases in size (_____ *decreases*).

3. The pleural cavity _____ *increases.*

4. Alveolar pressure becomes greater than atmospheric pressure.

5. Air flows out of the alveoli.

Some conditions or diseases can affect expiration.

• *Emphysema* is a disease in which the alveoli lose elasticity. How is gas exchange affected? _____
_____

• *Pneumothorax* is an opening in the thoracic wall; it can cause a pressure leak.

• *Atelectasis* is collapse of the lung or part of the lung; it obstructs the movement of air. What can cause atelectasis? _____

Forced expiration follows the conscious contraction of the *internal* intercostal muscles and abdominal wall muscles. These muscles _____ the thoracic cavity, pressure *increases* beyond normal, and more air is forced out of the lungs.

> **TIP!** In summary, the relaxation of muscles leads to changes in volume that leads to changes in pressure. To expire, your thoracic cavity volume must decrease so that pleural cavity pressure can increase.

Review Time!

I. *Using the figure below, describe how the contraction or relaxation of inspiratory muscles leads to changes in volume and pressure, and the movement of air into or out of the lungs.*

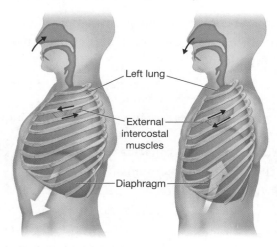

Left lung

External intercostal muscles

Diaphragm

During inspiration the diaphragm presses the abdominal organs downward and forward.

During expiration the diaphragm rises and recoils to the resting position.

A Action of rib cage during inspiration

B Action of rib cage during expiration

_____
_____
_____
_____
_____

II. *In the blank before each statement, indicate whether the description or action is part of inspiration (I) or expiration (E).*

_____ 1. Breathing in

_____ 2. Decreased pressure in the pleural cavity

_____ 3. Air flows out of the alveoli

_____ 4. Diaphragm and external intercostal muscles contract

_____ 5. Thoracic cavity expands as inspiratory muscles contract

_____ 6. Breathing out

_____ 7. Diaphragm and external intercostal muscles relax

_____ 8. Alveolar pressure is greater than atmospheric pressure

_____ 9. Thoracic cavity decreases in size and volume

_____ 10. Air rushes into the alveoli

Respiratory Volumes

LEARNING OBJECTIVE **8. Identify the respiratory volumes and how they are measured.**

Spirometry is the procedure used to measure respiratory volumes using a *spirometer.*

> **TIP!** For most of these respiratory volumes, you can breathe along with the descriptions as you read through the following list. A great way to practice is to read and practice the volumes together.

- **Tidal volume (TV)** = 500 milliliters; the air moved in and out of the lungs with each breath.
- **Inspiratory reserve volume (IRV)** = 3,100 milliliters; the amount of air forcibly inhaled over TV.
- **Expiratory reserve volume (ERV)** = 1,200 milliliters; the amount of air that can be forcibly exhaled after a TV.
- **Residual volume (RV)** = 1,200 milliliters; the volume of air remaining in the lungs after a forced expiration.
- **Vital capacity (VC)** = 4,800 milliliters = TV + IRV + ERV; the total amount of exchangeable air.
- **Total lung capacity (TLC)** = 6,000 milliliters = VC + RV
- **Anatomic dead space volume** = 150 milliliters; the air remaining in the passageways that never reaches the alveoli. The amount of air that actually reaches the alveoli during TV is about 350 milliliters.

Using the respiratory volumes' spirogram below, indicate the volume (in milliliters) for the following:

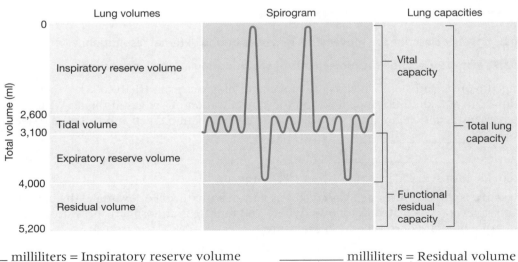

_____ milliliters = Inspiratory reserve volume

_____ milliliters = Tidal volume

_____ milliliters = Expiratory reserve volume

_____ milliliters = Residual volume

_____ milliliters = Vital capacity

_____ milliliters = Total lung capacity

Review Time!

I. *Provide a brief answer for each of the following questions about respiratory volumes.*

1. How much air, in milliliters, remains in the respiratory tract but never enters the alveoli during tidal breathing? _____

2. How much air, in milliliters, is forcibly exhaled after a tidal expiration?

   _____

3. Breathing in and out is termed _____

4. What volume is the sum of VC and RV? _____

5. What volume is the amount of air forcibly inhaled over the TV? _____

   _____

6. What volume is the sum of TV, IRV, and ERV? _____

7. Which volume is 500 milliliters? _____

8. What is the typical volume, in milliliters, for VC _____

9. What is the typical volume, in milliliters, for TLC? _____

10. Why do you think we can forcibly inhale 3,100 milliliters of air while we can only forcibly exhale 1,200 milliliters of air? What happens to the remaining air we don't exhale?

    _____

    _____

    _____

CONCEPT 4

Exchange of Gasses

Concept: Successful gas exchange requires the independent diffusion of oxygen and carbon dioxide between alveoli and the blood, and between the blood and body cells.

LEARNING OBJECTIVE 9. Describe the movements of gasses during external respiration.

LEARNING OBJECTIVE 10. Describe the movements of gasses during internal respiration.

Gas exchange involves diffusion, which is the movement of gasses from HIGH to LOW regions of concentration. The rate of diffusion depends on the concentration of the gas in the air we breathe. Of the following gasses in the air we breathe, we will only be dealing with oxygen and carbon dioxide:

- Nitrogen forms _____% of the air.
- Oxygen forms _____% of the air.
- Carbon dioxide forms _____% of the air.

Partial pressure is the pressure each gas creates as part of a mixture. For example, the partial pressure of oxygen at sea level is calculated as follows (where 760 mm Hg is atmospheric pressure at sea level and 21% is the partial pressure of oxygen in this mixture):

$$760 \text{ mm Hg} \times 21\% = 160 \text{ mm Hg}$$

Each gas diffuses until its partial pressure is equalized. Therefore, oxygen diffuses independently of carbon dioxide until the partial pressure for each gas becomes equalized. For example, most oxygen is bound to hemoglobin for transport in the blood, which does not affect the partial pressure of oxygen. Only the oxygen dissolved in the blood plasma determines the partial pressure. This is important becuase it allows an incredible volume of oxygen bound to hemoglobin to accumulate.

External Respiration

External respiration is _____.

It occurs across the respiratory membrane that exists between the alveoli and the bloodstream.

Transport of Oxygen

The partial pressure of oxygen is always *greater* in the alveoli than in blood plasma. The pressure gradient forces oxygen _____ the blood.

How is oxygen transported in the bloodstream?

- Bound to hemoglobin within the RBCs as _____ (98%)
- Dissolved in blood _____ (2%)

Transport of Carbon Dioxide

The partial pressure of carbon dioxide is *greater* in the blood plasma than in the alveoli. The pressure gradient forces carbon dioxide to move *out* of the blood into the air of the alveoli to be expired.

Internal Respiration

Internal respiration is _____.

It occurs between the capillaries in the body (other than the lungs) and body cells.

Transport of Oxygen

Oxygen moves along a _____ from the capillaries, to the interstitial fluid, and into the cytoplasm of cells. The partial pressure of oxygen is greater in the capillaries than in the cytoplasm of cells.

Transport of Carbon Dioxide

Carbon dioxide moves along a _____ from the cytoplasm of cells, to the interstitial fluid, and into the capillaries. The partial pressure of carbon dioxide is normally greater in the cytoplasm and least in the capillaries.

Carbon dioxide is transported in the bloodstream as follows:

- Bicarbonate ion (HCO_3^-), mainly within RBCs, is the most common method of transport (60 to 70%)
- Bound to _____ in RBCs (25%)
- Dissolved in the _____ (10%)

How is carbon dioxide transported as the bicarbonate ion?

- Carbon dioxide (CO_2) and water (H_2O) in the RBC combine to form _____ (H_2CO_3) with the help of an enzyme called *carbonic anhydrase*.
- Carbonic acid breaks apart (dissociates) into a bicarbonate ion (HCO_3^-) and a hydrogen ion (H^+).

$$\text{carbonic anhydrase}$$
$$CO_2 + H_2O \text{--------------------->} H_2CO_3 \text{--------->} HCO_3^- + H^+$$

Once this reaction is complete:

- Bicarbonate ions move from the RBC into the blood _____ until they reach the _____ of the lungs.
- Hydrogen ions stay in RBCs to temporarily combine with _____ molecules.

During external respiration:

- When bicarbonate ion reaches the pulmonary capillaries, the previous reaction is run in reverse to convert the ion into carbon dioxide for expiration.

- The carbon dioxide diffuses from RBCs into the _____. It diffuses across the respiratory membrane into the _____ where it can be exhaled.

$$HCO_3^- + H^+ \xrightarrow{\text{carbonic anhydrase}} H_2CO_3 \dashrightarrow CO_2 + H_2O$$

The removal of hydrogen ions provides an important buffering system. Hydrogen ions are removed from the blood:

1. When they combine with _____ of RBCs.
2. When they recombine with bicarbonate ions to form _____ acid. Recall that carbonic acid forms carbon dioxide and water.

Acidosis is the condition that results from a drop in blood pH. Hydrogen ion removal helps to prevent acidosis. An accumulation of carbon dioxide in the blood can overwhelm the buffering system by producing hydrogen ions faster than they can be removed. A person compensates by increased breathing.

How does increased breathing help restore blood pH balance? _____

_____

Review Time!

I. *Using the figure below, explain the movement of both carbon dioxide and oxygen along their respective partial pressure gradients.*

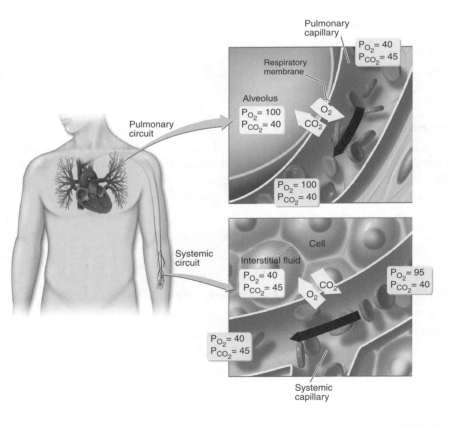

_____
_____
_____
_____
_____

II. Provide a brief answer for each of the following questions about the exchange of gasses.

1. Where does internal respiration occur? _____

2. Where does external respiration occur? _____

3. Define partial pressure. _____
_____

4. What are the two most important gasses in the air?
   1. _____
   2. _____

5. By what type of membrane transport do carbon dioxide and oxygen move? _____

6. How is most carbon dioxide transported? _____

7. How is most oxygen transported? _____

8. What is the role of an enzyme known as carbonic anhydrase? _____
_____

9. How does bicarbonate ion help to maintain blood pH balance? _____
_____

10. Define acidosis. _____
_____

CONCEPT 5

Control of Breathing

Concept: Breathing rate and depth are controlled by the respiratory center in the brain. They are influenced by factors that act upon the respiratory center.

LEARNING OBJECTIVE 11. Identify the main source of respiratory control and describe how it works.

LEARNING OBJECTIVE 12. Describe the factors that affect breathing in addition to the respiratory centers.

Respiratory Center

The **respiratory center** is a group of neurons in the _____ (medulla oblongata and pons) that control breathing. Breathing is rhythmic and involuntary. The **medullary rhythmicity center** houses two groups of neurons that extend the length of the medulla.

1. _____ **group** controls the basic rhythm of tidal breathing. How?
   • Neurons send impulses to the diaphragm and external intercostal muscles to contract.
   • One to three seconds later, the neurons stop. They are inactive during expiration.
   • Again, the neurons send another burst of impulses to promote another inspiration sequence.
   • This sequence promotes normal tidal breathing.

2. _____ **group** is *inactive* during normal tidal breathing. When are these neurons active?
   • Neurons in this group are activated when forceful inspiration and expiration are necessary.
   • Impulses are sent to the diaphragm and _____ muscles to stimulate forceful inspiration and to other thoracic and abdominal muscles to stimulate forceful expiration.

Pneumotaxic area is located in the _____ and houses neurons associated with the dorsal group to inhibit the rate of breathing.

- If *strong* nerve impulses are sent from the pneumotaxic area to the dorsal group, the duration of inspiratory bursts are inhibited. The breathing rate _____.
- If *weak* nerve impulses are sent, the inspiratory bursts are longer in duration, and the breathing rate _____. Expiration is permitted to proceed.

Apneustic areas are situated in the lower part of the pons. They *inhibit* expiration.

- If nerve impulses are sent to the dorsal group, inspiration is activated and prolonged.
- The apneustic neurons are only *active* when the neurons of the pneumotaxic area are *inactive*.

Factors That Affect Breathing

Breathing rate and the depth of breathing are also influenced by:

1. **Chemical changes in the blood** including oxygen, hydrogen ions, and particularly carbon dioxide.
   - In the nervous system, the **chemosensitive area** is located in the medulla oblongata. It monitors _____ levels in the arteries circulating the brain.
   - Outside the nervous system, **chemoreceptors** in the aorta and carotid arteries monitor low levels of _____, rising levels of _____, and rising levels of _____ ions. When carbon dioxide levels rise above normal levels, the respiratory center increases the rate of ventilation (known as *hyperventilation*) so we blow off the excess carbon dioxide.
2. **Degree of stretch by the lungs** is detected by **stretch receptors** in the walls of _____ and _____ . When overstretched during inspiration, these receptors send impulses to the respiratory center. Inspiration is inhibited and expiration follows to protect the lungs from overinflation.
3. **Mental state** can influence breathing involuntarily or voluntarily.
   - Involuntary increases in breathing rates can be initiated by _____ factors such as fear, stress, or pain.
   - Voluntary increases in breathing rates can also be initiated by the _____.
   - We can only stop breathing with limited control due to the buildup of carbon dioxide in the blood. What happens to carbon dioxide levels as you hold your breath? _____
   - How does your respiratory center respond? _____
   _____

Review Time!

I.   Provide a brief answer for each of the following questions about the control of breathing.

1. What parts of the brain stem house the respiratory center? _____
   _____
2. Which group of neurons promotes inspiration? _____
3. Which muscles are stimulated to contract during inspiration?_____
4. Which group of neurons promotes forceful breathing? _____
5. Which neurons are active during normal tidal breathing? _____
6. Which neurons are inactive during normal tidal breathing? _____
7. What is the function of the pneumotaxic area? _____
   _____
8. Which group—*the dorsal* or *the ventral*—is associated with the pneumotaxic area?
   _____

9. What is the function of the apneustic area? _____
_____

10. Explain how the pneumotaxic and apneustic areas work in coordination to control inspiration and the breathing rate. _____
_____
_____

11. Where are chemoreceptors located? _____

12. What do chemoreceptors monitor? _____

13. What conditions cause chemoreceptors to increase the breathing rate? _____
_____

14. What effect does the overinflation of the lungs having on breathing? _____
_____

15. Under what conditions would your respiratory center promote hyperventilation?
_____

16. Eight-year-old Quinn is so mad that he is holding his breath. Explain to his parents why they should *not* be concerned that he might be in grave danger. _____
_____
_____

15

The Digestive System

Tips for Success as You Begin

Read Chapter 15 from your textbook before attending class. Listen when you attend lecture and fill in the blanks in this notebook. You may choose to complete the blanks before attending class as a way to prepare for the day's topics. The same day you attend lecture, read the material again and complete the exercises after each section in this notebook. Spend time every day with this chapter as it will help you remember the role and responsibility of each digestive organ. As you learn about the digestive system, think about the structure (anatomy) for each organ as you consider its function (physiology). You also may want to review Chapter 2 for information as you read through the section on nutrition.

CONCEPT 1

Features of the Digestive System

Concept: The digestive system includes organs forming a long tube called the gastrointestinal (GI) tract and organs lying outside the tract known as accessory organs. Digestive processes include ingestion, mechanical digestion, propulsion, chemical digestion, and defecation. The serous membrane associated with digestive organs inferior to the diaphragm is called the peritoneum. The GI tract organs have a general design that includes four layers forming the wall of the tube.

Let's look at the organization of the digestive organs, the similarity of their structures, and their functions as part of the digestive system.

General Organization

LEARNING OBJECTIVE 1. Identify the two divisions of the digestive system and their organs.

The two main groups of the digestive system are:

1. **Gastrointestinal (GI) tract** (alimentary canal) is a hollow tube from the mouth to the anus. It consists of the mouth, pharynx, esophagus, stomach, small intestine, and large intestine. These organs digest _____, absorb _____, and form _____.

2. **Accessory organs** are located either within the GI tract or outside it and communicate by way of ducts (tubes). These organs (the teeth, tongue, salivary glands, pancreas, gallbladder, and liver) assist with the functions of the GI tract.

As we discuss the organs of the GI tract and the accessory organs, add labels to the illustration below. When you are done, you should be able to identify the organs listed below.

1. _____

2. _____

3. _____

4. _____

5. _____

6. _____

7. _____

8. _____

9. _____

10. _____

Esophagus	Mouth	Stomach
Gallbladder	Pancreas	Tongue
Large intestine	Pharynx	
Liver	Small intestine	

Digestive Processes

LEARNING OBJECTIVE 2. Describe the six functions of digestion.

The digestive system has six important roles.

1. **Ingestion** is the process of bringing food into the digestive system, usually through the

_____ .

2. **Propulsion** is the movement of food through the GI tract by *swallowing* (mouth and throat) and _____ (wave-like muscular contractions that pushes material through a tube).

3. **Mechanical digestion** is the breakdown of food particles by mechanical means, including _____ (*chewing*), mixing food with the tongue, churning and mixing in the stomach, and mixing in the small intestine.

4. **Chemical digestion** is the breakdown of large molecules of food into their building blocks by _____ and other chemicals.

5. **Absorption** is the transport of _____ from the lumen (cavity) of the GI tract, usually the small intestine, to blood or lymph.

6. **Defecation** is the elimination of _____ material from the large intestine as feces.

Review Time!

I. *Using the terms in the list below, write the appropriate process of the digestive system in each blank. You may use a term more than once.*

Absorption   Chemical digestion   Defecation   Ingestion

Mechanical digestion   Propulsion

1. Placing food in the mouth   _____

2. Elimination of indigestible material   _____

3. Movement of food through the GI tract   _____

4. Breakdown of large molecules of food using enzymes   _____

5. Mastication   _____

6. Swallowing   _____

7. Peristalsis   _____

8. Transport of food into blood or lymph   _____

9. Removal of feces by the large intestine   _____

10. Breakdown of food by mixing with the tongue   _____

Peritoneum

LEARNING OBJECTIVE   3. Describe the components of the peritoneum and the organs with which they are associated.

Recall from Chapter 4 that serous membranes are thin, moistened sheets of lubricating tissue. The peritoneum is a serous membrane located in the abdominal cavity. Its three major parts are:

1. **Parietal peritoneum** lines the wall of the abdominal cavity. It contains folds that suspend or anchor organs in the peritoneal cavity. The folds include:

    • **Falciform ligament** divides the _____ into two major lobes and connects the liver to the anterior abdominal wall and diaphragm.

    • **Lesser omentum** extends between the _____ margin of the stomach and liver; attaches to the anterior abdominal wall.

    • **Mesentery** suspends the _____ coils to one another and to the posterior abdominal wall.

    • **Greater omentum** is a double-layered fold of the visceral peritoneum of the _____. It hangs from the stomach over the abdomen and looks like a lacy apron draped over the lower abdomen. It is embedded with many lymph nodes that provide protection against infection.

2. **Visceral peritoneum (serosa)** covers the external surface of most digestive organs.

3. **Peritoneal cavity** is the space between the parietal and visceral membranes; it houses a small amount of serous fluid.

    • What is the function of serous fluid?_____

    _____

Wall Structure of the GI Tract

LEARNING OBJECTIVE 4. Describe the layers forming the walls of GI tract organs.

The wall structure is similar for the organs forming the major portion of the GI tract: esophagus, stomach, small and large intestines. The four layers of the wall from deep to superficial are:

1. _____
2. _____
3. _____
4. _____

Mucosa

The mucosa is a mucous membrane lining of the lumen of the GI tract.

Structure

- Inner layer that contacts the lumen of epithelium with _____ secreting cells
- Middle layer composed of loose (areolar) _____ tissue
- External layer contains a small amount of smooth _____

Functions

- *Protection* from _____ due to thickness of epithelium and mucus
- *Absorption* of _____
- *Secretion* of _____

Submucosa

The submucosa is external to the mucosa layer.

Structure

- Loose (areolar) _____ tissue
- Blood vessels
- Lymphatic vessels
- Nerve endings
- Small glands

Function: Nourish surrounding tissues and carry away _____.

Muscularis

The muscularis is _____ muscle that encircles the submucosa layer.

Structure

- Inner _____ layer of smooth muscle
- Outer _____ layer of smooth muscle
- *Sphincters* are formed at several points along the GI tract when the circular layer thickens.

Functions

- _____ act as valves to control food passage from one organ to the next.
- _____ *digestion* through the mixing and churning of food.
- *Peristalsis* propels food through the GI tract.

Serosa

Serosa is the visceral peritoneum, the outer covering of the GI tract.

Structure: Loose connective tissue with a single layer of flattened _____ cells.

Function: Secretion of _____ fluid reduces friction between contacting surfaces.

Review Time!

I. *Using the terms in the list below, write the appropriate layer of the GI tract wall structure in each blank. You may use a term more than once.*

   Mucosa   Muscularis   Serosa   Submucosa

   1. External to the muscularis layer   _____

   2. Inner circular and outer longitudinal smooth muscle layers _____

   3. Lines the lumen of the GI tract   _____

   4. Protects from invading microorganisms   _____

   5. Performs peristalsis   _____

   6. Forms sphincters   _____

   7. Secretes serous fluid   _____

   8. Nourishes surrounding tissues   _____

   9. Contains mucus-secreting cells   _____

   10. Visceral peritoneum   _____

CONCEPT 2

Upper Digestive Organs

Concept: The upper digestive organs include the mouth, pharynx, and esophagus of the GI tract, and the accessory organs including the tongue, teeth, and salivary glands. Together, they begin the processing of ingested food.

LEARNING OBJECTIVE 5. Describe the structure and function of the mouth, tongue, teeth, and salivary glands.

LEARNING OBJECTIVE 6. Describe the structure and function of the pharynx and esophagus.

The upper digestive organs are located above the diaphragm and include the mouth, pharynx, and esophagus of the GI tract. Accessory organs associated with the mouth include the tongue, teeth, and salivary glands.

Mouth

The **oral cavity** is the space within the mouth between the tongue and _____ (roof of the mouth). Accessory organs associated with the mouth include the tongue, teeth, and salivary glands.

Functions

• *Ingestion*

• *Mechanical digestion* of food into smaller particles by chewing (known as _____)

• _____ *digestion* of food using saliva

• *Prepares* food for swallowing

Associated Structures

1. **Lips** are the first structures to contact food.

   • Sensory receptors in the lips detect fine touch, temperature, and _____.

   • Skeletal muscle fibers form the lips and are covered by a thin layer of skin on the outside and _____ on the inside.

   • The reddish color is due to _____

2. **Cheeks** form the lateral walls of the mouth.
   - Skeletal muscle and fat form the cheeks; they are lined externally with _____
     and internally with _____ membrane.
   - **Oral vestibule** separates the teeth and both the cheeks and lips.
3. **Palate** forms the roof of the oral cavity.
   - **Hard palate:** The bony, _____ part of the palate covered with mucous membrane.
   - **Soft palate:** The muscular, _____ part of the palate covered with mucous membrane.
   - _____: Archway opening of the oral cavity into the pharynx.
   - **Palatine** _____: Lie partially embedded in mucous membrane along both sides of
     the archway.
   - **Uvula:** The finger-like projection extending from the archway. The uvula is drawn upward during
     swallowing to close the opening between the pharynx and the nasal cavity (internal nares).
     Why? _____

   > **TIP!** Have you ever watched a cartoon where a character is running directly toward you? You
   > likely have seen his or her *uvula* dangling from the back of the mouth—like a punching bag. Also,
   > when you open your mouth and say "ah," the palatine tonsils are the tonsils that you can see on
   > the lateral sides at the back of the mouth. (You cannot see the other tonsils—they were discussed
   > in an earlier chapter.)

Tongue

The tongue is an *accessory organ* situated within the mouth.

Structure

- The tongue is composed of skeletal muscle and covered with mucous membrane. The mucous
  membrane contains projections known as _____.
- Two sets of skeletal muscles, internal and external, change the shape of the tongue and move it.
- The **lingual frenulum** anchors the tongue to the _____.
- The tongue is also anchored to the pharynx and _____ bone at the posterior
  margin (where the lingual tonsils are located).

Functions

- *Mixes food* with saliva as it is chewed.
- _____ of speech.
- Papillae provide *friction* for handling food and contain _____.

Teeth

The teeth are *accessory organs* of the mouth.

Structure: Teeth are hard, corrosion-resistant, and resist breakage. A tooth has two regions.

1. **Crown** is the visible part of the tooth above the **gingivae** (gums). The crown is covered by the hardest
   substance in the body, _____. Enamel is a heavily mineralized substance produced by
   cells that die soon after the tooth erupts. Enamel cannot be replaced if cracked or damaged by decay.
   - _____ is a slightly harder substance than bone that lies beneath the
     enamel. It surrounds a central pulp cavity.
   - **Pulp cavity** contains connective tissue, blood vessels, and _____ (**pulp**).
     The pulp cavity extends through the roots to allow the passage of blood vessels and nerves.
   - **Root canals** are the narrow channels through which _____ and _____ travel.

2. **Root** is the part of the tooth buried below the gum line. The crown meets the root at the
   _____ of the tooth.
   • **Cementum** is a hardened connective tissue coat that covers the _____.
   • **Periodontal ligament** contains collagen fibers and anchors the tooth in the jaw.

As we discuss the different parts of a tooth, add labels to the illustration below. When you are done, you should have added the following labels.

1. _____

2. _____

3. _____

4. _____

5. _____

6. _____

7. _____

8. _____

9. _____

10. _____

Cementum	Enamel	Periodontal ligament	Root
Crown	Gingivae	Pulp in pulp cavity	Root canal
Dentin	Neck		

Functions

• *Chewing,* or *mastication,* by tearing and grinding food into smaller particles in preparation for swallowing.

• Mastication *increases particle surface area* for improved chemical digestion by enzymes.

Sets of teeth: Two different sets of teeth form during normal development.

1. **Deciduous teeth** are the first set of _____ *(how many?)* teeth that appear
   between 6 months and 24 months of age. As the second set of teeth develops, the roots of the deciduous
   teeth are absorbed. This primary dentition loosens and falls out between the ages of 6 and 12 years.

2. **Permanent teeth** are the second set of _____ *(how many?)* teeth that
   replace the deciduous teeth. By the end of adolescence, all of these teeth have emerged except for
   wisdom teeth (third molars), which emerge between the ages of 17 and 25 years.
   • How many teeth are present in a full set of permanent teeth?_____
   • Why might the number vary from person to person?_____
   _____

Different Shapes of Teeth

The shapes of the teeth reflect their roles in chewing food.

• _____ are pointed chisels that *cut* food.

- _____ (cuspids) are the cone-shaped eye teeth that *tear* food.
- _____ (bicuspids) have broad, flattened surfaces that *grind* and *crush* food.
- _____ have broad, flattened surfaces that *grind* and *crush* food.

As we discuss the different shapes of the teeth, add labels to the illustration below. When you are done, you should be able to identify the teeth listed below.

1. _____
2. _____
3. _____
4. _____

| Canines | Molars |
| Incisors | Premolars |

Salivary Glands

The salivary glands are a collection of *accessory organs* surrounding the mouth.

Function: Salivary glands secrete **saliva** which contains mostly _____ and some solutes (mucus and two primary enzymes). Water dissolves soluble food molecules for taste. Saliva secretion is stimulated by involuntary nerve impulses from the brain when you see, smell, taste, or think of food. Two important substances found in saliva are:

- Lysozyme is an enzyme that _____
  _____

- **Salivary amylase** is a second enzyme that _____
  _____

> **TIP!** The suffix -ase means enzyme. When you encounter this suffix, use it as a clue to mean enzyme. For example, amyl*ase* is an enzyme that breaks down starch (amyl).

Three pairs of salivary glands produce most of the saliva that enters the mouth. *Buccal glands* are part of the mucous membrane lining the mouth that secrete a small amount of saliva.

1. **Parotid glands** are the largest salivary glands located in front of and slightly below each ear, between the skin of the cheek and the _____ muscle. Saliva rich in salivary amylase is secreted.

2. **Submandibular glands** are located along the inner surface of the jaw (mandible) in the floor of the mouth. Secretions contain viscous (thick) mucus.

3. **Sublingual glands** are under the _____. Secretions are rich in mucus.

Digestion in the Mouth

Both chemical and mechanical digestion begins in the mouth. The mixing of food with saliva through mastication creates a moistened, mucus-covered mass of food known as a **bolus**.

- **Mechanical digestion** involves the mastication of food. The two functions of mastication are:

  1. _____

  2. _____

- **Chemical digestion** of food using salivary amylase. Salivary *amylase* breaks down _____ and _____. *Maltose,* a disaccharide, is produced from the breakdown of these molecules.

As we discuss the parts of the mouth, add labels to the illustration below. When you are done, you should be able to identify the parts of the mouth listed below.

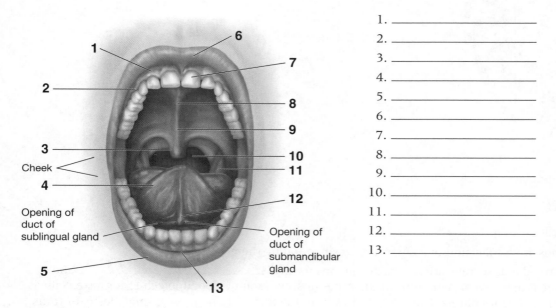

1. _____
2. _____
3. _____
4. _____
5. _____
6. _____
7. _____
8. _____
9. _____
10. _____
11. _____
12. _____
13. _____

Fauces	Lingual frenulum	Soft palate	Upper central incisor
Gingivae (gums)	Oral vestibule	Superior lip	Uvula
Hard palate	Palatine tonsil	Tongue	
Inferior lip	Right upper canine		

Pharynx

The pharynx is located behind the oral cavity, extending from the internal nares of the nasal cavity to the larynx.

Structure: Walls of skeletal muscle lined with _____; three segments (nasopharynx, oropharynx, and laryngopharynx).

Function: *Swallowing* is the main digestive role of the pharynx. Describe the process of swallowing, beginning with the tongue pushing the bolus of food from the oral cavity into the pharynx:

_____

_____

_____

Esophagus

The esophagus is a 25-centimeter (10 inches) long muscular tube that extends from the pharynx, through the esophageal hiatus in the diaphragm, to the stomach (beneath the diaphragm). The esophagus is behind the trachea in the neck and upper thorax.

Structure of the wall of the esophagus (from deep to superficial)

- **Mucosa** is the inner layer composed of _____ squamous epithelium. How does this epithelium provide protection? _____

  _____

- **Submucosa**
- **Muscularis** begins as skeletal muscle, then transitions into _____ muscle. *Circular* and *longitudinal* layers create peristaltic waves to push food to the stomach from the proximal to the distal end of the esophagus. The **lower esophageal sphincter (LES)** is a thickened part of the circular fibers near the union of the _____ with the _____ that remains closed unless peristaltic waves open it. A leaky LES can cause *heartburn* as acidic stomach juices leak irritate the lining of the esophagus.
- **Connective tissue**, *not* _____, forms the outer layer.

Review Time!

I.   *Provide a brief answer for each of the following questions about the upper digestive organs.*

1. List the accessory organs associated with the mouth. _____

   _____

2. What is the function of the lingual frenulum? _____

   _____

3. What is the difference between the oral cavity and the oral vestibule? _____

   _____

4. What are the two parts of a tooth?
   1. _____
   2. _____

5. What part of the tooth cannot be replaced because the cells die shortly after the tooth emerges?

   _____

6. How could you visually determine the difference between the incisors, canines, and premolars?

   _____

   _____

   _____

7. Where is the neck of the tooth located? _____

   _____

8. What is the function of the periodontal ligament? _____

   _____

9. List the three pairs of salivary glands and their secretions.

  1. _____

  2. _____

  3. _____

10. What is the function of salivary amylase? _____
_____

11. What does saliva contain? _____
_____

12. What type of mechanical digestion is performed by the mouth? _____

13. What is a bolus? _____

14. What is the function of the pharynx? _____

15. What is the name of the opening in the diaphragm through which the esophagus travels?
_____

16. What is the function of the muscularis layer of the esophageal wall?_____
_____

17. From what layer of the esophageal wall is the lower esophageal sphincter formed?
_____

18. What is the function of the pharynx?_____

19. What type of tissue forms the mucosa layer of the esophagus?_____
_____

20. How does the tissue forming the muscularis layer of the esophagus change?
_____
_____

CONCEPT 3

Lower Digestive Organs

Concept: The lower digestive organs include the stomach, small intestine, and large intestine of the GI tract, and the liver, gallbladder, and pancreas as accessory organs. They each contribute one or more important functions to the digestive process to bring it to completion.

LEARNING OBJECTIVE 7. Describe the structure and function of the stomach and pancreas.

LEARNING OBJECTIVE 8. Describe the structure and function of the liver and gallbladder.

LEARNING OBJECTIVE 9. Describe the structure and function of the small and large intestine.

The lower digestive organs are located inferior to the _____ and include the stomach, small intestine, and large intestine of the GI tract. What accessory organs are included?
_____

Stomach

The **stomach** unites with the distal end of the _____. It is a temporary storage container for food and an important site for mechanical and chemical digestion.

Structure of the Stomach

Features of the Stomach

- Holds up to _____ (*how many?*) liters of food (in most people) in this sac-like pouch.
- **Rugae** are deep folds of the inner linings that appear when the stomach is empty. When do they disappear? _____
- **Greater curvature** is the convex lateral margin. The *greater omentum* extends from the greater curvature.
- **Lesser curvature** is the concave _____ margin. The *lesser omentum* extends from the lesser curvature.

Four Regions of the Stomach

1. **Cardia** surrounds the opening near the heart that receives food from the _____.
2. **Fundus** expands and bulges above the _____ and is a temporary holding area for food.
3. **Body** is between the fundus and pylorus and is the main portion of the stomach.
4. **Pylorus** is the inferior end. The **pyloric sphincter** is formed from the _____ layer of the wall and serves as a valve to control food movement to the small intestine.

Layers of the Wall of the Stomach

1. **Mucosa** is modified in the stomach to contain:
   - **Gastric pits** are millions of openings into the stomach lining; they are lined with _____. The gastric pits lead into tube-like gastric glands.
   - **Gastric glands** secrete chemicals called **gastric juice**. Gastric glands contain secretory cells such as zymogenic (chief), parietal, and mucous cells.
   - **Zymogenic (chief) cells** secrete _____
   - **Parietal cells** secrete _____ and intrinsic factor necessary for vitamin B_{12} absorption.
   - **Mucous cells** secrete _____
2. **Submucosa**
3. **Muscularis** has a third layer of muscle fibers that run in an oblique direction. This additional muscle layer provides the stomach with the ability to _____ _____.
4. **Serosa**

Functions of the Stomach

Mechanical digestion is accomplished by the churning and mixing actions provided by muscularis of the stomach wall.

Chemical digestion is provided by gastric juice that contains several enzymes such as **pepsin**.

- What cells produce the inactive form of pepsin, known as **pepsinogen**? _____.
- What activates pepsinogen into pepsin for protein digestion? _____ _____
- Why doesn't the stomach digestive itself? _____ _____
- What happens if that defensive layer is not enough? _____ _____

Absorption is limited to water, certain salts, glucose, alcohol, aspirin, and some lipid-soluble drugs.

Propulsion is accomplished by peristalsis of the stomach wall. The semi-fluid paste of small food particles and gastric juice ready to enter the small intestine are known as **chyme**. As chyme presses against the pyloric sphincter, _____

_____

- Rank these meals (1 thourhg 3; 1 = fastest) in terms of how quickly they move through the stomach:
  _____ meal rich in carbohydrates
  _____ meal rich in fats
  _____ meal rich in proteins

Release of intrinsic factor by _____ cells of the gastric glands.
- What vitamin depends on intrinsic factor for absorption in the small intestine?
  _____

- Why is this vitamin required for survival?_____
  _____

- What form of anemia results due to lack of this vitamin?_____

Regulation of Stomach Functions
The activities of the stomach are regulated by:
- **Involuntary control centers of the brain (hypothalamus, medulla)**
- **Hormones (gastrin)**

The _hypothalamus_ stimulates the secretion of gastric juices as soon as you see, smell, hear, or think of food. Once food enters the stomach, a reflex continues gastric secretions. As the stomach wall stretches, impulses are send to the _medulla oblongata_ and back to the secretory cells in the gastric pits. These cells release a hormone, **gastrin**. What does gastrin stimulate?
  1. _____
  2. _____

As chyme enters the small intestine, the activities of the stomach must be slowed to prevent damage by its acidic gastric juice. To accomplish this, the mucosa of the small intestine releases two hormones, **secretin** and **cholecystokinin (CCK)**. Both hormones:
- Inhibit _____
- Stimulate the secretion of _____ and bile into the small intestine

> **TIP!** Remember that hormones are released by an organ to travel in the bloodstream to a set of target tissues or a target organ. Secretin and CCK are released by the small intestine into the bloodstream. They will travel to their target organs.

Acid in the upper part of the small intestine and pressure in the walls of the small intestine as it fills trigger reflexes that cause the pyloric valve to close. This action protects the small intestine by

_____

_____

Review Time!

I.   Using the terms in the list below, label the parts of the stomach.

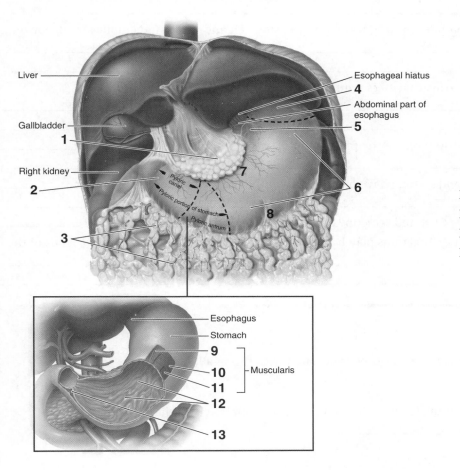

1. _____
2. _____
3. _____
4. _____
5. _____
6. _____
7. _____
8. _____
9. _____
10. _____
11. _____
12. _____
13. _____

Body of stomach	Greater omentum	**On cutaway**	Oblique layer
Cardiac portion of stomach	Lesser curvature	**(boxed image):**	Pyloric valve
Fundus of stomach	Lesser omentum	Circular layer	Rugae
Greater curvature	Pylorus	Longitudinal layer	

II. Provide a brief answer for each of the following questions about the stomach.

1. Name the four regions of the stomach.

   1. _____
   2. _____
   3. _____
   4. _____

2. Describe how the mucosa and muscularis layers of the stomach wall are modified.

   _____
   _____
   _____

3. List the items absorbed through the mucosa of the stomach. _____
_____

4. Name the two sphincters that enclose the stomach. _____
_____

5. What kind of meal empties most quickly from the stomach and what kind empties most slowly?
_____
_____

6. Name two reasons intrinsic factor is required for survival.
   1. _____
   2. _____

7. What effect does gastrin have on the production of gastric juice?_____
_____

8. What effect do CCK and secretin have on peristalsis in the stomach? _____
_____

9. What organ produces CCK and secretin?_____

10. What role does the hypothalamus play in the secretion of gastric juices from gastric glands of the stomach?_____
_____

Pancreas

The pancreas is an *accessory organ* that is closely associated with the small intestine.

Structure of the Pancreas

The pancreas is located behind the stomach in the upper abdominal cavity. It has three parts:

- **Head:** Near the _____
- **Body:** The middle portion
- **Tail:** Touches the spleen

The **acini** are exocrine secretory cells that form the majority of the organ. A small portion of the cells are endocrine pancreatic islets that release insulin and glucagon (Chapter 11). The acini release a mixture of enzymes called **pancreatic juice** into a centrally located **pancreatic duct.** These juices eventually make their way into the small intestine.

Functions of the Pancreas

The pancreas releases alkaline, enzyme-rich pancreatic juice into the _____ of the small intestine. *What is the function of this juice?* _____
_____.

Regulation of Pancreatic Secretions

The activities of the pancreas are regulated by:

- **Involuntary control centers of the brain**
- **Hormones:** Secretin and _____

While the hypothalamus stimulates the stomach mucosa to secrete gastric juice, it also stimulates acini cells in the pancreas to release pancreatic juice. The hormonal control of pancreatic juice release is by secretin and CCK.

1. Secretin is released into the blood in response to acidic chyme entering the small intestine from the stomach.

   • Once secretin reaches the pancreas, what does it stimulate the pancreas to release?

   _____

   _____

   • What is the function of these ions? _____

   _____

2. CCK is released into the blood in response to fats and proteins entering the small intestine from the stomach.

   • Once CCK reaches the pancreas, what does it stimulate the pancreas to release?

   _____

   _____

These enzymes complete the chemical digestion of carbohydrates, lipids, and proteins.

Review Time!

I.   Provide a brief answer for each of the following questions about the pancreas.

   1. Where is the pancreas located? _____

   _____

   2. With what organ is the pancreas closely associated? _____

   _____

   3. What do acini cells produce? _____

   What do the pancreas islets produce? _____

   _____

   _____

   4. Which hormone tells the pancreas to release bicarbonate-rich pancreatic juice?

   _____

   _____

   5. Which hormone tells the pancreas to release enzyme-rich pancreatic juice?

   _____

   _____

   6. What stimulates the release of CCK from the small intestine?_____

   _____

   7. What effect do CCK and secretin have on the secretion of gastric secretions from the stomach?

   _____

   _____

   8. What influence does the hypothalamus have on the pancreas?_____

   _____

   9. Why is alkaline, bicarbonate-rich pancreatic juice needed in the small intestine?

   _____

   _____

10. Marjorie has diabetes mellitus and has heard that her pancreas does not work *at all*. Did she receive correct information about her pancreas? Explain. You may need to refresh your knowledge of the endocrine role of the pancreas from Chapter 10. _____

_____

_____

Liver

The liver is located on the upper right side of the abdominal cavity; it presses against the diaphragm sitting superior to it. Although it is an *accessory organ* of the digestive system, it is also critically important for its roles in metabolism and regulation.

Structure of the Liver

The liver is enclosed by fibrous connective tissue that divides it into two main sections: **right lobe** and smaller **left lobe**. The _____ separates the right and left lobes and suspends the liver from the diaphragm and anterior abdominal wall. How is the lesser omentum attached to the liver?

_____

Lobule Organization

- **Liver lobules** are the structural and functional subunits of the liver.
- **Hepatocytes** are liver cells that are arranged in columns toward a **central vein**. These columns are separated from adjacent columns by channels, called *sinusoids,* lined with endothelial cells. Hepatocytes secrete _____.
- **Sinusoids** are filled with blood received from the hepatic artery and the hepatic portal vein. The blood passes through the sinusoids and drains into the central vein. Phagocytic cells known as _____ cells remove bacteria traveling in the blood from the digestive tract.

Bile Flow

- **Bile canaliculi** are tiny tubes that run parallel to the _____; they carry **bile**.
- **Bile** is a yellowish-green fluid secreted by the hepatocytes. Bile contains water, bile salts, bile pigments (biliverdin and bilirubin), cholesterol, and electrolytes. The bile salts and bile pigments are breakdown products of _____ blood cell destruction. What part of bile is the only active participant in the preparation of fats for chemical digestion? _____

_____

Bile is carried from bile canaliculi in the *opposite direction* to blood flowing through the sinusoids. Blood flows *to* the central vein. Bile flows *away* from the central vein.

- **Hepatic duct** is a larger duct that collects bile and emerges from the _____.
- **Cystic duct** collects bile stored in the gallbladder. The cystic duct unites with the hepatic duct to form the common bile duct.
- **Common bile duct** is formed from the union of the _____ duct and _____ duct.
- **Hepatopancreatic ampulla** is a small tube formed from the union of the _____ duct and the _____ duct. This tube unites with the duodenum of the small intestine.

> **TIP!** Think of the organization of the lobules of hepatocytes, sinusoids, and central vein as a bicycle tire. The lobules of hepatocytes are arranged like the spokes of the tire around the central vein. Blood flows toward the central vein. Bile, however, flows away from the central vein. Use the plentiful clues to help you keep the pathway of bile straight. Cystic means "bladder" while hepatic means "liver."

Functions of the Liver

The functions of the liver include:

1. **Secretion of bile.** The primary digestive function of the hepatocytes is to secrete bile. Bile salts are not enzymes. Instead, they break apart clumps of lipids into tiny drops, a process known as *emulsification*.
   - How does emulsification benefit digestion? _____
   _____
   _____
   - Bile salts promote the absorption of vitamins _____,
   _____, _____, and
   _____ in the small intestine.

2. **Metabolism of sugar.** The liver plays a role in blood sugar (glucose) homeostasis under the direction of hormones from the pancreas.
   - The two hormones secreted by the pancreas that regulate blood sugar levels are
   _____ and _____ .

3. **Metabolism of lipids.** The liver plays a role in the metabolism of lipids. It packages lipids for storage or transport that are bound to small proteins called _____.
   - **High-density lipoproteins** (HDLs) transport cholesterol *from* cells to the liver, where it becomes part of bile. HDLs are _____ lipoproteins because they are used in cell repair and growth and do not tend to accumulate in body spaces where they are not needed.
   - **Low-density lipoproteins** (LDLs) transport cholesterol *to* cells outside the liver for membrane or hormone synthesis.
   - **Very low-density lipoproteins** (vLDLs) come from the liver and transport
   _____ made in the liver *to* adipose tissue for storage.

   > **TIP!** HDLs are beneficial lipoproteins and LDLs can lead to health problems. Keep in mind that "H" are *h*elpful lipoproteins and "L" are *l*ousy lipoproteins in terms of the functions.

4. **Metabolism of proteins.** The liver converts amino acids into products that can be used or removed as waste. Amino acids are necessary for the synthesis of _____
   _____

5. **Storage.** The liver stores glycogen; vitamins _____,
   _____, and _____; and iron.

6. **Filter.** The liver filters and removes unwanted substances from the bloodstream.
   - What do Kupffer cells do? _____
   _____

7. **Clean.** Hepatocytes detoxify harmful substances that travel through the liver in the bloodstream
   (such as _____ and _____) by changing their composition.
   - If the hepatochytes are unable to change a substance's harmful form, what happens to the substance?
   _____
   _____
   - How is the storage of toxins damaging to the liver?_____
   _____
   _____

Gallbladder

Where is the gallbladder located?_____

_____

Structure: The gallbladder is lined internally with epithelium, which is supported by connective tissue and an external layer of smooth muscle.

Function: The gallbladder stores and concentrates bile secreted by the liver. The gallbladder receives bile from the liver from the _____ duct, which travels between the hepatic duct and the gallbladder. After a meal, the gallbladder contracts to send bile to the small intestine along this pathway:

Gallbladder → Cystic duct → Common bile duct → Hepatopancreatic ampulla →
Duodenum of small intestine

Review Time!

I. *Using the terms in the list below, label the parts of the liver and gallbladder.*

1. _____
2. _____
3. _____
4. _____
5. _____
6. _____
7. _____
8. _____

Cystic duct	Gallbladder	Hepatic duct	Left lobe
Falciform ligament	Hepatic artery	Inferior vena cava	Right lobe

II. *Place a number from 1 to 6 in the blank before each statement to indicate the correct order of the flow of bile from the liver to the small intestine.*

_____ Common bile duct

_____ Hepatopancreatic ampulla

_____ Hepatocytes

_____ Hepatic duct

_____ Duodenum of small intestine

_____ Bile canaliculi

III. Using the terms in the list below, label the parts of the pancreas.

1. _____
2. _____
3. _____
4. _____
5. _____
6. _____
7. _____
8. _____
9. _____
10. _____

Body of pancreas	Duodenum (small intestine)	Hepatic ducts	Pancreatic duct
Common bile duct	Gallbladder	Hepatopancreatic duct	Tail of pancreas
Cystic duct	Head of pancreas		

IV. Provide a brief answer for each of the following questions about the liver and gallbladder.

1. What is the name of the ligament that separates the right and left lobes of the liver?

_____

_____

2. Name two blood vessels that carry blood into the liver.

1. _____

2. _____

3. What are Kupffer cells? What is their function?_____

_____

_____

4. What components of bile are responsible for the chemical digestion of lipids?_____

_____

5. What ducts join to form the hepatopancreatic ampulla?_____

_____

6. Differentiate between the functions of HDLs and LDLs. _____

_____

7. Describe the role of the hepatocytes in cleansing the blood that travels through the liver.

_____

_____

_____

8. Discuss how the storage of toxins can damage the liver._____

_____

9. What is the function of the gallbladder?_____

_____

10. Trace the flow of bile from the gallbladder to the small intestine soon after a meal.

_____

_____

_____

Small Intestine

The small intestine is the body's *most important* digestive organ. It performs both chemical and mechanical digestion and is the *main site* of _____.

Structure of the Small Intestine

The small intestine:

- Extends from the _____ to the large intestine for about 6 meters (20 feet).
- Has a diameter of about 2.5 centimeters (1 inch).
- Is suspended in the abdominal cavity by the _____ which anchors it to the posterior abdominal wall.
- Is framed by the large intestine laterally and superiorly.

Three Segments of the Small Intestine

- **Duodenum** is the first portion. It is approximately 25 centimeters (10 inches) in length. It receives chyme from the stomach through the _____ valve.
- **Jejunum** is the middle region. It extends for 2.5 meters (8 feet) to the third and the last segment.
- **Ileum** is the last segment. It is about 3.6 meters (12 feet) in length. The ileum unites with the _____ at the **ileocecal valve.** The ileocecal valve regulates the flow of material from the ileum to the large intestine.

Modifications of the Layers of the Small Intestine Wall

1. **Mucosa** has modifications for chemical digestion and the absorption of nutrients.
   - **Villi** are tiny, 1 millimeter projections of the mucosa that come into contact with the contents of the small intestine. What is the function of the villi? _____

   _____

     - **Lacteal** is a lymphatic vessel that is present within each villus along with a blood capillary. These vessels carry absorbed nutrients.
     - **Microvilli** are thousands of tiny projections covering each villus. How do the villi and microvilli affect absorption? _____

     _____

   - **Intestinal glands** are situated between the bases of adjacent villi. They release a colorless secretion of water and mucus with a neutral pH.

• In what part of the small intestine are these glands most numerous? _____
• What function does this secretion serve? _____

_____

2. **Submucosa** of the small intestine differs from other organs.
   • **Peyer patches** are lymphatic nodules which protect the body from infectious microorganism that may penetrate the intestinal wall.
   • **Brunner glands** are mucous glands. They are only found in what part of the small intestine?

   _____

   What is the function of the mucus secreted by these glands?_____
   _____

3. **Plicae circulares** (circular folds) are created by deep, permanent folds of the mucosa and submucosa.
   • Why do these folds exist? _____
   _____
   _____

Functions of the Small Intestine

The three main functions of the small intestine are:

1. **Chemical digestion**
   • Pancreatic enzymes from the pancreas break down a wide spectrum of _____.
   • Intestinal enzymes of the _____ also break down a wide variety of foods.
   • Bile from the liver emulsifies _____.

2. **Absorption**
   The small intestine is the *main site* of nutrient absorption. Nutrients and water move across the mucosa lining into blood vessels and lacteals of the villi. The increased surface area of the villi and microvilli increase the effectiveness of the small intestine.
   • **Carbohydrate digestion and absorption.** Carbohydrate digestion begins in the _____ and is completed in the small intestine. Nearly 100% of usable simple sugars, known as monosaccharides, are moved into the lining epithelium of villi by facilitated diffusion or active transport. Once inside the epithelial cells, the monosaccharides are transported by

   _____

   _____

   • **Protein digestion and absorption.** Protein digestion begins in the _____ by pepsin and is completed in the _____ by pancreatic and intestinal enzymes. Amino acids are absorbed by *active transport* across the intestinal lining, then by *diffusion* into the blood capillaries.
   • **Lipid digestion and absorption.** Lipid digestion is completed by bile salts and enzymes within the _____ (*which organ?*). Most lipids consumed in the diet are triglycerides which are broken down into fatty acids and glycerol. Once absorbed into the lining epithelium, the lipids are resynthesized into fat droplets called _____ which move to the lacteals. Lacteals carry the droplets to the bloodstream.
   • **Water and electrolyte absorption.** Two-thirds (2 liters) of the water entering the small intestine is absorbed into the capillaries by _____. Electrolytes (such as sodium, potassium, chlorine, hydrogen, iron, calcium) are moved into the lining epithelium by *active transport* and *diffusion*.

3. **Propulsion**

Propulsion of chyme through the small intestine is provided by _____.
The peristaltic waves continue then pause in a slow propulsion that takes 3 to 10 hours to move
chyme through the small intestine. If the chyme is moved too quickly so that water, electrolytes, and
nutrients cannot be normally absorbed, what condition results?_____

Review Time!

I.   *Provide a brief answer for each of the following questions about the small intestine.*

1. What are the three segments of the small intestine?

   1. _____

   2. _____

   3. _____

2. What are the two modifications of the mucosa? Explain the functions of these two modifications.

   _____

   _____

   _____

3. Describe the function of the plicae circulares. _____

   _____

   _____

4. What are the two valves (sphincters) that enclose the small intestine at each end?

   _____

   _____

5. How are the intestinal glands and Brunner glands functionally similar? Do these glands differ and
   if so, how?_____

   _____

   _____

6. Name and briefly describe the three functions of the small intestine. _____

   1. _____

   2. _____

   3. _____

7. Describe the role of pancreatic enzymes and bile in chemical digestion in the small intestine.

   _____

   _____

   _____

   _____

8. Where within the GI tract does carbohydrate digestion begin? Where is carbohydrate digestion
   completed?_____

   _____

9. Where within the GI tract does protein digestion begin? Where is protein digestion completed?

   _____

   _____

10. What does peristalsis accomplish in the small intestine?_____

   _____

Large Intestine

The large intestine is the last organ of the GI tract. It extends 1.5 meters (5 feet) from the small intestine at the ileocecal valve to the anus.

• Which organ has a larger diameter: the *small* intestine or the *large* intestine?_____

Structure of the Large Intestine

The large intestine has four main segments:

1. **Cecum** is connected to the _____ of the small intestine by the ileocecal valve. The **vermiform appendix** is attached to the cecum's lower margin.
    • What type of tissue is housed in the appendix? _____
    • What is appendicitis? _____
    _____
    • How can appendicitis lead to peritonitis?_____
    _____
    _____

2. **Colon** is the longest segment of the large intestine.
    • **Ascending colon** continues from its union with the _____ (*which organ?*) up the right side of the abdominal cavity to a point below the liver. At the right colic (hepatic) flexure, the ascending colon becomes the transverse colon.
    • **Transverse colon** extends across the abdomen to a point just below the _____ (*which organ?*) at the left corner of the abdominal cavity. At the left colic (splenic) flexure, the transverse colon becomes the descending colon.
    • **Descending colon** continues down the left side of the _____ cavity. Once inside the pelvic cavity, it becomes the sigmoid colon.
    • **Sigmoid colon** is an S-shaped turn of the colon. It continues on as the rectum.
3. **Rectum** is situated against the _____ in the pelvic cavity. It is a straight tube that converges with the anal canal.
4. **Anal canal** opens to the exterior at the **anus**. The anus has an internal, involuntary sphincter composed of _____ muscle and an external, voluntary sphincter composed of _____ muscle. Both sphincters are normally closed until defecation.

> **TIP!** The order of the four regions of the colon of the large intestine is logical: ascending, transverse, then descending, and last the sigmoid colon.

Modifications of the Layers of the Large Intestine Wall

1. **Mucosa** lacks the villi seen in the small intestine, but it does have folds in the mucosa and submucosa similar to the small intestine's plicae circulares. Mucus-secreting cells are common in the large intestine.
    • Why is mucus beneficial?_____
    _____
    _____
    • The **anal columns** are parallel ridges or folds in the mucosa of the anal canal. What function do these columns serve?_____
    _____

2. **Submucosa**
3. **Muscularis** is different from other organs. The outer longitudinal layer of smooth muscle does not cover the entire organ. Instead, it is arranged in three bands.
   - These bands, the **taenia coli,** extend the entire length of the colon and contract to gather the colon into pouches called **haustra.** What is the function of the haustra?

   _____

   _____

Functions of the Large Intestine

The large intestine has two major functions:

1. **Water absorption.** Indigestible food wastes travel through the large intestine as the mucosa absorbs water and electrolytes. As the chyme moves toward the rectum, **feces** are formed.
   - What is found in feces?_____

   _____

   _____

   - The bacterial population of the large intestine is called the *intestinal flora.* What are the benefits of these bacteria?_____

   _____

   _____

   - What gasses are produced by the intestinal flora?

   _____

   _____

2. **Defecation.** Defecation is the propulsion of feces through the large intestine and out the anus. Propulsion of food wastes through the large intestine is slower than it is through the small intestine.
   - How long does it take material to pass through the colon?_____
   - The peristaltic contractions of the large intestine only travel a short distance before stopping, then resuming elsewhere. What is the function of these gentle waves that occur only several times a day?

   _____

   _____

Defecation reflex: This reflex begins when the rectum becomes full of feces and receptors in the wall are stimulated. Peristalsis intensifies and the internal sphincter relaxes.

- If the external (voluntary) sphincter relaxes, what happens?_____

_____

_____

- If the external sphincter is not relaxed, what happens?_____

_____

_____

Review Time!

I.   *Using the terms in the list below, label the parts of the large intestine.*

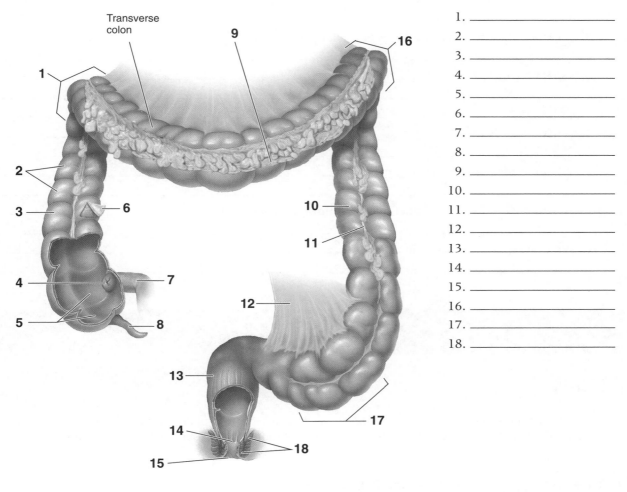

1. _____
2. _____
3. _____
4. _____
5. _____
6. _____
7. _____
8. _____
9. _____
10. _____
11. _____
12. _____
13. _____
14. _____
15. _____
16. _____
17. _____
18. _____

Anal canal	Descending colon	Left colic (splenic) flexure	Taenia coli
Anal sphincters	Greater omentum	Mesentery	Vermiform appendix
Anus	Haustra	Rectum	Visceral peritoneum
Ascending colon	Ileocecal valve	Right colic (hepatic) flexure	
Cecum	Ileum	Sigmoid colon	

II.   *Provide a brief answer for each of the following questions about the large intestine.*

   1. Name the four segments of the large intestine.

      1. _____
      2. _____
      3. _____
      4. _____

   2. Trace the pathway of indigestible food wastes through the large intestine until the feces are defecated. _____
   _____
   _____

3. What is the function of the anal columns?_____
_____

4. How is the muscularis layer of the large intestine wall modified?_____
_____
_____

5. What are the two main functions of the large intestine?_____

6. What do feces contain?_____
_____
_____

7. What are intestinal flora?_____
_____

8. What are the benefits of intestinal flora?_____
_____

9. Where are feces stored until elimination through defecation?_____
_____

10. What initiates the defecation reflex?_____
_____

CONCEPT 4

Nutrition

Concept: Adequate nutrition is necessary to maintain health in order to provide nutrients for metabolism, growth, and repair. It requires the intake of all nutrients on a regular basis, especially essential nutrients.

LEARNING OBJECTIVE 10. Explain why the body requires energy to sustain life.

LEARNING OBJECTIVE 11. Identify the basic classes of nutrients and define essential nutrients.

Metabolism is the production of energy from glucose, mainly, to enable enzymes to perform work. Energy is used for the creation of new molecules, growth, repair, and reproduction of cells.

Nutrition is the process of providing fuel to cells, including the modification, absorption, and utilization of food substances, or nutrients, by the body.

Nutrients include carbohydrates, lipids, proteins, vitamins, minerals, and water. Where do we get nutrients from? _____
_____

Essential nutrients must be obtained through the diet. Some 50 essential nutrients include certain amino acids, 2 lipids, B-complex vitamins, vitamin C, water, and minerals.
_____

Metabolism

Define metabolism. _____
_____

Anabolism and catabolism are two metabolic processes.

1. **Anabolism** is a process that *uses* energy for body functions.
2. **Catabolism** is a process that *releases* energy from the breakdown of nutrients. Energy released from these reactions builds molecules of ATP for _____

Cellular respiration is a catabolic process that results in the production of energy (ATP) for cells to power their activities.

- What is the nutrient molecule preferred by all cells to power cellular respiration?

_____

- Why is this particular sugar preferred? _____

Two Cellular Respiration Pathways

1. **Anaerobic respiration** is a pathway of cellular respiration that does not require _____. The process of cellular respiration begins with anaerobic respiration, then may continue on to aerobic respiration (next). We start with *glycolysis,* used during strenuous exercise and when no oxygen is available:

   - Glucose, a six-carbon molecule, is broken down to produce two pyruvic acids, a three-carbon compound. How many molecules of ATP are produced? _____
   - If *no* oxygen is available, the pyruvic acid is converted into _____.
   - When oxygen is available, the lactic acid is converted back to pyruvic acid.

2. **Aerobic respiration** is a pathway that begins when oxygen is available. We start with pyruvic acid from the anaerobic pathway just discussed:

   - Pyruvic acid is broken down to form acetyl coenzyme A (acetyl Co-A).
   - Hydrogen ion transfer produces _____ ATP molecules along with carbon dioxide and water.

Have you kept track of how many ATP molecules have been produced from *one* glucose molecule? Enter the total here: _____

Carbohydrates

- **Building blocks:** Simple sugar subunits
- **Function:** Energy source for cellular activities. The body can also break down tissue proteins and fats to fuel cellular activities if the diet is low in carbohydrates.
- **Metabolism:** Digestion begins in the _____ when polysaccharides are broken down into disaccharides. Digestion is completed in the _____ when disaccharides are broken down into monosaccharides for absorption into the bloodstream.
- **Dietary requirements:** _____ (*how many?*) grams of carbohydrates per day are required to spare protein and maintain blood glucose levels, although current recommendations call for 125 to 175 grams per day with an emphasis on complex carbohydrates.

EXAMPLE

- **Monosaccharides** (simple sugars or "one sugar")
- **Disaccharides** (two simple sugar subunits)
- **Polysaccharides** (complex carbohydrates or "many sugars," starches, fiber—"roughage" for facilitation of movement of food through the digestive tract, for increasing the bulk of the stool, and facilitating defecation)

Lipids

- **Building blocks:** Triglycerides (fats) are the most abundant source of dietary lipids and consist of a _____ attached to three fatty acid chains.
- **Function:** Lipids serve as a backup fuel source to _____ metabolism; provide insulation from outside temperature changes; provide padding for protection; help the body absorb fat-soluble vitamins; and provide the building blocks for creation of cell membranes.
- **Metabolism:** Lipid metabolism produces ketone bodies, which are potentially toxic waste products. What situations might cause the body to produce ketone bodies from fat metabolism for fuel and result in *ketoacidosis*? _____
  _____
- **Dietary requirements:** Lipids represent _____% of the calories in an average American diet, much from saturated fats which may contribute to cardiovascular disease. Saturated fats should account for 10% or less of the total lipid intake; daily cholesterol should be no more than 250 milligrams.

EXAMPLE OF LIPIDS

Two Types of Triglycerides

- **Saturated fats** are triglycerides that contain single bonds between carbon atoms, are solid at room temperature, and are found in animal products and a few plant foods, such as
  _____
  _____

- **Unsaturated fats** are triglycerides that contain one or more double bonds between carbon atoms, are liquid at room temperature, and found in plant sources such as _____
  _____

Two Essential Fatty Acids

Two *essential fatty acids* (linoleic acid and alpha-linoleic acid) are needed for the synthesis of certain phospholipids used in the construction of cell membranes. They may protect against *atherosclerosis*. Explain what atherosclerosis is (you may need to review Chapter 12). _____
_____

Cholesterol

Cholesterol is not used for energy, but is used as a structural component of bile salts, steroid hormones, and cell membranes.

Proteins

- **Building blocks:** Amino acids
- **Function:** Cell structure and function; in certain situations, proteins can be used for fuel
- **Metabolism:** Lipids can be broken down by liver cells to produce glucose in a process called _____ when carbohydrate and lipid sources are inadequate for fuel requirements for cells. The metabolism of proteins produces a toxic waste product called _____. How does the body handle this waste?_____ _____ _____

- **Dietary requirements:** Protein requirements depend on age, body weight, and metabolic rate. Generally, 0.8 grams of protein per kilogram of body weight are needed on a daily basis. Why do pregnant and nursing women need more protein?_____

EXAMPLE

There are eight *essential amino acids* that the body cannot synthesize. These eight amino acids may be obtained from any animal source since animal proteins are nutritionally complete. What should a strict vegetarian eat to obtain these eight essential amino acids since plant proteins are nutritionally incomplete?_____ _____

Vitamins

12. Discuss the roles of vitamins and minerals in your diet.

Vitamins are organic compounds that are not used for energy or structural building blocks. Your body uses them for:
- Metabolism
- Cell membrane transport
- _____ formation
- Vision

Vitamins are either fat soluble or water soluble.

- **Fat-soluble vitamins** bind lipids and are absorbed with lipid products during digestion. These vitamins are not easily damaged by cooking and food processing. Fat-soluble vitamins are vitamin _____ (must be obtained from food); vitamin D (must be obtained from food); vitamin _____ (synthesized from cholesterol in skin exposed to sunlight); and vitamin _____ (synthesized by bacteria in the intestine).

- **Water-soluble vitamins** must be obtained in the food you eat and absorbed with water across the intestinal wall, except for vitamin B_{12}. What is needed for vitamin B_{12} absorption? _____ _____

The water-soluble vitamins are *not* stored in the body. They are excreted in urine if they are not needed. They are damaged during food processing and cooking. Water-soluble vitamins are the B-complex vitamins and vitamin C.

Minerals

Minerals are *inorganic* molecules and include:

- Calcium, phosphorus, and magnesium, which are needed for _____
  _____
- Sodium, chloride, and potassium, which are needed for _____
  _____
- Sulfur, a component of _____
- Trace minerals

Water

Water is the major component of cells and forms most of the fluids of the body (interstitial fluid, plasma, saliva, and cerebrospinal fluid). It is required as a:

- Solvent for dissolving molecules
- Medium of transport
- Lubrication of surfaces
- Heat absorber

The body loses water through three mechanisms: _____.

How much water do you need on a daily basis?_____

Review Time!

I. *Provide a brief answer for each of the following questions about nutrition.*

1. Define nutrition. _____
   _____
   _____

2. How do we obtain essential nutrients? _____
   _____

3. What chemical reactions make ATP from glucose? _____
   _____
   _____

4. How does anaerobic respiration differ from aerobic respiration? _____
   _____
   _____

5. How many ATP are made from one glucose during aerobic respiration? _____
6. Why should our diets include fiber? _____
   _____
   _____

7. On what basis do monosaccharides differ from disaccharides and polysaccharides?
   _____
   _____
   _____

8. Dieting and diabetes mellitus force the body to turn to fats for ATP production. What are the toxic products of this process? _____

9. Why do we need the two essential lipids in our diets? _____
_____
_____

10. Why should we limit our intake of saturated fats? _____
_____
_____

11. Describe the differences between saturated and unsaturated fats. Provide at least two differences.
_____
_____
_____
_____

12. How do animal and plant sources differ as sources of amino acids? _____
_____
_____
_____

13. How many essential amino acids are there? _____

14. Which class of vitamins can be stored in the body? _____

15. List the fat-soluble vitamins. _____
_____

16. What vitamins can be synthesized by the body? _____
_____

17. Which type of vitamin is damaged by cooking or food processing? _____
_____

18. What are minerals? How are they different from vitamins? _____
_____
_____
_____
_____

19. Which minerals compose the bones and teeth?_____
_____
_____

20. Why do you need fat in your diet for the absorption of vitamins A, D, E, and K?
_____
_____
_____
_____

21. Why should people with diabetes mellitus be concerned about ketoacidosis?
_____
_____
_____
_____

22. What diet would you recommend to a strict vegetarian so all eight essential amino acids are obtained? _____

_____

_____

_____

23. Why should we drink between 8 and 12 cups of water per day? _____

_____

_____

24. Rank the following nutrients in the order that the body would prefer to use them to make ATP: protein, starch, saturated fat. _____

25. Explain how glycolysis differs from gluconeogenesis. _____

_____

_____

_____

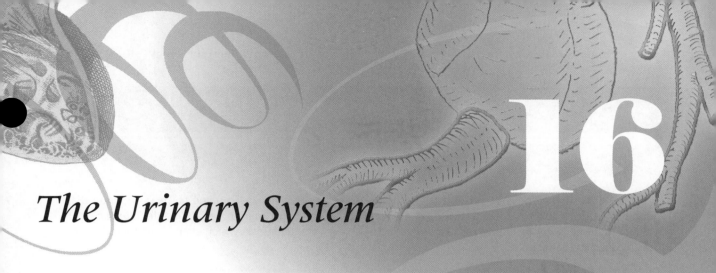

The Urinary System

16

Tips for Success as You Begin

Read Chapter 16 from your textbook before attending class. Listen when you attend lecture and fill in the blanks in this notebook. You may choose to complete the blanks before attending class as a way to prepare for the day's topics. The same day you attend lecture, read the material again and complete the exercises after each section in this notebook. Frequent review of the material in this chapter will help you understand the various roles of the kidneys. Try teaching what you learn in this chapter to someone else—you'll be surprised how much you'll retain!

Introduction to the Urinary System

The urinary system's functions are to:
- Maintain purity and homeostatic balance of body fluids
- Recycle usable materials
- Remove metabolic wastes, toxins, excess ions, and water as urine (known as **excretion**)
- Regulate fluid and electrolyte levels
- Help regulate blood pressure
- Control red blood cell production in red bone marrow

The urinary system's organs are the:
- _____
- _____
- _____
- _____

CONCEPT 1

Kidney Structure

Concept: The two kidneys are located against the posterior abdominal wall outside of the peritoneum. Each kidney includes a solid interior composed of an outer renal cortex and an inner renal medulla, which contain many functional subunits known as nephrons. The nephrons produce urine, which eventually drains into a basin called the renal pelvis.

LEARNING OBJECTIVE   1. Identify the structural features of the kidneys.

External Anatomy

Kidneys are fist-sized and the shape of a kidney bean. Their indented margin faces the midline of the body.

Location: Lumbar region against the posterior abdominal wall. The kidneys are *retroperitoneal,* that is, they are external to the peritoneum.

- The right kidney is lower than the left kidney. Why? _____

Coverings: Several layers of connective tissue externally support both kidneys.

- **Renal fascia** includes _____ fibers that anchor the kidney and adrenal gland to surrounding tissues.

- **Adipose capsule** is deep to the renal fascia and provides the kidney with a cushioning layer of

  _____.

- **Renal capsule** is a layer of _____ connective tissue that forms the outer wall of the kidney.

Internal Anatomy

The major parts of the kidney are:

- **Hilum** is the concave margin of the kidney that faces the body's midline. It is the point at which the _____, renal vein, nerves, and _____ unite with the kidney.

- **Renal sinus** is visible when the kidney has been cut open. It is a space filled with fat, connective tissue, and the **renal pelvis**.

- **Renal pelvis** is a membrane-lined basin that extends into the _____.

- **Calyces** are funnel-shaped channels that collect _____ from the kidney tissue and direct it into the renal pelvis.

The three regions of the kidney are:

- **Renal pelvis** (previously described)

- **Renal medulla** is characterized by the presence of cone-shaped renal pyramids. The tip, or apex, of each pyramid points toward the renal pelvis where it is surrounded by a calyx. Tubules of the _____ give the pyramids a striped appearance. The base of the pyramid borders the cortex.

- **Renal cortex** is an outer layer with a light, granulated appearance formed by the functional units of the kidney called **nephrons**. **Renal columns** are portions of _____ tissue that extend between the renal pyramids.

As we discuss the parts of the kidney, ureter, and associated structures, add labels to the illustration below. When you are done, you should be able to identify the parts and structures listed below.

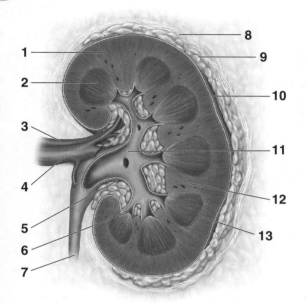

1. _____
2. _____
3. _____
4. _____
5. _____
6. _____
7. _____
8. _____
9. _____
10. _____
11. _____
12. _____
13. _____

Coverings
  Renal fascia
  Adipose capsule
  Renal capsule

Regions
  Cortex
  Renal column
  Medulla
  Renal pyramid
  Renal pelvis

Other structures
  Calyx
  Renal artery
  Renal sinus
  Renal vein
  Ureter

Blood Supply

LEARNING OBJECTIVE   2. Describe the blood vessels associated with the kidneys.

The kidneys have a vast blood supply. We will follow blood flow into the kidney through the arterial pathway.

• **Renal artery** branches from the abdominal aorta.
• **Segmental** (lobar) **arteries** (5) branch off the renal artery and enter the renal sinus.
• _____ **arteries** branch off the segmental arteries and extend between the renal pyramids.
• _____ **arteries** branch off the interlobar arteries and curve over the outer margin of the pyramids.
• _____ **arteries** branch from the arcuate arteries into the renal cortex.
• **Afferent arterioles** are branches of the interlobular arteries. They lead to the nephrons.

> **TIP!** Notice the naming scheme for these vessels: after the renal artery, the segmental or *lobar* arteries branch or segment into a longer word, the *interlobar* arteries. The *arcuate* arteries "arch" over the pyramids. Now, we move to an even longer word—the *interlobular* arteries. Finally, the interlobular arteries move us to the afferent arterioles leading into the glomerulus. Afferent means "toward."

The venous pathway parallels the arterial pathway with similar names. Blood is emptied into the **renal vein** as it exits the kidney. The renal vein delivers blood to the inferior vena cava. Recall that the inferior vena cava takes blood to _____.

Nephron Structure

LEARNING OBJECTIVE 3. Identify the components of the nephron.

LEARNING OBJECTIVE 4. Describe the flow of blood through the nephron.

The **nephron** is the functional subunit of the kidney. A single nephron occupies both the cortex and medulla of the kidney. The two parts of the nephron are:

1. **Renal corpuscle** is the expanded, bowl-shaped end. Parts of the renal corpuscle are:
   - **Glomerular** (Bowman's) **capsule** is a bowl-shaped structure that partly surrounds the glomerulus, a capillary network. The outer wall is composed of _____ while the inner wall closely follows the twists of the glomerulus.
   - **Glomerulus** is a capillary network surrounded by the _____. Some features of the glomerulus are:
     - _____ are large pores in the endothelial walls of the glomerulus.
     - **Podocytes** are specialized cells that form the inner wall.
     - **Filtration** _____ are gaps that are found between adjacent podocytes.
     - **Filtration** _____ includes the podocytes and their filtration slits, an underlying basement membrane, and fenestrations of the glomerular wall.
2. **Renal tubule** is composed of several, continuous segments:
   - **Proximal convoluted tubule (PCT)** is a segment *closest* to the glomerular capsule. Its coils start in the cortex and then plunge into the _____ in a renal pyramid.
   - **Loop of Henle** (renal loop) is a segment that descends into the medulla, and then makes a U-turn back into the cortex. The _____ travels down into the medulla while the _____ returns to the cortex.
   - **Distal convoluted tubule (DCT)** is a segment coiled in the cortex.
   - **Collecting duct** is a larger segment that collects urine and channels it from the cortex to the medulla to the renal pelvis.

   > **TIP!** The PCT is proximal (closest) to the glomerulus. The DCT is distal (farther) from the glomerulus. Thus, the names. If you have to identify these tubules on a model or image, trace the tubule as it leaves the capsule and travels toward the collecting duct.

Blood Supply to the Nephron

- **Afferent arteriole** carries blood *into* the nephron.
- **Glomerulus** is a capillary network that receives blood from the _____ arteriole.
- **Efferent arteriole** drains blood *from* the glomerulus.
- **Peritubular capillaries** are a second capillary network that receives blood from the _____ arteriole. These capillaries are porous and low pressured, well suited to their function of picking up materials. They are closely associated with the renal tubule and carry blood to the _____ pathway.

The diameter of the efferent arteriole is smaller than the afferent arteriole. How does that impact the blood flow? _____

The slow flow of blood out of the efferent arteriole causes blood to stall in the glomerulus. High pressure is created in the glomerulus, which is needed to force fluids and solutes out of the bloodstream and into the glomerular capsule during a process called filtration.

Juxtaglomerular Apparatus

LEARNING OBJECTIVE 5. Describe the juxtaglomerular apparatus and its primary product.

The **juxtaglomerular apparatus** is a region where the _____ convoluted tubule contacts the _____ arteriole.

- **Macula densa** are _____ cells from the DCT.
- **Juxtaglomerular cells** are modified _____ cells from the afferent arteriole.

These specialized cells regulate the (1) rate of urine formation and (2) blood pressure.

As we discuss the structure of the nephron, add labels to the illustration below. When you are done, you should be able to identify the structures listed below.

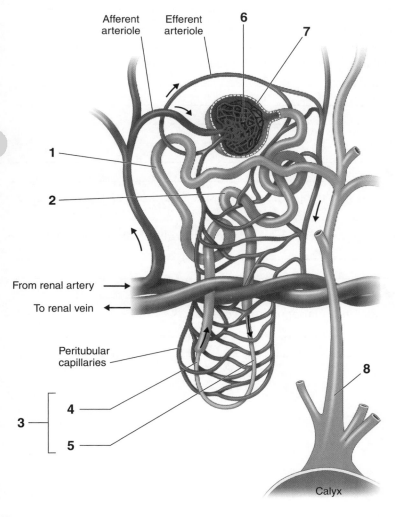

1. _____
2. _____
3. _____
4. _____
5. _____
6. _____
7. _____
8. _____

Renal corpuscle
  Glomerulus
  Glomerular capsule

Renal tubule
  PCT
  DCT

Loop of Henle (including descending limb and ascending limb)
Collecting duct

Review Time!

I.   *Provide a brief answer for each of the following questions about kidney structure.*

1. What are the four organs of the urinary system?

     1. _____

     2. _____

     3. _____

     4. _____

2. What are the three layers that surround each kidney?

     1. _____

     2. _____

     3. _____

3. Name the three regions of the kidney.

     1. _____

     2. _____

     3. _____

4. What is the functional subunit of the kidney? _____

5. Trace the flow of blood from the renal artery until you reach the glomerulus.

     _____

     _____

     _____

6. What are the two parts of the nephron?

     1. _____

     2. _____

7. What segment of the renal tubule is closest to the glomerular capsule? _____

     _____

8. How does the structure of the efferent arteriole ensure blood pressure will remain high in the glomerulus? _____

     _____

9. What vessels receive blood from the efferent arteriole? _____

10. What two regulatory roles do the juxtaglomerular apparatus cells play?

     1. _____

     2. _____

CONCEPT 2

Kidney Function

Concept: The nephrons of the kidneys process blood by glomerular filtration, tubular reabsorption, and tubular secretion. The result is the formation of urine, which is the means for eliminating urea and uric acid, and for maintaining fluid, electrolyte, and pH homeostasis. The kidneys also play a role in blood pressure regulation.

The primary functions of the kidneys are to:

1. Remove unwanted substances from the bloodstream by the formation of urine.
2. Maintain _____ and _____ homeostasis.
3. Regulate blood pressure.
4. Regulate pH of body fluids.

Urine Formation

The kidneys filter:

- 1,200 milliliters of blood every minute of which 120 milliliters of blood are pushed into renal tubules.
- 180 liters (45 gallons) of blood every day of which 99% is reabsorbed. The remaining 1% (1 to 2 liters per day) is released as **urine**. Urine contains _____

_____

The three main processes involved in urine formation are:

1. Glomerular filtration
2. Tubular reabsorption
3. Tubular secretion

Glomerular Filtration

LEARNING OBJECTIVE   6. Describe the process of glomerular filtration and the importance of the net filtration pressure (NFP).

Glomerular filtration is the movement of blood plasma across the filtration membrane of the renal corpuscle.

- Do you recall what constitutes the filtration membrane? _____

_____

- What can travel across the filtration membrane, forming the **filtrate**? _____

_____

_____

- What can *not* travel across the filtration membrane? _____

_____

_____

- Why are certain items restricted from crossing the filtration membrane? _____

_____

_____

- Where does filtrate travel after it is pushed across the filtration membrane? _____

_____

How are fluids pushed across the filtration membrane of the glomerulus? High hydrostatic pressure within the glomerulus is the force of blood pushing against the glomerular walls. Narrowing of efferent arteriole makes the hydrostatic pressure unusually high in the glomerulus.

Hydrostatic pressure must overcome two forces:

1. Osmotic pressure created by the solutes in the blood within the glomerulus. This osmotic pressure *pulls* fluids back into the glomerulus.

2. Pressure of filtrate within the glomerular capsule (filtrate pressure). This pressure *pushes* fluids back into the glomerulus.

NFP is the net force of _____ mm of mercury (Hg) that *pushes* plasma through the filtration membrane to become filtrate.

Glomerular filtration rate (GFR) is the rate of filtration determined by the amount of NFP present during one minute. The average value is _____ milliliters per minute (7.5 liters per hour).

• When GFR _____, filtrate volume increases, and urine volume increases.

• When GFR _____, filtrate volume decreases, and urine volume decreases.

GFR is influenced by:

• Volume of blood in the glomerulus

• Systemic blood pressure

Renal autoregulation changes the _____ of the afferent arterioles, which alters the volume of blood flowing into the glomerulus.

Tubular Reabsorption

LEARNING OBJECTIVE 7. Describe the process of tubular reabsorption and tubular secretion.

Tubular reabsorption is a reclamation process that returns needed materials to the blood stream. Concentration of wastes in the urine increases.

• How are urine and filtrate different? _____
_____
_____

How are items reabsorbed from filtrate into the bloodstream? Items are moved from the renal tubule into the blood stream by active transport or passive transport. For instance, items such as amino acids and glucose move by _____ transport while water moves by _____.

What is the pathway of reabsorption? Substances move (1) through the single cell layer of the renal tubule wall, (2) to a space filled with interstitial fluid, (3) to the endothelial wall of the peritubular capillaries, and (4) into the bloodstream.

At what point in the renal tubule does reabsorption occur? Reabsorption varies along the length of the tubule, based on the permeability of the cells lining the tubule.

• **PCT** is the main site of _____ reabsorption by osmosis. Glucose, amino acids, and ions are reabsorbed and water follows.

• **Loop of Henle, descending limb** absorbs more water and less solutes while the **ascending limb** absorbs less water and more solutes. Filtrate becomes dilute by the time it enters the DCT.

• **DCT** and **collecting duct** reabsorb more solutes by active transport and water by osmosis.

Tubular Secretion

Tubular secretion occurs when items not filtered at the _____ are removed from the blood. Movement of the items is *opposite* to reabsorption: items are moved from the peritubular capillaries into the renal tubule to join the filtrate.

What is removed from the blood via tubular secretion?

• Harmful substances that were not removed from the blood during filtration (such as penicillin)

• _____ that have been reabsorbed along with needed materials (such as urea and uric acid)

• Excess potassium ions

• Excess _____ ions as a way to control blood pH

> **TIP!** Glomerular filtration means blood plasma and solutes are moved from blood into the glomerular (Bowman's) capsule. Tubular reabsorption means fluid and solutes (now known as filtrate) are moved from the renal tubule into the bloodstream (peritubular capillaries). Tubular secretion is opposite of tubular reabsorption. During tubular secretion, items to be removed from the body are moved from the bloodstream (peritubular capillaries) into the renal tubule.

Review Time!

I. *Provide a brief answer for each of the following questions about kidney function.*

1. What are the three main processes involved in urine formation?

   1. _____

   2. _____

   3. _____

2. How much blood is filtered by the glomerulus every minute (in milliliters)?

   _____

3. How are filtrate and blood plasma similar and how are they different? _____

   _____

   _____

   _____

4. Explain how pressure remains high in the glomerulus so that filtration can occur.

   _____

   _____

   _____

5. Define NFP. _____

   _____

   _____

6. What is the main determinant of GFR? _____

   _____

7. Explain the function and benefit of renal autoregulation. _____

   _____

   _____

8. In general, how do solutes in the renal tubule rejoin blood flow? _____

   _____

   _____

9. Where in the renal tubule is water mainly reabsorbed? _____

   _____

10. What is reabsorbed in the descending limb of the loop of Henle? In the ascending loop?

    _____

    _____

    _____

11. How do solutes in the peritubular capillaries join filtrate in the renal tubule without being filtered by the glomerulus? _____
_____
_____

12. What types of items are secreted into the renal tubule? _____
_____

13. What region of the renal tubule is most active in tubular secretion? _____
_____

14. Explain how tubular reabsorption and tubular secretion are opposite processes.
_____
_____

Regulation of Urine Concentration and Volume

LEARNING OBJECTIVE 8. Describe the processes that regulate urine volume and blood pressure.

The kidneys function to maintain constant blood composition and volume. They accomplish this by adjusting the amount of water and solutes filtered, reabsorbed, or secreted. If the kidneys cannot regulate urine concentration and volume, *renal failure* can occur. Adjusting urine volume and concentration is a method for adjusting blood pressure. We will look at how blood pressure can be regulated by antidiuretic hormone (ADH); renin, angiotensin, and aldosterone; atrial natriuretic peptide (ANP); and sympathetic stimulation.

Antidiuretic Hormone

ADH is released by the _____ pituitary gland. This hormone targets the DCT and the collecting duct to reabsorb _____ from filtrate when blood volume and blood pressure are low. ADH operates by negative feedback.

• By reabsorbing more water from filtrate, ADH decreases urine production. As a result, urine becomes more concentrated with solutes and is a deeper yellow color. In turn, blood volume and blood pressure
_____.

• Decreased ADH production means an increased urine output and the urine is light colored. In turn, blood volume and blood pressure _____.

In summary:
• What triggers ADH release? _____
• Where is ADH produced? _____
• What is the function of ADH? _____
_____
• What effect does ADH have on blood volume and blood pressure? _____
_____

Renin, Angiotensin, and Aldosterone

When blood pressure decreases, such as through hemorrhage (loss of blood) or heart failure, the kidneys help increase and return blood pressure to normal. They do so through the following processes:

• Juxtaglomerular cells (in the juxtaglomerular apparatus) release into the bloodstream an
_____ called renin.

• Renin performs conversions in the liver of plasma proteins, forming angiotensin I.

• **Angiotensin I** is converted by angiotensin-converting enzyme (ACE) to angiotensin II.

- **Angiotensin II** vasoconstricts virtually all arterioles in the body; thus, systemic blood pressure _____ (*increases* or *decreases*)
- Aldosterone is secreted when angiotensin II contacts the adrenal gland. Aldosterone targets the kidneys to _____.
_____

- Blood volume and blood pressure increase while urine output decreases. The urine is deep yellow and more concentrated with _____.

Chronic hypertension (chronic high blood pressure) is treated with ACE inhibitors.

- What does this medication prevent from happening? _____
_____
_____

- How does it lower blood pressure? _____
_____
_____

In summary:

- What triggers renin release to start this chain of events? _____
_____

- What is the function of renin? _____

- What influence does angiotensin II have on blood pressure? _____

- What is the function of aldosterone? _____

- What is the role of ACE? _____

- What effect does aldosterone have on blood volume and blood pressure? _____
_____

> **TIP!** Keep the mechanism in order: renin → angiotensin I → angiotensin II (with the help of ACE) → aldosterone.

Atrial Natriuretic Peptide

ANP is released by the _____ atrium of the heart when blood pressure in that chamber *increases*. ANP decreases the kidney's ability to reabsorb water and solutes. As a result, more urine is made while blood volume and blood pressure decrease.

> **TIP!** What's an easy way to remember the function of this hormone? *Atrial* tells us where the hormone is made (right atrium of the heart). *Natriuretic* tells us two things: *natri-* means sodium while *-uretic* is related to urine production. This hormone is produced by the right atrium of the heart and releases sodium in the urine.

In summary:
- What triggers ANP release? _____
- Where is ANP produced? _____
- What is the function of ANP? _____
- What effect does ANP have on blood volume and blood pressure? _____

Sympathetic Stimulation

Nerve impulses from the sympathetic nervous system (part of the autonomic nervous system) cause
_____ of smooth muscles in the walls of afferent arterioles. These arterioles
vasoconstrict and reduce the volume of blood passing through the glomeruli. *Exercise* or *excitement* normally
causes sympathetic stimulation.

> **TIP!** Remember the "e" words such as exercise or excitement promote sympathetic stimulation.

- How is NFP affected during sympathetic stimulation? _____
- How is urine production affected during sympathetic stimulation? _____
_____

Urea and Uric Acid

LEARNING OBJECTIVE 9. Explain how urea and uric acid are formed and how they are excreted.

Urea and uric acid are nitrogen-containing wastes resulting from the metabolism of
_____ and _____ in cells.
- What happens if these items are allowed to accumulate in body tissues? _____
_____
_____

When amino acid metabolism occurs in the _____ from the proteins in
our diet, ammonia is released as a by-product. Ammonia is converted into **urea** and released into the
bloodstream. Although urea enters the renal tubule by filtration, 50% of it is reabsorbed by *diffusion* with
water and other solutes. The remaining 50% is excreted in the urine.
Uric acid is produced by the metabolism of certain _____. It is also filtered and
reabsorbed by *active transport,* but only a small portion is removed by secretion into the renal tubule.

Maintenance of Body Fluids

LEARNING OBJECTIVE 10. Identify the role of the kidneys in maintaining body fluid composition and pH.

Organs that maintain the balance of water and electrolytes include skin, liver, organs of the GI tract, and
kidneys. The kidneys have the *greatest* immediate effect on fluid balance. How? The kidneys process large
volumes of blood continually by glomerular filtration, tubular reabsorption, and tubular secretion.
The blood that has traveled through the kidneys is transported to _____, and
blood plasma is exchanged with interstitial fluids. Cells receive those interstitial fluids through exchanges.
Although the kidneys only deal with blood, they influence fluids in other body compartments.

Regulation of pH

Blood and body fluid pH is controlled by:
- Buffers
- _____ system
- Kidneys

The pH of body fluids should be between 7.35 and 7.45.

• _____ is a condition that arises when the pH declines below 7.35.

• _____ is a condition that arises when the pH rises above 7.45.

The kidneys help regulate the pH of body fluids by adjusting pH, primarily through tubular secretion.

To lower and restore blood pH when it is too high (alkalosis):

• Hydrogen ions are moved by active transport from the bloodstream to the renal filtrate when blood pH declines. Hydrogen ions are secreted into the renal tubule.

• Bicarbonate ions are reabsorbed and moved from the renal tubule to the _____.
  Recall that bicarbonate ions combine with hydrogen ions to form carbonic acid.

To raise and restore blood pH when it is too low (acidosis):

• _____ ion tubular secretion slows.

• _____ ion tubular reabsorption slows.

Review Time!

I. *Provide a brief answer for each of the following questions about the regulation of urine concentration and volume.*

1. What part of the nephron is targeted by ADH? _____

2. How does ADH help restore low blood volume and low blood pressure? _____
_____
_____

3. What effect does ADH have on urine volume? _____

4. What part of the brain releases ADH? _____

5. What part of the nephron is targeted by aldosterone? _____

6. What effect does aldosterone have on blood pressure and blood volume?
_____
_____

7. Explain how renin is involved in the restoration of low blood volume and low blood pressure.
_____
_____

8. Why is ACE critical to the formation of angiotensin II? _____
_____
_____

9. How does angiotensin II help maintain blood pressure? _____
_____
_____

10. How are ADH and aldosterone similar in their functions? How does each hormone perform its job?
_____
_____
_____
_____

11. Explain how ANP maintains blood pressure. _____
_____

12. How are ANP and aldosterone functionally opposite of one another? _____
_____
_____

13. Where is ANP made? What triggers its secretion? _____
_____
_____

14. What happens to urine volume during sympathetic stimulation? _____
_____

15. Why would a person with increased blood pressure take a medication called an ACE inhibitor?
_____
_____
_____

16. Explain how the kidneys regulate fluid balance among various compartments.
_____
_____
_____
_____

17. Explain how the kidneys regulate pH balance when acidosis is encountered.
_____
_____
_____

18. What hormone is involved in regulation of water and fluid balance on a daily basis?
_____

19. How do the kidneys regulate pH of bodily fluids? _____
_____

20. Why does a person with diseased kidneys have difficulty maintaining blood pH?
_____
_____
_____

21. Alcohol inhibits ADH production. Do you think drinking alcohol on a hot summer day is a wise way to replenish lost fluids? Explain. _____
_____
_____
_____

II. *Provide a brief answer for each of the following questions about urea and uric acid.*

1. What is the source of urea in the body? _____
_____

2. What is the source of uric acid in the body? _____
_____

CONCEPT 3

Ureters, Urinary Bladder, and Urethra

Concept: The ureters carry newly formed urine from the kidneys to the urinary bladder. The urinary bladder is an expandable saclike organ that stores urine until voiding. The urethra is a single tube that carries urine to the exterior during voiding, or micturition, which combines involuntary and voluntary activities.

LEARNING OBJECTIVE 11. Identify the structure and function of the ureters, urinary bladder, and urethra.

The pathway of urine from its production in the kidney to the exterior of the body is as follows:
- Nephrons
- Renal pelvis
- Calyces
- Ureters
- _____
- Urethra

Ureters

The ureters are paired, tubular organs.

Location: The ureters arise from the renal _____ of each kidney, extend inferiorly along the side of the vertebral column posterior to the peritoneum, and curve to unite with the urinary _____.

Structure: Three layers construct the wall of the ureter.
1. Inner layer is a mucous membrane; the mucus protects cells from exposure to _____.
2. Middle layer is a smooth muscle and elastic connective tissue that contracts with peristaltic waves to propel urine through the ureter.
3. Outer layer is a protective fibrous connective tissue.

Function: The ureters transport urine from the _____ to the _____.

Urinary Bladder

The urinary bladder is a hollow, muscular organ.

Location: The urinary bladder is located at the floor of the pelvic cavity posterior to the symphysis pubis. It is retroperitoneal. What does it mean to be *retroperitoneal*? _____
_____

Structure: The **fundus** of the urinary bladder is the round, dome-shaped portion and the **neck** is the region that narrows to unite with the urethra. The urinary bladder is typically full when 500 milliliters (1 pint) of urine has collected. The **trigone** is the triangular region outlined between the openings of the two _____ and the _____. The wall of the urethra has four layers:
1. The innermost layer is a mucous membrane. Stretchy transitional epithelium forms the epithelium of the mucous membrane. _____ protects the cells of the bladder from urine exposure.

2. The second layer is a connective tissue supporting the mucous membrane.

3. The third layer is a smooth muscle formed by the _____ and _____ layers of the **detrusor muscle**. This muscle helps with urination.

4. The outermost layer is a fibrous connective tissue except where _____ covers the superior surface of the bladder.

Function: The urinary bladder temporarily stores urine.

> **TIP!** Ever wonder why we just don't call it the "bladder?" We learned in the previous chapter about a different bladder called the gallbladder. A full bladder may not just mean urine!

Urethra

The urethra is a muscular tube.

Location: The urethra location and length differs between males and females.

- **Females:** Urethra is 3 to 4 centimeters (1.5 inches) long and bound to the anterior wall of the female's vagina by connective tissue. The external urethral orifice (urinary meatus or external opening) is situated between the vaginal opening and the clitoris.

- **Males:** Urethra is 20 centimeters (8 inches) long and extends from the urinary bladder to the end of the penis. It passes through the _____ gland (which may enlarge around the urethra later in life). The male urethra also transports reproductive fluids (semen).

Structure: Two sphincters are situated at the junction of the bladder and the urethra.

- **Internal urethral sphincter** prevents stored urine in the bladder from entering the urethra. It is an _____ sphincter.

- **External urethral sphincter** is voluntarily controlled since it is composed of _____ muscle.

Function: The urethra drains urine from the urinary bladder and transports it to the body's exterior.

Micturition

LEARNING OBJECTIVE 12. Describe the process of micturition.

Micturition is also known as _____ or _____.

This process combines involuntary and voluntary activities:

- Stretch receptors are activated when the urinary bladder has collected more than _____ (*how many?*) milliliters of urine. Stretch receptors send sensory nerve impulses to the spinal cord.

- Spinal cord sends motor impulses to the bladder along a _____ reflex arc.

- Detrusor muscle contracts and the internal sphincter relaxes.

- Urine is pushed through the internal sphincter into the urethra as contractions intensify and you feel the urge to void. You have the choice to voluntarily *stop* urine flow by closing the _____ muscle. Inhibition of urination occurs via a sympathetic pathway from the brain to the detrusor muscle.

- If you choose to urinate, what must happen to the external sphincter muscle and detrusor muscle?

_____

_____

Review Time!

I. *Using the terms in the list below, write the appropriate organ of the urinary system in each blank. You may use a term more than once.*

Ureter   *Urinary bladder*   *Urethra*

1. Temporarily stores urine   _____
2. Transports urine to the exterior of the body   _____
3. Longer in males than in females   _____
4. Detrusor muscle forms part of the wall   _____
5. Surrounded by the prostate gland in males   _____
6. Transports reproductive fluids in males   _____
7. Receives urine from the renal pelvis   _____
8. Holds 500 milliliters of urine when full   _____
9. Has a region known as the trigone   _____
10. Two muscular sphincters control urine flow   _____

II. *Place a number from 1 to 6 in the blank before each statement to indicate the correct order of the flow of urine from the kidney to the exterior.*

_____ Calyces   _____ Ureters
_____ Nephron   _____ Urethra
_____ Renal pelvis   _____ Urinary bladder

III. *Using the terms in the list below, label the parts of the urinary system.*

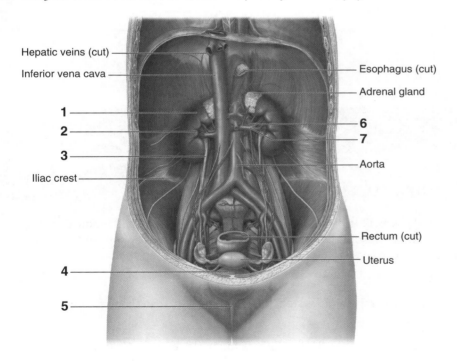

1. _____
2. _____
3. _____
4. _____
5. _____
6. _____
7. _____

Kidney   Ureter
Renal artery   Urethra
Renal hilum   Urinary bladder
Renal vein

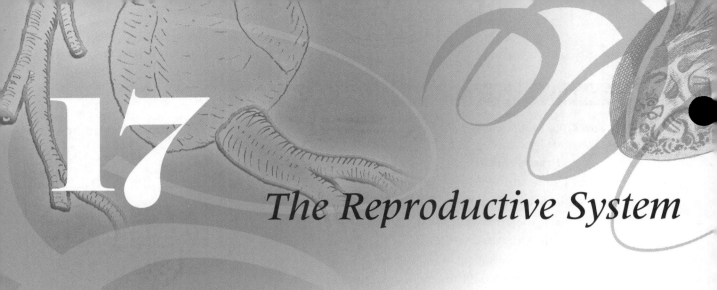

The Reproductive System

Tips for Success as You Begin

Read Chapter 17 from your textbook before attending class. Listen when you attend lecture and fill in the blanks in this notebook. You may choose to complete the blanks before attending class as a way to prepare for the day's topics. The same day you attend lecture, read the material again and complete the exercises after each section in this notebook. As you study these systems, consider the similarities and differences between the male and female reproductive tracts and the processes of gamete production.

Introduction to the Male and Female Reproductive Systems

What are gonads and what hormones do they secrete? _____
_____

What are gametes? _____
_____

CONCEPT 1

Organs of Male Reproduction

Concept: The male reproductive organs include the testes, which secrete testosterone and produce sperm; a series of ducts that transport the sperm to the outside; and several accessory organs that nourish and support the sperm along their journey. Sperm is conveyed into the female by an external organ, the penis.

LEARNING OBJECTIVE 1. Identify the organs of the male system based on their structural and functional features.

Gonads are called _____. They produce the male sex hormone called _____ and the male gametes called _____. Ducts transport, store, and support sperm while accessory glands secrete fluids to support sperm and provide a fluid medium in which they are transported.

Testes

A testis is one of the two paired organs (testes) found in the scrotum outside the abdominal cavity. The outside of the body an ideal location for the testes because _____
_____

Structure

Each testis is:

- About 4 centimeters (1.5 inches) long by 2.5 centimeters (1 inch) wide.
- Enclosed in fibrous connective tissue that subdivides it into about 250 compartments known as
  _____.

Seminiferous tubules (1 to 4) are in each lobule.

- **Interstitial cells** (cells of Leydig) are between the seminiferous tubules; they secrete
  _____.

- **Germinal epithelium** lines the walls of the seminiferous tubules. This epithelium is made of two types of cells:
  1. _____ *cells* that provide nourishment and support for the germ cells.
  2. _____ *cells* produce new sperm cells by *spermatogenesis*.
- **Rete testis** is a small set of tubes on the posterior edge of the testis. These tubes are formed from the
  _____. The rete testis gives rise to the efferent ductules.
- **Efferent ductules** are formed from the rete testis. The efferent ductules form a single tube known as
  the _____.

Spermatogenesis

LEARNING OBJECTIVE 2. Describe the process of spermatogenesis and its results.

Spermatogenesis is the production of sperm cells by the testes. It occurs in the
_____ tubules by meiosis.

> **TIP!** Remember that spermatogenesis is the process of sperm production. "Genesis" means beginning.

Do you recall how cell division occurs during mitosis and meiosis? Complete the missing information for this comparison chart.

	Mitosis	Meiosis
Purpose	Growth, tissue repair, and cell replacement	
In what types of cells does this process occur?	Most body cells	Only in the male and female gonads
Number of daughter cells produced	2	
Genetic information	Daughter cells are genetically identical to each other and to the parent cell	Daughter cells are genetically different from each other and the parent cell
Number of chromosomes	Full chromosome number (diploid)	One-half the chromosome number as the parent cell (haploid)

Spermatogenesis relies on the descent of the testes into the scrotum soon before or at birth. During adolescence (age 12 to 14), spermatogenesis in the testes begins. The steps of spermatogenesis follow and are also illustrated below:

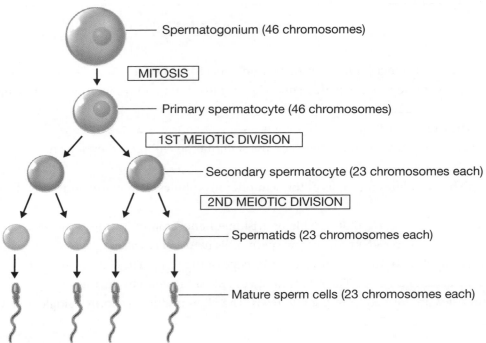

- **Spermatogonia** are stem cells that divide by *mitosis.* Two cells are produced. One cell remains as a spermatogonium. Why? _____
The other cell, a **primary spermatocyte**, will continue through the process of meiosis.
- **Primary spermatocyte** divides by meiosis to produce two secondary spermatocytes.
- **Secondary spermatocyte** continues the meiotic division to produce two spermatids.
- **Spermatids** contain _____ (*how many*) chromosomes. Spermatids mature into sperm while still part of the germinal epithelium. Where is the germinal epithelium located?

_____

- **Sperm cell (spermatozoan)** has a head, a midpiece, and a _____. Sperm break away from the germinal epithelium and continue development as they travel toward the epididymis.

> **TIP!** To keep the process straight, remember that spermatogonia give rise to primary (fist) spermatocytes, and then secondary (second) spermatocytes form.

Spermatogenesis continues throughout the lifetime of a male, and millions of sperm will be produced each day. If sperm cell production is insufficient to fertilize an egg, *male infertility* or *sterility* may be encountered. These conditions may be caused by _____

_____.

Review Time!

I. *Provide a brief answer for each of the following questions about the male reproductive system.*

1. What gametes are produced by the male gonads? _____

_____

2. What is the benefit of the location of the testes for sperm production? _____

_____

_____

3. What cells produce testosterone in the testes? _____

4. What role do the seminiferous tubules play in the male reproductive system?

_____

_____

5. What route do sperm travel from the seminiferous tubules to the epididymis?

_____

_____

_____

6. Compare the processes of mitosis and meiosis:

   a. How many daughter cells are made by mitosis? _____

   b. How many daughter cells are made by meiosis? _____

   c. What is the purpose of mitosis? _____

   _____

   d. What is the purpose of meiosis? _____

   _____

   e. Are the daughter cells produced by mitosis genetically *identical* or genetically *different*?

   _____

   f. Are the daughter cells produced by meiosis genetically *identical* or genetically *different*?

   _____

   _____

7. Around what age do male testes begin the process of spermatogenesis?

_____

8. Why does one of the cells resulting from the spermatogonium return to the stem cell line?

_____

_____

9. What changes occur to transform a spermatid into a sperm? _____

_____

10. How many chromosomes are found in a sperm? _____

Male Ducts

LEARNING OBJECTIVE 3. Describe the tubes that carry fluids through the male system.

Sperm travel from the testes to ducts that store, support, and transport it to the urethra. These ducts include:

* _____
* _____
* _____

Epididymis

The epididymis is a comma-shaped organ located on the posterior of each _____.

Structure: Single, threadlike tube that stretches 6 meters (20 feet) from the efferent ductules to the

_____.

Function: Maturation of sperm so that they can independently move their _____ and fertilize the egg.

Ductus Deferens (Vas Deferens)

Structure: Each ductus deferens travels from each _____.

* From the epididymis, the ductus deferens travels through the _____ an opening in the abdominal wall to the lateral wall of the pelvic cavity.
* The ductus deferens crosses the lateral wall of the pelvic cavity, and loops over the back of the urinary bladder to the ejaculatory duct.
* The ejaculatory duct carries sperm through the prostate gland and into the _____.

Function: Carries sperm from the epididymis to the urethra.

Spermatic cord consists of the:

* Ductus deferens
* _____ artery and veins
* Lymph vessels
* Testicular nerve
* **Cremaster muscle** is bands of skeletal muscle that form the outer layer of the spermatic cord. It elevates the testes when the external temperature is cold to limit the temperature range of developing

  _____.
* Connective tissue

Which part of the spermatic cord is cut when sterilization is performed (called a vasectomy)?

_____

Does a vasectomy interfere with a male's ability to produce sperm or testosterone?

_____

_____

Urethra

The urethra travels from the urinary bladder some 20 centimeters (8 inches) to the distal end of the penis.

Structure: Mucous membrane with mucous glands lines a thick layer of smooth muscle. The **external urethral orifice (urinary _____)** is the opening of the urethra at its distal end.

Function: Transports urine during _micturition_ and male reproductive fluids during _ejaculation_. Control mechanisms prevent the passage of both fluids at the same time.

Review Time!

I. *Provide a brief answer for each of the following questions about male ducts.*

1. List the structures for the pathway of sperm through the ducts from their production until they leave the body via the urethra. _____
_____
_____

2. What tube empties into the ductus deferens? _____

3. Which tube carries both urine and male reproductive fluids? _____

4. Which tube is housed as part of the spermatic cord? _____

5. Which tube connects the ductus deferens to the urethra? _____

6. Name the opening of the urethra. _____

7. How does the scrotum respond to cold temperatures? _____
_____
_____

8. Can urine and male reproductive fluids travel in the urethra simultaneously?
_____
_____

9. When sperm exit the epididymis, are they fully functional? _____
_____

10. Where are sperm transported if they are in the efferent ductules? _____
_____

Male Accessory Glands

LEARNING OBJECTIVE 4. Identify the male accessory glands and describe their secretions.

The male accessory glands include the:

- Seminal vesicles
- _____ gland
- _____ glands

Function: Provide a liquid, nutritious medium for the support of sperm cells. **Semen** is a mixture of sperm cells and seminal fluids. Volume released is between 2 and 7 milliliters and _____ million sperm.

> **TIP!** Use the clues built into the names of these accessory glands. Seminal vesicles produce fluids that contribute to semen (seminal). Bulbourethral tells you exactly where this gland is located: it is a small bulb that connects directly to the urethra.

Seminal Vesicles

The **seminal vesicles** are glands located at the base of the bladder.

Structure: Each gland houses saclike structures. The secretions join the ductus deferens. The union of the seminal vesicles and the ductus deferens forms the _____ duct.

- Into what duct does the ejaculatory duct empty semen? _____

Function: Sugar-rich (fructose) secretions nourish and activate sperm.

Prostate Gland

The **prostate gland** is located at the lower part of the urinary bladder around the urethra. It may enlarge and constrict the urethra in men over 50 years of age, a condition known as *benign prostatic hyperplasia (BPH).*

- How does BPH affect urination? _____

_____

Structure: Walnut-sized and shaped gland. Its secretions eventually reach the urethra.

Function: Secretion is an alkaline, thick, milky fluid that aids sperm motility during fertilization.

Bulbourethral Glands

The bulbourethral glands (Cowper glands) are located inferior to the prostate gland.

Structure: Pea-sized glands.

Function: Thick, clear mucus drains into the _____ from this gland. The mucus is thought to be a lubricant for sexual intercourse.

External Structures

LEARNING OBJECTIVE 5. Describe the external male structures.

The external structures are external genitalia. In males, they are the _____ and

_____ .

Scrotum

The **scrotum** hangs below the abdominal wall.

Structure: Saclike pouch of skin that is divided into left and right chambers by a septum (wall). The chambers are lined with serous membrane to reduce the friction between the testis and the wall. The **dartos muscle** is an involuntary muscle that lines the inner wall of the scrotum.

Function: Each chamber houses a _____ . The dartos muscle assists the cremaster muscle in pulling the testes closer to the abdominal wall for warmth.

Penis

The **penis** is an external cylindrical organ.

Structure: The penis contains the distal portion of the urethra. It is covered with a layer of skin; internally there are _____ (*how many*) columns of spongy erectile tissue. During erection, the spongy tissue fills with blood and the penis enlarges and becomes firm.

- **Corpora cavernosa** are two of the three columns. They form the dorsal and lateral columns of the penis.
- **Corpora spongiosum** is the third column. It forms the ventral portion of the penis and the **glans penis**, a cap over the penis. The skin of the glans penis is thin, hairless, and supplied with sensory receptors. Foreskin or _____ covers the glans penis at birth and is often removed by *circumcision* soon after birth.
- *Through which column does the urethra travel?* _____
- *What is the benefit of circumcision?* _____

_____

Function: When erect, the penis can be inserted into the female vagina during sexual intercourse.

Review Time!

I. *Using the terms in the list below, label the sagittal view of the male reproductive organs.*

1. _____
2. _____
3. _____
4. _____
5. _____
6. _____
7. _____
8. _____
9. _____
10. _____
11. _____

Bulbourethral gland   Penis   Testes in scrotum

Ductus deferens   Prostate gland   Urethra

Ejaculatory duct   Rectum   Urinary bladder

Epididymis   Seminal vesicle

II. *Provide a brief answer for each of the following questions about male accessory glands and external structures.*

1. Where is the dartos muscle located? What is its function? _____
_____
_____

2. What secretion is released by the bulbourethral gland? _____
_____

3. What secretions do the seminal vesicles contribute to semen? _____
_____

4. Why is it beneficial that prostate gland secretions are alkaline? _____
_____
_____

5. Where is the prostate gland located? Why might this gland cause urination problems later in life?
_____
_____
_____

6. Which gland(s) secrete fluid into the ejaculatory duct? _____

7. What are the two tubes that form the ejaculatory duct? _____
_____

8. What are the two male external structures (genitalia)? _____
_____

9. What happens to the columns of spongy tissue of the penis during erection?
_____
_____
_____

10. What part of the penis is removed during circumcision? _____
_____

III. *Using the terms in the list below, write the appropriate structure or organ of the male reproductive system in each blank. You may use a term more than once*

Bulbourethral gland   *Ductus deferens*   *Epididymis*   *Penis*

Prostate gland   *Scrotum*   *Seminal vesicles*   *Testes*

Urethra

1. Site of spermatogenesis   _____
2. Gland that secretes mucus as a lubricant for sexual intercourse   _____
3. Duct that transports both urine and semen   _____
4. Gland that contributes sugary secretions to semen   _____
5. Saclike pouch of skin that houses testes outside the body   _____
6. Duct connecting the epididymis to the urethra   _____
7. Gland that secretes a thick, milky fluid   _____
8. Duct that passes through the inguinal canal   _____
9. Produces testosterone   _____
10. Covered by a loose fold of skin called foreskin or prepuce   _____
11. Inner wall is lined with the dartos muscle   _____
12. Gland that secretes thick mucus into the urethra   _____
13. Duct housed within the spermatic cord   _____
14. Gland that encircles the urethra   _____
15. Gland that produces testosterone   _____

CONCEPT 2

Physiology of Male Reproduction

Concept: The functions of the male system include the generation and release of sperm, which are accomplished by neural and hormonal mechanisms.

LEARNING OBJECTIVE   6. Describe the processes of erection, emission, and ejaculation.

Male reproductive physiology is influenced by two mechanisms:

1. _____ *(nervous system) mechanisms* are involved in erection, orgasm, and ejaculation.
2. _____ *mechanisms* play a role in development of reproductive structures, regulation of reproductive functions, development of secondary sex characteristics, and sexual behavior.

Neural Mechanisms

Erection is the first step in sexual arousal. It occurs when autonomic impulses originate either from the hypothalamus or from a reflex in response to sensory stimuli.

1. _____ impulses cause arteries supplying the penis to dilate (enlarge).
2. Blood flows into the erectile tissue spaces of the penis.
3. As erectile tissue swells with blood, veins are compressed from transporting blood out of the penis.
4. Since more blood enters than leaves the penis, it swells and becomes erect.

Emission occurs when _____.

1. Sympathetic impulses travel to the walls of the ducts.
2. Peristaltic contractions of the testicular ducts, the epididymides, the ductus deferentes, and the ejaculatory ducts provide propulsion for the sperm to pass through quickly.

Ejaculation occurs as semen is forced through the _____ due to rhythmic contractions of skeletal muscles situated at the base of the penis. Ejaculation releases:

- _____ gland secretions
- Seminal vesicle secretions
- _____ gland secretions
- Sperm
- Small amount of testicular fluid

After ejaculation, _____ impulses cause constriction of arteries supplying the penis; so more blood exits than enters. The penis returns to its flaccid state.

Male orgasm (male climax) is the combination of sensory impulses, erection, emission, and ejaculation that results in a pleasurable experience.

Hormonal Mechanisms

LEARNING OBJECTIVE   7. Describe the hormonal effects on male reproduction.

Hormones that influence male reproduction arise from:
- Hypothalamus
- Anterior pituitary gland
- _____

Hypothalamic and Pituitary Influences

In adolescence, as a child nears puberty:

1. **Gonadotropin-releasing hormone (GnRH)** is secreted by the _____ to target the anterior pituitary gland.
2. **Luteinizing hormone (LH)** and **follicle-stimulating hormone (FSH)** are secreted by the anterior pituitary gland. These two hormones are *gonadotropins,* meaning they stimulate the gonads (testes).
   - **LH** (also known as interstitial cell-stimulating hormone, or ICSH) promotes the development of interstitial cells in the testes. At maturation, these cells secrete _____.
   - **FSH** prepares the _____ walls to respond to testosterone. Once responsive, cells stimulate spermatogenesis in the presence of FSH and testosterone.

> **TIP!** Releasing hormones are always produced by the hypothalamus, such as GnRH. Since LH is also known as ICSH, remember that ICSH stimulates the interstitial cells to secrete testosterone.

Testosterone

Androgens are _____

Testosterone is the most abundant and functionally important androgen. What part of the testes secretes testosterone? _____

- At what age does puberty onset for a male? _____
- What changes, known as *secondary sex characteristics,* are seen in a young male who undergoes puberty due to the influence of testosterone? _____

_____

_____

_____

- Explain how the hypothalamus controls the rate of secretion of testosterone by the testes.

_____

_____

_____

_____

Review Time!

I.   *Provide a brief answer for each of the following questions about neural and hormonal mechanisms of control over the male reproductive system.*

1. What is the difference between erection and ejaculation? _____

_____

_____

2. Which branch of the autonomic nervous system is responsible for erection?

_____

_____

3. Which branch of the autonomic nervous system is responsible for emission?

_____

_____

4. What events are parts of male orgasm (male climax)? _____

_____

_____

_____

5. Describe the role played by the sympathetic nervous system in returning the penis to its original, flaccid state after male orgasm. _____

_____

_____

_____

6. Which hormone stimulates the anterior pituitary gland to release LH? Where is this hormone made? _____

_____

_____

7. What two gonadotropins are released by the anterior pituitary in response to GnRH?

_____

_____

_____

8. Which gonadotropin stimulates interstitial cells to release testosterone? _____

_____

9. How does the hypothalamus respond to low levels of testosterone in the blood?

_____

_____

_____

_____

10. What effect does a high level of testosterone have on the development of secondary sex characteristics during puberty? _____

_____

_____

_____

CONCEPT 3

Organs of Female Reproduction

Concept: The female reproductive organs produce and transport the eggs, promote the success of fertilization by receiving the penis, and support the offspring during prenatal development.

LEARNING OBJECTIVE 8. Identify the organs of the female reproductive system based on their structural and functional differences.

Female gonads are called _____. They produce female sex hormones and female gametes.

Ovaries

Female gonads or **ovaries** are paired organs located against the lateral walls of the pelvic cavity. They are supported by ligaments attached to the pelvic wall and the uterus.

Structure

From superficial to deep, each ovary is covered by:

- _____ (single layer)
- _____ (single layer of epithelial cells)
- _____ (protective shell around the ovary)

Two interior regions of the ovary:

- **Cortex** (outer region) consists of dense connective tissue and **ovarian follicles** each of which contains a single _____ (ovum or egg cell), the female gamete.
- **Medulla** (inner region) consists of loosely arranged connective tissue that receives blood vessels, lymph vessels, and nerves. The medulla is continuous with the **ovarian ligament**. What does this ligament attach the ovary to? _____

Oogenesis

LEARNING OBJECTIVE   9. Describe the process of oogenesis, follicle development, and ovulation.

As you study the process of oogenesis, consider how it varies from the production of male gametes during spermatogenesis. **Oogenesis** is the process of oocyte formation by the female ovaries. It begins at puberty and continues on a monthly menstrual cycle until around age 50.

1. **Primary oocytes** are present in the ovary at _____. A **primordial follicle** constructed of a single layer of cells surrounds each primary oocyte. Oogenesis pauses until _____ when hormonal changes stimulates some (about 20) primary oocytes to begin dividing by meiosis each month. Only one primary oocyte completes division and becomes two cells.

2. **Secondary oocyte** and a **first polar body:** The small first polar body completes the second division of meiosis and produces two more very small cells that die and are reabsorbed. The secondary oocyte does not yet divide; it is ready to be fertilized by a sperm cell.
   - If fertilized, the secondary oocyte undergoes the _____ division to produce a **second polar body** and a **zygote**.
   - The zygote is the fertilized egg which develops into an _____. The second polar body degenerates.

Follicle Development

At puberty, the rise of FSH promotes changes occur in the stalled primordial follicles, as described next and shown in the illustration.

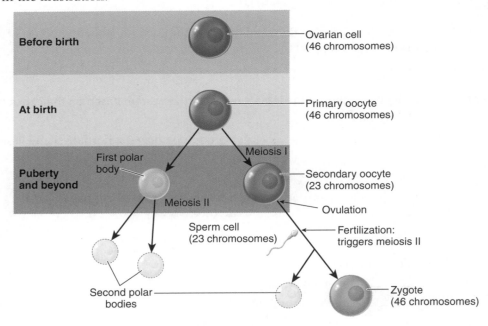

- **Primordial follicle** surrounds the primary oocyte as they sit stalled during childhood.
- **Primary follicle** develops once the flattened cells of the primordial follicle enlarge starting at puberty. The primary follicle surrounds the primary _____, which is now preparing for its first meiotic division to form a secondary follicle.
- **Secondary follicle** enlarges and secretes estrogen, the primary female sex hormone. The follicles have progressed through rapid mitotic division and became multiple layers around the oocyte. An **antrum** (cavity) appears between the oocyte and the follicle cells and is filled with clear fluid. The presence of the antrum is the indicator that the follicle is now a _____ follicle. Follicle cells secrete the substance that forms the **zona pellucida.** What is the zona pellucida? _____.
- **Graafian follicle** is a mature follicle that bulges from the surface of the ovary like a blister. The Graafian follicle will be ovulated with the secondary oocyte.

Ovulation

Ovulation occurs about _____ (*how many?*) days after development when the Graafian follicle is expelled from the surface of the ovary. The follicle ruptures and the secondary oocyte is released into the peritoneal cavity. Some protective follicle cells remain around the secondary oocyte, called the **corona radiata**. A current sweeps the secondary oocyte to the uterine tube where _____ may occur.

- **If no fertilization occurs**, the oocyte degenerates in 5 days. The **corpus luteum** is the remnant of the follicle cells that stay in the ovary and are transformed into a yellow glandular mass. The corpus luteum secretes two hormones: _____ and _____. Without fertilization, the corpus luteum lasts 10 to 12 days, and then degenerates.
- **If fertilization does occur**, pregnancy occurs, and the corpus luteum enlarges. The hormonal secretions of the corpus luteum maintain the pregnancy for the initial 3 months until the _____ takes over hormone production.

Female Accessory Organs

Uterine Tubes

The **uterine tubes** (**fallopian tubes**, oviducts) extend between the ovary and the uterus.

Structure: The uterine tubes are 10 centimeters (4 inches) long and 1 centimeter in diameter. Important parts of the tube are:

- **Fimbriae** are fringed, fingerlike projections that nearly touch the surface of the _____. Their cilia collect and sweep the oocyte during ovulation into the tube.
- **Infundibulum** is the typical site of fertilization. Cilia transport the embryo to the uterus.

Function: _____.

_____

Uterus

The uterus is located near the pelvic cavity floor between the urinary bladder and rectum.

Structure: This pear-shaped organ is suspended by ligaments that tilt it downward into the vagina. It has two main regions:

1. **Body** is the upper, dome-shaped region that receives the uterine tubes. The space within the body is known as the _____.
2. **Cervix** is the lower, narrow region. The space within the cervix is known as the **cervical canal**. The cervical canal opens into the vagina by way of the **external os.**

The three walls of the uterus are:

1. **Perimetrium** is the outermost layer which consists of a thin layer of _____ (serous membrane).

2. **Myometrium** is composed of smooth muscle and elastic connective tissue.

3. **Endometrium** is the vascular, innermost lining. What tissue composes the endometrium? _____ What glands are embedded in this layer?_____.
   What happens to the endometrium during menstruation each month?
   _____

> **TIP!** Use the prefixes to help you remember each layer of the wall of the uterus. Peri- means around, myo- means muscle but you can also remember the "m" for middle layer, and endo- indicates the inner layer.

Function: The uterus provides support for the developing embryo and fetus. Its smooth muscle contracts to push the fetus out during birth.

Vagina

The vagina is a thin-walled tube that extends from the cervix of the _____ to the outside.

Structure: The walls of the vagina form pockets around the cervix at the **fornix** while it opens to the outside at the **vagina orifice**. The **hymen** is a thin, vascular, mucosa barrier that may extend across the vaginal orifice.

The walls of the vagina are:

- Outer layer of elastic _____ that allows for expansion during intercourse or childbirth.
- Inner mucous membrane consists of stratified epithelium for protection. This mucous membrane lacks _____, so the vagina relies on secretions such as those from the external **vestibular glands** for lubrication.

Function: The main functions of the vagina are:

- Receive the _____ during sexual intercourse
- Serve as the birth canal during _____
- Serve as a passageway during menstruation

External Structures

Structures external to the vagina are the female external genitalia, including the structures of the **vulva**:

- **Mons pubis** is a rounded area over the symphysis pubis that is covered with pubic hair after puberty.
- **Labia majora** are two narrow folds of skin that are hair-covered after puberty. They extend from the mons pubis and are the female equivalent, or *homologue*, to the _____.
- **Labia minora** are two thin, hair-free folds of skin that are covered with mucous membrane rich with oil glands.
- **Vestibule** is a region formed by the outer margins of the labia _____. The vestibule houses, from upper (anterior) to lower (posterior):
  - **Clitoris** is the female homologue to the _____. It is composed of erectile tissue and the **glans** is supplied with sensory nerve endings. But, unlike the penis, there is no corpus spongiosum in the clitoris and the urethra does not pass through the clitoris as it does in the penis. A hood of tissue called the **prepuce** covers part of the clitoris. The prepuce is formed by the union of labia _____.
  - External urethral orifice
  - Vagina orifice

• **Perineum** is the region between the vestibule (upper border) and the anus. The perineum may tear between the vaginal orifice and the anus during childbirth, or an _____ may be performed surgically to widen the birth canal.

> **TIP!** Notice the hints built into the terminology when studying the female external genitalia. "Mons" means mound. The labia majora are the major hair-covered, thick folds of skin and the minora are the smaller hair-free, thin folds of skin.

Mammary Glands

Mammary glands are organs that produce milk for infant nourishment. They are located in the _____ (or *mammae*).

Structure: The breasts of both males and females contain an **areola**, an external, heavily pigmented region that contains a centrally elevated **nipple**. What two hormones promote breast enlargement by fat accumulation and glandular development? _____

Mammary gland structure:

• **Lobes** (15 to 20) are found in each adult female mammary gland. They radiate around the nipple.

• _____ are small chambers within each lobe. They house alveolar glands.

• **Alveolar glands** produce milk during lactation (process of milk production). The milk travels through ducts that open to the outside at the nipple.

Review Time!

I.   *Using the terms in the list below, label the sagittal view of the female reproductive organs.*

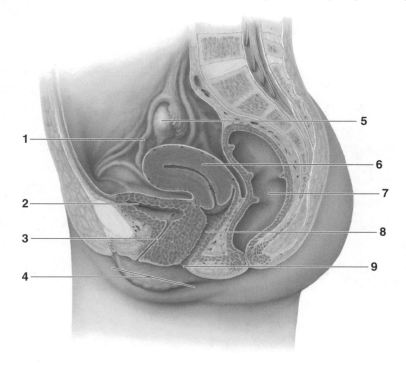

1. _____
2. _____
3. _____
4. _____
5. _____
6. _____
7. _____
8. _____
9. _____

Ovary	Urinary bladder	Vagina
Rectum	Uterine tube	Vaginal orifice
Urethra	Uterus	Vulva

II. *Using the terms in the list below, label the anterior view of the female reproductive organs.*

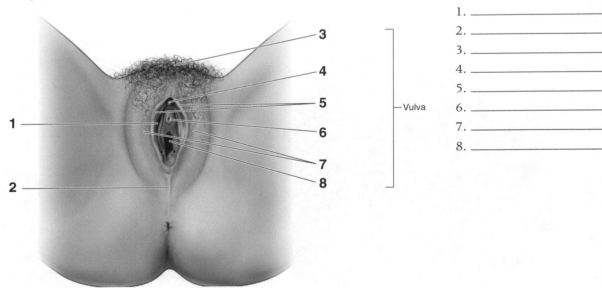

1. _____
2. _____
3. _____
4. _____
5. _____
6. _____
7. _____
8. _____
9. _____
10. _____
11. _____
12. _____
13. _____
14. _____

Body of uterus
Cervical canal
Cervix
Fimbriae
Fornix

Infundibulum
Layers of the wall of the uterus
    (including endometrium,
    myometrium, and perimetrium)
Ovarian ligament

Ovary
Uterine cavity
Uterine tube
Vagina

III. *Using the terms in the list below, label the female external structures.*

1. _____
2. _____
3. _____
4. _____
5. _____
6. _____
7. _____
8. _____

External urethral orifice
Glans of clitoris
Labia majora

Labia minora
Mons pubis
Perineum

Vaginal orifice
Vestibule

IV. *Using the terms in the list below, write the appropriate structure or organ of the female reproductive system in each blank. You may use a term more than once.*

Clitoris	*Endometrium*	*Mammary glands*	*Myometrium*	*Ovary*
Perimetrium	*Uterine tube*	*Uterus*	*Vulva*	*Vagina*

1. Region between the upper border of the vestibule and the anus _____

2. Organs that produce milk _____

3. Tube lined with ciliated mucous membrane _____

4. Homologue to the male penis _____

5. Outermost layer of the uterine wall _____

6. Birth canal _____

7. Body and cervix are the two main regions _____

8. Superficial layer of the uterine wall sloughed off during menstruation _____

9. Releases a secondary oocyte once every 28 days _____

10. Female gonads _____

11. Infundibulum and fimbriae are parts of this organ _____

12. Hymen covers the opening of this tube _____

13. Organ where an embryo and fetus develop _____

14. Produces female gametes _____

15. Smooth muscle layer of the uterine wall _____

V. *Provide a brief answer for each of the following questions about the female reproductive system.*

1. What cell is released from the ovary during ovulation? _____

_____

2. What critical role does the corpus luteum play if pregnancy occurs? _____

_____

_____

3. Where does fertilization usually occur within the female reproductive system?

_____

_____

4. How is oogenesis similar to spermatogenesis? _____

_____

_____

5. How are oogenesis and spermatogenesis different? _____

_____

_____

_____

_____

6. What makes the corona radiate similar to the Graafian follicle? _____

_____

_____

7. How does the uterine tube collect the ovulated oocyte from the ovary?

_____

_____

_____

8. Where is the cervix situated? _____
_____

9. What is the female homologue to the penis? _____

10. What is the female homologue to the scrotum? _____

11. Which layer of the uterus wall is sloughed off during menstruation? _____
_____

12. How is the clitoris structurally similar to the penis? How is it structurally different?
_____
_____
_____
_____

13. Since the vagina lacks glands, how is it lubricated? _____
_____
_____

14. What structures are enclosed by the vestibule? _____
_____
_____
_____

15. What do the alveolar glands produce? _____
_____

CONCEPT 4

Physiology of Female Reproduction

Concept: The female system produces oocytes on a regular, monthly cycle for the purpose of fertilization. This cyclic process is regulated by hormones, while neural mechanisms govern the sexual response.

1. *Neural (nervous system) mechanisms* govern physiologic responses to sexual stimulation.
2. _____ *mechanisms* control reproductive organ development, ovulation, menstruation, and maintain pregnancy.

Neural Mechanisms

LEARNING OBJECTIVE   10. Describe the neural mechanisms that influence female reproduction.

Female orgasm involves the stimulation of sensory nerves of the vulva and the vagina.

1. The sensory nerves send impulses to the _____.
2. Parasympathetic reflex dilates vessels in erectile tissues of the vulva.
   - The clitoris enlarges as its erectile tissues fill with blood when stimulated.
   - The vaginal walls swell with blood as it prepares for entry of the penis.
   - Mucus secretion increases from vestibular glands for lubrication.
3. Blood flow increases to the breasts and face.

4. As female orgasm begins, rhythmic, peristaltic contractions of the muscles associated with the perineum, walls of the vagina, walls of the uterus, and uterine tubes occur.

   • What is the purpose of these contractions? _____

   _____

   _____

Hormonal Mechanisms

11. **Identify the roles of hormones in female sexual development.**

Hormones that stimulate organ development and regulate the cycles that influence female reproduction arise from:

1. Hypothalamus

2. _____ (*anterior* or *posterior?*) pituitary gland

3. Ovaries

Development of Reproductive Cycles and Puberty

In adolescence, as a child nears puberty:

1. **Gonadotropin-releasing hormone (GnRH)** is secreted by the _____ to target the anterior pituitary gland.

2. **LH** and **FSH** are secreted by the anterior pituitary gland. These two hormones are _____, meaning they stimulate the gonads (ovaries).

   • **FSH** acts upon the primary follicles of the ovary and promotes their maturation. Follicle cells produce increasing levels of estrogen and progesterone.

   • **LH** promotes further secretion of estrogen and progesterone from the follicle cells.

   TIP! Remember the name connection: FSH stimulates the follicles of the ovaries to mature.

Menarche begins at some point between the ages 10 and 15 when increased estrogen and progesterone levels initiate the first episode of menstrual bleeding.

• List four body changes associated with puberty and presence of estrogen in a female:

   1. _____

   _____

   2. _____

   _____

   3. _____

   _____

   4. _____

   _____

Progesterone is another major female reproductive hormone secreted by the degenerating mature follicle cells of the corpus luteum. What are the effects of progesterone on a female?

   1. _____

   _____

   2. During pregnancy: _____

   _____

Menstrual Cycle

LEARNING OBJECTIVE 12. Explain the hormonal events that maintain the ovarian and menstrual cycles.

The **menstrual** (uterine) **cycle** is on average a 28-day cycle that begins at puberty and continues until around age 50. The endometrium is the uterine layer affected in response to changing levels of ovarian hormones.

Menses is menstrual bleeding caused by sloughing off of part of the _____. The phases of the cycle and their main events are:

1. **Menstruation** marks day 1 of the menstrual cycle. Increased _____ promotes the regeneration of the endometrium within the few days after onset of menstruation.

2. **Proliferative phase** is characterized by rapid growth of the endometrium in response to increasing estrogen levels. Why do estrogen levels increase?
   - GnRH levels stimulate more FSH and LH from the pituitary gland.
   - FSH and LH stimulate the development of _____ in the ovary.
   - Estrogen levels increase in response. Estrogen causes growth of the _____.
   - Positive feedback increases GnRH levels.
   - FSH and LH levels surge on day _____; the rise in LH stimulates ovulation.

3. **Secretory phase** is the time period after ovulation.
   - Follicle cells are converted to a corpus luteum in the ovary which secretes two hormones: _____ and _____.
   - Progesterone decreases LH and FSH levels.
   - Progesterone promotes further development of the endometrium by stimulating cell growth and the secretion of nourishing fluid.
   - Around day 21 or 22 (7 to 8 days after ovulation), the endometrium is ready to receive the early embryo.
   - **If fertilization does not occur**, the _____ degenerates (day 24 of the cycle). Progesterone and estrogen levels decline and the arterioles of the endometrium constrict. The endometrium separates from the outer layer of the endometrium and flows out of the uterus.

4. **Menstruation** occurs again by around day 28. A new cycle starts again.

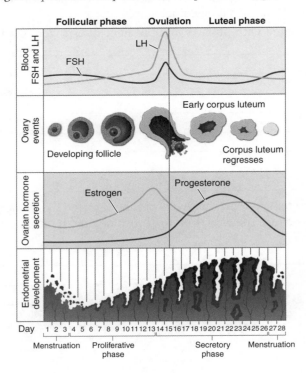

Menopause

At approximately what age does a female experience menopause? _____

What is *premenopause* or *female climacteric*? _____

_____

_____

What happens in the ovary to promote menopause?

• Follicles are less sensitive to _____ and _____; fewer follicles are
  stimulated to mature and secrete estrogen. Fewer corpora lutea are produced to secrete progesterone.

• Estrogen and progesterone levels decrease, leading to a decrease in the size of the uterus, reduction in
  vestibular gland secretions, thinning of all epithelial tissues.

• "Hot flashes" are temperature fluctuations that often accompany these changes.

Review Time!

I.   *Provide a brief answer for each of the following questions about the physiology of female reproduction.*

1. Describe the secondary sex changes that occur at puberty when estrogen is present.

   _____

   _____

   _____

   _____

2. What significant event happens at menarche? Around what age does menarche occur?

   _____

   _____

   _____

   _____

3. What significant event happens at menopause? Around what age is a female premenopausal?
   Around what age does a female experience menopause? _____

   _____

   _____

   _____

4. What type of feedback mechanism promotes ovulation? _____

5. What hormone is responsible for the release of FSH and LH from the anterior pituitary gland?

   _____

   _____

6. During the secretory phase, what does progesterone promote? _____

   _____

7. What role does the corpus luteum play during the secretory phase of the menstrual cycle to
   prepare the uterus for a fertilized egg? _____

   _____

   _____

8. What happens to the corpus luteum if the ovulated oocyte is not fertilized?

_____

_____

_____

9. What hormone is secreted by the corpus luteum to maintain pregnancy?

_____

_____

10. Explain the role of the parasympathetic nervous system in female orgasm.

_____

_____

_____

18

Human Development and Inheritance

Tips for Success as You Begin

Congratulations! You are close to completing your survey of the human body. Read Chapter 18 from your textbook before attending class. Listen when you attend lecture and fill in the blanks in this notebook. You may choose to complete the blanks before attending class as a way to prepare for the day's topics. The same day you attend lecture, read the material again and complete the exercises after each section in this notebook. To make learning easier for the section on genetic inheritance, try completing the genetics problems after each section. You may want to review material from Chapter 12 so you have a grasp on the fetal shunts and blood flow pattern.

Introduction to Human Development and Inheritance

In this chapter, you'll cover human development—the continuous process of body change, and explore the basic concepts of genetic inheritance.

There are two periods of human development:

1. **Prenatal development** refers to the changes that occur prior to birth called *embryology*.
2. **Postnatal development** refers to the changes that occur after birth, such as body growth, puberty, and old age.

CONCEPT 1

Prenatal Development

Concept: Prenatal development involves the differentiation of early embryonic cells that lead to tissue and organ development. Once these structures have arisen, they undergo rapid growth until birth.

The prenatal period begins at _____ and continues to
_____. Two periods exist.

1. _____ *period* lasts 8 weeks.
2. _____ *period* continues beyond the embryonic period to about 38 weeks or birth.

Fertilization

LEARNING OBJECTIVE 1. Describe the process of fertilization and the changes it induces.

Fertilization is the union of an egg cell (oocyte or ovum) and sperm cell. The journey of sperm to encountering the egg begins with the release of sperm into the vagina, then progresses through the uterus, and into the uterine tubes.

To consider the window of time during which fertilization can occur, we must look at how long these cells can survive.

- The oocyte is capable of being fertilized up to _____ hours after ovulation.
- Most sperm degenerate 24 hours after ejaculation, although some may survive for several days in the female's reproductive tract.
- For fertilization to occur, sexual intercourse must occur between _____ days before and _____ day after ovulation.

During fertilization:
- Sperm cell penetrates the follicle cells of the **corona radiata** and through the _____ before reaching the cell membrane of the oocyte.
- The head of the sperm releases an enzyme (_____) that aids in penetration of the oocyte's cell membrane. Biochemical changes of the zona pellucida prevent further sperm cells from attaching once a sperm's head has penetrated the membrane.
- Oocyte completes the second _____ division once the sperm cell has entered the oocyte.
- The haploid nucleus of the oocyte joins with the haploid nucleus of the sperm cell.
- The diploid **zygote**, a fertilized cell, results.

What is the difference between haploid and diploid? Recall that chromosomes are DNA. DNA is housed in the nucleus of a cell.

- **Haploid** means that each nucleus contains *half* the chromosome complement (23 chromosomes).
- **Diploid** means that each nucleus contains the full complement of chromosomes (_____ chromosomes or 23 pairs of chromosomes).

> **TIP!** Haploid sounds like "half"—indeed a haploid cell has half the normal number of chromosomes that a diploid cell would have. Likewise, remember that "di" means two, so diploid cells have twice the chromosomes as haploid cells (two sets of 23 chromosomes for a total of 46 chromosomes).

In vitro fertilization occurs outside the woman's body in a lab environment when the oocyte is fertilized, then transferred into the mother's _____ through artificial implantation.

The First Eight Weeks of Life

Embryonic period is the first _____ weeks following fertilization.

Early Cell Division

Cleavage is a process of successive mitotic divisions that occur while the zygote is traveling down the uterine tube on its way to the uterus.

- **Morula:** _____ days after fertilization, this small ball of cells arrives in the uterine cavity and undergoes cell division and change, called _____.
- **Blastocyst** forms after the morula. It has two distinctive regions separated by fluid.
  1. **Trophoblast** is the outer layer of cells separated from the inner layer by fluid. The trophoblast contributes to the _____.
  2. **Inner cell mass** is the inner layer of cells. It becomes the _____.
- **Blastocyst cavity** (blastocele) is one large, fluid-filled cavity.

Implantation

Implantation occurs _____ days after fertilization and after freely floating in the uterine cavity when the trophoblast contacts the inner wall (endometrium) of the uterus. The trophoblast burrows and the blastocyst eventually becomes completely buried in the endometrium.

During the second week of development, differentiation occurs:

• The _____ differentiates into two layers with the outer layer forming fingerlike processes (extensions) that penetrate the endometrium.

• The embryo (formerly the inner cell mass) forms three **germ layers** which are the layers of early cells that will become (or differentiate into) tissues and organs of the body by the end of the second week. The three germ layers are:

1. _____

2. _____

3. _____

During the third week of development, three membranes are formed:

1. Trophoblast forms the **chorion**, a membrane later associated with the fetus. The chorion forms the embryonic portion of the _____.

2. **Amnion** is the second membrane developed; it expands the fluid-filled amniotic cavity until it envelopes the _____.

3. **Yolk sac** arises from the endoderm to form another cavity.

Development of Body Form

From the third to the eighth week, the body form of the embryo changes to appear more animal-like.

Foldings lead to the formation of a head fold and a tail fold. As a result, the following are formed:

• _____ (head cavity)

• Hindgut (tail cavity)

• _____ (formed by endoderm) becomes the GI tract

Umbilical cord forms from the folding to connect the embryo to the endometrium with portions of the yolk sac and a fourth membrane, the _____.

Amniotic sac is formed from the amnion that envelops the embryo. The amniotic sac holds **amniotic fluid**.

Review Time!

I.   Provide a brief answer for each of the following questions about prenatal development.

1. What cell division process must the oocyte complete for the sperm's nucleus to fuse with it?

_____

_____

2. What happens to the oocyte and sperm nuclei during fertilization? _____

_____

3. What chromosome number does the zygote have? _____

_____

4. Explain the difference between haploid and diploid. _____

_____

_____

5. How long does an oocyte live? During what window of time can fertilization occur?

   _____

   _____

6. What is the time period for embryonic development? For fetal development?

   _____

7. When does the zygote undergo cleavage? What does cleavage achieve?

   _____

   _____

   _____

8. How is a zygote different from a morula? How does the morula become a blastocyst?

   _____

   _____

   _____

   _____

9. What is differentiation? _____

   _____

10. What arises from the trophoblast? _____

    _____

11. What does the inner cell mass become? _____

    _____

12. Name the three germ layers formed through differentiation of the embryo.

    1. _____

    2. _____

    3. _____

13. Provide a function for each of these membranes: chorion, amnion, yolk sac, and allantois.

    _____

    _____

    _____

    _____

    _____

    _____

14. What does folding of the embryo accomplish? _____

    _____

    _____

15. What forms the umbilical cord? _____

    _____

Development of Organs

LEARNING OBJECTIVE 2. Describe the events of the embryonic period of development, from formation of the zygote to organogenesis.

Organogenesis is the process of organ development. At what point of development (in weeks) do most organs appear? _____

- Some organs arise as outpockets of cells or directly from the midgut.
- The heart arises from the mesoderm around day _____ as two tubes fuse to form a single heart.
- The kidneys arise from the _____ and the brain arises from the _____.

External features also emerge, such as:

- The head enlarges as the brain develops; it is well formed by the end of the seventh week.
- Arm buds, then leg buds appear.
- _____ regresses.

Development of the Placenta

LEARNING OBJECTIVE   3. Explain how the placenta develops and identify its roles in maintaining pregnancy.

The **placenta** first appears during week _____. Both mother and embryo contribute to the placenta.

- _____ contributes the chorion. The chorion sends fingerlike projections, called **chorionic villi**, into the endometrium.
- *Maternal contribution* is the **lacunae**, pools of maternal blood, and the **decidua**, modified endometrial tissue.

Does the blood from the embryo mix with the mother? No, an embryonic capillary wall, basement membrane, and chorion create the *placental blood barrier*. This barrier prevents the mixing of embryonic and maternal blood.

The embryo receive nourishment from the mother through the **umbilical cord**, a stalk that connects the embryo to the placenta. The cord contains:

- _____ (*how many?*) umbilical arteries (originate from the embryo's iliac arteries), which carry blood from the embryo to the mother.
- One umbilical vein, which carries blood from the mother to the embryo

> **TIP!** Think about these three vessels in reference to the embryo's heart. Arteries carry blood away from the heart; the umbilical arteries carry blood away from the embryo's heart to its mother. Veins return blood to the heart; the umbilical vein carries blood from the mother to the embryo.

The placenta is an endocrine gland. It secretes:

- **Human chorionic gonadotropin (HCG)** when it develops during the _____ month. It takes over HCG production from the _____, which produced HCG in the mother's ovary during the second and third months.
- Estrogen
- Progesterone

Growth of the Fetus

LEARNING OBJECTIVE   4. Identify the main events during the fetal period of development.

The embryo become the fetus at _____ weeks. *What marks this transition from the embryo to the fetus?* Bone ossification begins during the fetal period and continues until birth.

By the start of the fetal period:

- Most organs and organ systems have developed.
- The heart is beating.
- Blood is flowing.
- The brain neurons are forming _____.
- _____ are filtering blood.

Changes continue during the fetal period:

- Growth is the most notable feature of the fetal period. It is accomplished by mitosis of cells in all tissues and organs.
- **Lanugo** is fine, soft hair that covers the skin along with a waxy coat of sloughed epithelial cells that protect the fetus from _____.
- Fat accumulates to insulate and provide a nutrient reserve.

The fetus can survive outside the mother at _____ weeks

The fetus is considered full term at _____ weeks

Review Time!

I. Using the terms in the list below, label the illustration of a full-term pregnancy.

1. _____
2. _____
3. _____
4. _____
5. _____
6. _____
7. _____
8. _____
9. _____

Alveolar glands and ducts	Fetus at full term	Urethra
Amniotic sac	Placenta	Vagina
Cervical canal	Umbilical cord	Wall of uterus

II. Provide a brief answer for each of the following questions about growth and development of the embryo and fetus.

1. When does organogenesis occur? _____
   _____

2. What organs form from cell outpockets? _____
   _____

3. What organs form from the midgut? _____
   _____

4. How does the heart form? From what germ layer does it form? By how many days?
   _____
   _____
   _____

5. How does the brain develop? From what germ layer does it form? _____
_____
_____

6. What external features develop during the first 8 weeks? _____
_____
_____

7. Discuss the fetal and maternal contributions to the placenta. _____
_____
_____

8. Name the three vessels carried in the umbilical cord. How do they connect mother and fetus?
_____
_____
_____

9. Discuss the production of HCG by the corpus luteum and the placenta ._____
_____
_____

10. What is the placental blood barrier? What is its function? _____
_____
_____

11. At how many weeks of development does the fetal period begin? _____
12. What is the most noticeable change that occurs during the fetal period? _____
_____

13. What is lanugo? _____
_____

14. At what point is the fetus considered full-term? What might you expect to see if the fetus is born at this point? _____
_____
_____

15. At what point is the fetus capable of surviving outside its mother? _____
_____

CONCEPT 2

Parturition

Concept: Parturition is a process regulated by the hypothalamus, which results in the birth of a child through three successive stages.

LEARNING OBJECTIVE 5. Describe the events resulting in childbirth.

Parturition is the birthing processing. Leading up to this event:

• The placenta increases production of estrogen.
• Braxton Hicks contractions are minor contractions of the uterine wall induced by increasing estrogen levels.

What leads to the process of labor when the fetus moves through the birth canal in response to uterine contractions?
- Stretch of the uterine wall initiates nerve impulses that signal the hypothalamus.
- Hypothalamus signals the posterior pituitary to release a hormone, _____.
- Oxytocin targets the myometrium to strengthen its rhythmic contractions.
- Positive feedback loop ensures that more oxytocin is released to promote more uterine contractions.
- Once contractions increase in frequency and strength, *labor begins.*
- **Labor** is the movement of the fetus through the birth canal in response to

_____

During the **first stage** of labor:
- Myometrial contractions push the fetus against the _____ of the uterus.
- Amniotic sac (the bag of waters) ruptures. (Often, it is said the "water has broken.")
- Cervical canal dilates in response to pressure.
- Fetus head is pushed into the _____.
- As cervical dilation progresses, the uterine contractions become more intense. What type of feedback mechanism is this? _____
- Cervix dilates to 10 centimeters and effaces (thins) for 1 to 24 hours.

During the **second stage** of labor:
- _____ feedback mechanism enlists the abdominal muscles to assist uterine contractions.
- Crowning of the newborn occurs when the head penetrates the _____.
- This stage may last several minutes to several hours.

During the **third stage** of labor:
- Placenta exits with another wave of contractions.
- Continued uterine contractions limit blood loss.

After labor and delivery of the fetus and placenta is complete:
- Progesterone and estrogen levels decline due to the loss of the _____.
- Menstrual cycle returns 8 to 12 weeks after parturition among women who are not breastfeeding. Breastfeeding delays the return of the menstrual cycle another month or two.

Review Time!

I. *Provide a brief answer for each of the following questions about parturition.*

1. What is parturition? _____

_____

2. What are Braxton Hicks contractions? _____

_____

3. What does oxytocin promote during labor? _____

_____

4. What are cervical dilation and effacement? _____

_____

5. What are the major events of the first stage of labor? _____

_____

_____

6. What are the major events of the second stage of labor? _____

_____

_____

7. What is "crowning"? _____
_____

8. What type of feedback mechanism promotes expulsion of the fetus? _____
_____

9. What major event occurs during the third stage of labor? What limits blood loss?
_____
_____
_____

10. Provide a time line for the first, second, and third stages of labor. _____
_____
_____
_____
_____

CONCEPT 3

Postnatal Development

Concept: The cycle of life proceeds from birth to death as postnatal development. During this period of life, changes occur in the body in definable stages that are more gradual than those of prenatal development.

Postnatal development begins at birth and continues until death. The five stages are:
1. Infancy
2. Childhood
3. Adolescence
4. Adulthood
5. Old age

Lactation

LEARNING OBJECTIVE 6. Describe the process of lactation and how it is regulated.

Lactation is milk production by the _____ glands.
• Why doesn't lactation occur during pregnancy? _____
_____
_____

Prolactin stimulates milk secretion. Prolactin is usually kept in check by progesterone and estrogen, which are secreted as long as the placenta is present. After birth, the loss of the placenta allows an increase in prolactin to stimulate milk production. During the first days following birth, _____ is produced.
• What does colostrum contain? _____
• Why is colostrum important? _____

Milk production occurs by the following process:

- Neural stimulation is provided by the suckling newborn, sound of a crying baby, or the anticipation of a scheduled feeding. This stimulation promotes the release of *oxytocin* from the _____.
- Oxytocin stimulates *milk letdown:* contractile cells around the _____ contract, forcing milk to eject through ducts and flow out the nipples.
- Both *prolactin* and *oxytocin* continue milk production and release as long as nursing continues.
- If nursing is stopped for more than a few days, what happens? _____

_____

_____

Stages of Life

LEARNING OBJECTIVE 7. Identify the primary stages of life.

What is the life expectancy of males? _____.

What is the life expectancy of females? _____.

List the five stages of life.

1. _____: First year of life
2. _____: Toddlerhood until onset of puberty at age 10 to 12 years
3. _____: Puberty until 16 to 20 years
4. _____: End of adolescence to 65 years
5. _____: After 65 years

Infancy

LEARNING OBJECTIVE 8. Describe the circulatory changes that occur immediately after birth.

Neonates, or newborns, experience three major circulation changes due to life in an air-filled rather than a fluid-filled environment.

1. **Foramen ovale** is a fetal shunt that must close upon birth. The foramen ovale is an opening in the interatrial septum that shunts blood away from the _____ in fetal circulation. When the infant breathes air, muscular spasms close this shunt permanently and a slight depression, called fossa ovalis, remains.
2. **Ductus arteriosus** is a fetal shunt that bypasses blood flow to the _____. It is a channel connecting the pulmonary trunk to the aorta. It also closes upon birth and is converted to a small ligament.
3. **Ductus venosus** is a fetal shunt that delivers blood to the fetal inferior vena cava by way of the umbilical vein. The umbilical vein carries blood to the liver, but the ductus venosus bypasses the digestive function of the _____ and carries the blood on to the inferior vena cava.

> **TIP!** Recall from Chapter 12 that the foramen ovale means oval-shaped hole while *fossa ovalis* means oval-shaped depression. For the other two fetal shunts, use the clues built into the words to help you. *Ductus arteriosus* connects two arteries—the pulmonary trunk and the aorta. *Ductus venosus* connects two veins—the umbilical vein to the inferior vena cava.

Additionally, during the first year of life, important changes occur, such as:

- Rapid brain growth and development
- Muscle growth and coordination
- Bone development
- Growth of most body tissues and internal organs

Childhood

What is the time period for childhood? _____

When is a child classified as a toddler? _____

How much weight will the average toddler gain? _____

How many inches will the average toddler grow? _____

What characterizes the toddler years?

• Slower body growth

• _____ stores diminish

• Muscles and bones lengthen and straighten

• _____ in the brain become established

• Body proportions become closer to those of adults

Adolescence

Puberty marks the beginning of **adolescence**.

When is the onset of puberty in a male? _____

When is the onset of menstruation in a female? _____

At what age is the maximum height or stature reached by males? _____

At what age is the maximum height or stature reached by females? _____

What physiologic changes characterize adolescence?

• Sex hormones are produced in high amounts.

• _____ organs reach maturity.

• _____ characteristics appear.

• Onset of puberty is accompanied by a growth spurt, then a slow growth period.

Adulthood

What marks the beginning of **adulthood**? _____
_____

Adulthood is the longest period of life.

What characterizes adulthood?

• Lack of vertical growth

• Effects of aging accumulate (increased fat deposition, gradual muscle loss, decline in metabolic rate, and thinning of the skin)

Diet, psychological stress, and exercise affect health and influence longevity

Old Age

Senescence—old age—is the last stage in human development.

At what age does old age begin? _____

What characterizes old age?

• _____ fragility

• Loss of posture, muscle atrophy, and slowing of nervous responses.

• Skin continues to thin and lose elasticity and becomes more heavily pigmented in some areas.

• _____ weakens with age.

Review Time!

I.   *Provide a brief answer for each of the following questions about postnatal development.*

1. Describe how prolactin and oxytocin work together to promote lactation. _____
    _____
    _____
    _____

2. What stimulates the release of prolactin? _____
    _____
    _____

3. List the five stages of life.
    1. _____
    2. _____
    3. _____
    4. _____
    5. _____

4. List the three changes that occur in the circulation of a neonate that occur in response to breathing air.
    1. _____
    2. _____
    3. _____

5. What do the following fetal shunts bypass?
    1. Foramen ovale _____
    2. Ductus venosus _____
    3. Ductus arteriosus _____

6. What changes characterize the childhood years? _____
    _____
    _____
    _____

7. When does puberty occur for males? For females? _____
    _____

8. What changes characterize adulthood? _____
    _____
    _____

9. When does old age begin? _____
10. What changes are expected during old age? _____
    _____
    _____

CONCEPT 4

Genetic Inheritance

Concept: Inheritance is determined by genes, and may be predicted through the study of genetics.

LEARNING OBJECTIVE 9. Correlate the patterns of inheritance with the structure of DNA and genes.

Genetics is a study of inherited traits and their variations. Recall that nuclei house chromosomes. Chromosomes are DNA. DNA provides a molecular map of the body's structure and function. Genes are specific sequences of DNA that code for proteins. The combination of genes occurs when a male gamete (sperm) joins with a female gamete (oocyte).

Chromosomes and Genes

Homologous chromosomes are pairs of chromosomes that carry genes determining the same trait. One chromosome of the pair comes from the father's sperm while the other comes from the mother's oocyte. There are 23 pairs of chromosomes, or _____ total chromosomes—the diploid number— in cells of the human body.

Alleles are genes that carry the same trait and occupy the same position on homologous chromosomes.

> **TIP!** Alleles are alternate forms of genes: *alt*ernate resembles *all*ele.

- **Homozygous** is the term used to describe the situation when alleles for a trait are _____.
- **Heterozygous** is the term used to describe the situation when alleles for a trait are _____.

EXAMPLE

Homologous chromosomes carry a gene for hair color. If both the homologous chromosomes code for blonde hair, that person is homozygous for that trait. However, if one chromosome codes for blonde hair while the allele on the other chromosome codes for black hair, that person is heterozygous for that trait.

> **TIP!** Use the prefix to help you remember each situation: the prefix "homo" in homozygous means "same" while the prefix "hetero" in heterozygous means "different."

Genes and their physical expression are termed differently as well:
- **Genotype** for any particular trait is determined by the individual's genes.
- **Phenotype** is the physical expression of the genes (actual trait). It refers to _____.

EXAMPLE

A genotype of *AA* produces a phenotype of normal pigmentation in the skin while a genotype of *aa* produces a phenotype of albinism. Albinism is an inherited condition involving the absence or reduction of melanin, a brown pigment responsible for coloration of the skin, hair, and eyes.

> **TIP!** Use the first few letters of each term, genotype and phenotype, to help you keep them organized: genotype has the word "gene" as a prefix. *Gen*otypes are determined by *gene*s. Phenotype has "ph" for physical expression as part of the word. *Ph*enotypes are the *ph*ysical expressions of genes.

Dominant-recessive Inheritance

The expression of a phenotype is the result of the interaction of the alleles.

- **Dominant allele** is expressed, if present as one of the alleles, in the phenotype.
- **Recessive allele** is only expressed if _____.
- **Carrier** is a person who has an abnormal allele and can pass it along to offspring.

> **EXAMPLE**
>
> Albinism is carried on recessive alleles, like most genetic disorders. If a person inherits only one abnormal allele, that person will not express the disorder but can pass it along to offspring. To express the disorder, the person must inherit two recessive alleles for albinism.

Punnett square is a chart used to show possible combinations of alleles for a single trait that would result from the combining of male and female gametes. Punnett squares only predict a _____ of inherited traits and cannot predict actual outcomes.

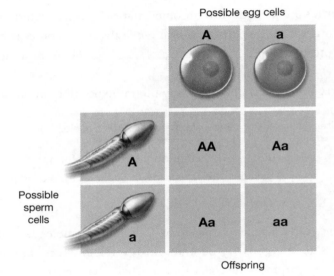

> **TIP! Punnett Square Tutorial:** If you are asked to complete a Punnett square, draw and divide a box into four possibilities. These four boxes will represent the possible genotypes of offspring. To the left of the box, place each one of the two alleles for the male sperm by an individual box, as shown in the figure. Above the box, place each one of the two alleles for the female egg above an individual box, also shown in the figure. When you combine the alleles to form the genotype of a possible offspring, look UP and to the LEFT to obtain the allele from each parent. Write down those two alleles. Complete all four boxes in the same manner (look to the box above and to the left) to determine the possible genotypes of the offspring.

> **EXAMPLE**
>
> Let's discuss albinism again. This skin disorder is carried on the recessive allele. If two heterozygous parents have a child, each parent has a genotype of Aa. The possible genotypes of the offspring are:
> - Two of four children may be heterozygous genotype (Aa)
> - Two of four children may be homozygous genotype (AA and aa)
>
> The chance of producing an albino child (aa) is one in four (or 25%).

Review Time!

I. *Using the information in the table below, answer the questions below and on the next page about genotypes and phenotypes.*

Traits Determined by Dominant-recessive Inheritance

Dominant Phenotype	Recessive Phenotype
Feet with normal arches	Flattened arches (flat feet)
Astigmatism	Normal vision
Freckles on the skin	Absence of freckles
Ability to roll the tongue in U shape	Inability to roll the tongue
Unattached (free) earlobes	Attached earlobes
Widow's peak hairline	Straight hairline
Polydactyly (extra digits)	Normal number of digits
Huntington's disease (brain deterioration)	Absence of Huntington's disease
Achondroplasia (one form of dwarfism)	Absence of achondroplasia
Absence of cystic fibrosis	Cystic fibrosis
Normal heart	Congenital heart block
Ability to digest lactose (milk sugar)	Lactose intolerance

1. Lactose intolerance is carried on a recessive allele. _____

    1. If a person inherits two recessive alleles, what is her genotype? _____

    2. If a person inherits only one recessive allele, what is her phenotype? _____

2. Astigmatism is carried on the dominant allele while normal vision is recessive.

    1. What is the genotype of a person who inherits two recessive alleles? _____

    2. What is the phenotype of a person who inherits one dominant allele and one recessive allele? _____

3. A widow's peak hairline is carried on the dominant allele while a straight hairline is recessive.

    1. What is the genotype of a person with a straight hairline? _____

    2. What are two possible genotypes of a person with a widow's peak?_____

    3. What phenotype does a person have if two recessive alleles are inherited? _____

4. What is the possibility of flat feet if both parents are heterozygous for the trait? Set up and solve a Punnett square to answer this question. _____

5. What is the possibility of cystic fibrosis if one parent is a carrier but the other parent is normal? Set up and solve a Punnett square to answer this question. _____
_____
_____
_____

6. What is the possibility of congenital heart block if both parents have a normal heart, but are carriers? Set up and solve a Punnett square to answer this question. _____
_____
_____
_____

7. What is the possibility of rolling the tongue if both of the parents have the genotype *tt*? Set up and solve a Punnett square to answer this question. _____
_____
_____
_____

II. *Provide a brief answer for each of the following questions about genes and dominant-recessive inheritance.*

1. How many total chromosomes do most of our body cells have? _____

2. How many pairs of *homologous chromosomes* do most of our cells have?
_____

3. What do we call genes that code for the same trait and are carried on homologous chromosomes?
_____
_____

4. What is the difference between homozygous and heterozygous alleles? _____
_____
_____
_____

5. Define genotype. _____
_____

6. Define phenotype. _____

7. What does it mean for a person to be a "carrier" of a trait? _____
_____
_____

8. Which allele, the *dominant* or the *recessive* allele, is expressed in the phenotype if it is present?
_____

Sex-linked Inheritance

Sex chromosomes are only one pair of the 23 pairs of chromosomes we have. Sex chromosomes are *not homologous* to one another. The other 22 pairs are called **autosomes**.

- Females have _____ for their sex chromosomes.
- Males have _____ for their sex chromosomes.

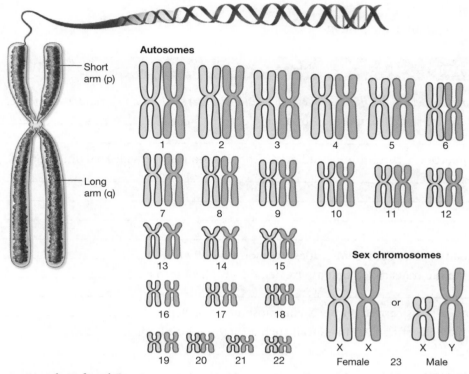

What makes a person male or female?

Sex is determined by the presence or absence of the Y chromosome. A gene on the Y chromosome called the SRY gene (sex-determining region of the Y), switches on the transformation of embryonic gonadal tissue into testes. If there is no Y chromosome, what does the embryonic gonadal tissue become?

_____

Sex-linked traits are carried on the sex chromosomes:

- If the trait is carried on the X chromosome, it is known as _____.
- If the trait is carried on the Y chromosome, as is rarely, it is known as _____.

Genetic Screening

LEARNING OBJECTIVE   10. Explain how genetic screening works and why it is important.

Why perform genetic screening?

Many inherited diseases may be preventable if identified early.

Genetic screening can be performed:

- Before pregnancy
- During pregnancy
- At birth

How genetic screening is performed depends on the time at which it is performed.

1. Before pregnancy:
   - Blood analysis to determine the presence of a mutated gene sequence
   - **Pedigree analysis** to determine the presence of a genetic trait through several generations

2. During pregnancy:
  - **Amniocentesis** involves sampling the amniotic fluid for genetic analysis

3. At birth:
  - Newborns are screened with blood tests for anatomical and metabolic disorders, or retardation.

How is a genetic disease handled if diagnosed after birth?

- Surgical repair
- Genetic counseling on management

Review Time!

I. *Provide a brief answer for each of the following questions about sex-linked inheritance and genetic screening.*

  1. What are the sex chromosomes for a female? For a male? _____
  _____

  2. What makes sex chromosomes different from autosomes? Provide two differences.
  _____
  _____
  _____
  _____

  3. How many pairs of autosomes does a person typically have? _____

  4. What are the traits called that are carried on sex chromosomes? _____
  _____

  5. Sex-linked traits carried on the X chromosome are called _____

  6. Can a male inherit an X-linked trait such as hemophilia? Explain. _____
  _____
  _____
  _____

  7. Can a female inherit an X-linked trait such as hemophilia? Explain. _____
  _____
  _____
  _____

  8. Sex-linked traits carried on the Y chromosome are called _____

  9. Can a male inherit a Y-linked trait, such as the hairy ear trait? Explain. _____
  _____
  _____
  _____

  10. Can a female inherit a Y-linked trait, such as the SRY gene? Explain. _____
  _____
  _____
  _____

  11. Which type of sex-linked trait is rare, X-linked or Y-linked? _____

  12. When is the best time to perform genetic screening to prevent inherited disease: *before* pregnancy,
  during pregnancy, or at *birth*? _____
  _____

II. *Using the information in the table below, answer the following questions about sex-linked traits.*

X-linked Traits in Humans

Trait	Description of Disease
Cleft palate	Incomplete fusion of the bony palate
Color blindness	Can vary from an inability to distinguish red from green (the most common form) to total inability to perceive colors
Deafness	Lack of hearing; includes three types of deafness by X-linkage
Duchenne muscular dystrophy	Progressive degeneration of muscle tissue. Onset is at age 6 and progresses until death, usually before age 20
Ectodermal dysplasia	Absence of teeth and sweat glands
Hemophilia	Lack of certain blood-clotting factors, resulting in uncontrolled loss of blood when injured
Ichthyosis	Rough, scaly skin originating at birth
Lesch–Nyhan syndrome	Enzyme deficiency resulting in mental retardation, loss of muscular control, and self-mutilating behavior
Retinitis pigmentosa	Degeneration of the retina of the eye resulting in blindness
Testicular feminization syndrome	Males born with female external genitals, breast development, and blind vagina (XY genotype)

1. Explain how a male inherits color blindness.

   _____

   _____

   _____

   _____

2. Marjorie is deaf; however, her husband is not deaf. Do you think their sons *or* their daughters are more likely to be deaf? Explain.

   _____

   _____

   _____

   _____

3. Julie and Steve want to have children. Julie has normal vision. Steve has retinitis pigmentosa, a trait carried on his X-chromosome. How would you advise them? _____

   _____

   _____

   _____

Congratulations

What an accomplishment! You have completed this workbook and your anatomy and physiology class! I hope you have gained a new appreciation and insight into the human body and its mechanisms!

Figure Credits

Chapter 1

Pages 4, 10, and 11. Modified with permission from: Nath JL. *Using Medical Terminology,* 2nd ed. Baltimore, MD: Lippincott Williams & Wilkins, 2013.

Page 13. Modified with permission from: McConnell TH. *The Nature of Disease Pathology for the Health Professions.* Baltimore, MD: Lippincott Williams & Wilkins, 2007.

Chapter 2

Pages 17, 22 and 23. Modified with permission from: Premkumar K. *Anatomy & Physiology: The Massage Connection.* Baltimore, MD: Lippincott Williams & Wilkins, 2012.

Chapter 5

Page 80. Modified with permission from: Porth CM. *Essentials of Pathophysiology Concepts of Altered Health States,* 2nd ed. Philadelphia, PA: Lippincott Williams & Wilkins, 2007.

Page 83. Modified with permission from Anatomical Chart Co.

Pages 86 and 89. Modified with permission from: Cohen BJ. *Memmler's The Human Body in Health and Disease,* 11th ed. Baltimore, MD: Lippincott Williams & Wilkins, 2009.

Chapter 6

Pages 94, 107, 108, 109, and 110. Modified with permission from: McConnell TH, Hull KL. *Human Form, Human Function: Essentials of Anatomy & Physiology.* Baltimore, MD: Lippincott Williams & Wilkins, 2011.

Page 112. Modified with permission from: Tank PW, Gest TR. *Lippincott Williams & Wilkins Atlas of Anatomy.* Baltimore, MD: Lippincott Williams & Wilkins, 2009.

Page 113. Modified with permission from: McConnell TH, Hull KL. *Human Form, Human Function: Essentials of Anatomy & Physiology.* Baltimore, MD: Lippincott Williams & Wilkins, 2011.

Pages 114, 115, 118, 119, 120, 121, 124, 125, 126, and 127. Modified with permission from: Tank PW, Gest TR. *Lippincott Williams & Wilkins Atlas of Anatomy.* Baltimore, MD: Lippincott Williams & Wilkins, 2009.

Chapter 8

Pages 182 and 189. Modified with permission from: Tank PW, Gest TR. *Lippincott Williams & Wilkins Atlas of Anatomy.* Baltimore, MD: Lippincott Williams & Wilkins, 2009.

Chapter 9

Page 211. Modified with permission from: McConnell TH, Hull KL. *Human Form, Human Function: Essentials of Anatomy & Physiology.* Baltimore, MD: Lippincott Williams & Wilkins, 2011.

Chapter 10

Page 216. Modified with permission from Anatomical Chart Co.

Chapter 11

Page 235. Reprinted with permission from: McConnell TH, Hull KL. *Human Form, Human Function: Essentials of Anatomy & Physiology.* Baltimore, MD: Lippincott Williams & Wilkins, 2011.

Chapter 12

Pages 252 and 253. Modified with permission from Anatomical Chart Co.

Page 258. Modified with permission from: McArdle WD, Katch FI, Katch VL. *Essentials of Exercise Physiology,* 2nd ed. Baltimore, MD: Lippincott Williams & Wilkins, 2000.

Chapter 13

Page 281. Modified with permission from: Nath JL. *Using Medical Terminology: A Practical Approach.* Baltimore, MD: Lippincott Williams & Wilkins, 2006.

Chapter 14

Page 298 and 303. Modified with permission from Anatomical Chart Co.

Page 310. Modified with permission from: Premkumar K. *Anatomy & Physiology: The Massage Connection.* Baltimore, MD: Lippincott Williams & Wilkins, 2012.

Chapter 15

Page 315. Modified with permission from: Werner R. *Massage Therapist's Guide to Pathology,* 4th ed. Baltimore, MD: Lippincott Williams & Wilkins, 2009.

Pages 320, 321, 322, 327, 333, and 339. Modified with permission from Anatomical Chart Co.

Chapter 16

Pages 349 and 363. Modified with permission from: Tank PW, Gest TR. *Lippincott Williams & Wilkins Atlas of Anatomy.* Baltimore, MD: Lippincott Williams & Wilkins, 2009.

Chapter 17

Page 371. Modified with permission from Anatomical Chart Co.

Page 376. Modified with permission from: Nath JL. *Using Medical Terminology.* Baltimore, MD: Lippincott Williams & Wilkins, 2006.

Pages 379 and 380 (top). Modified with permission from Anatomical Chart Co.

Page 380 (bottom). Modified with permission from: McConnell TH, Hull KL. *Human Form, Human Function: Essentials of Anatomy & Physiology.* Baltimore, MD: Lippincott Williams & Wilkins, 2011.

Chapter 18

Page 392. Modified with permission from Anatomical Chart Co.